POX ROMANA

TURNING POINTS IN ANCIENT HISTORY

Barry Strauss, Series Editor

Turning Points in Ancient History presents accessible books, by leading scholars, on crucial events and key moments in the ancient world. The series aims at fresh interpretations of both famous subjects and little-known ones that deserve more attention.

The books provide a narrative synthesis that integrates literary and archaeological evidence.

Pox Romana: The Plague That Shook the Roman World, Colin Elliott

Rome Is Burning: Nero and the Fire That Ended a Dynasty, Anthony A. Barrett

1177 B.C.: The Year Civilization Collapsed, Eric H. Cline

COLIN ELLIOTT

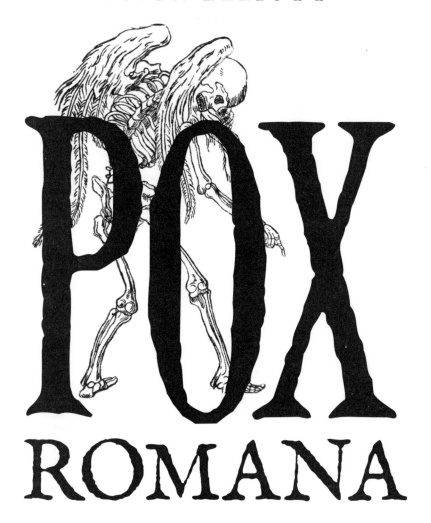

POX
ROMANA

THE PLAGUE THAT SHOOK
the ROMAN WORLD

PRINCETON UNIVERSITY PRESS
PRINCETON & OXFORD

Published by Princeton University Press
41 William Street, Princeton, New Jersey 08540
99 Banbury Road, Oxford OX2 6JX

press.princeton.edu

Library of Congress Cataloging-in-Publication Data

Names: Elliott, Colin P., 1982- author.
Title: Pox romana : the plague that shook the Roman world / Colin Elliott.
Other titles: Plague that shook the Roman world
Description: Princeton : Princeton University Press, [2024] | Series: Turning points
    in ancient history | Includes bibliographical references and index.
Identifiers: LCCN 2023011011 (print) | LCCN 2023011012 (ebook) |
    ISBN 9780691219158 (hardback) | ISBN 9780691220697 (ebook)
Subjects: LCSH: Plague—Rome—History—2nd century.
Classification: LCC RC178.R6 E45 2024 (print) | LCC RC178.R6 (ebook) |
    DDC 614.5/7320937—dc23/eng/20230315
LC record available at https://lccn.loc.gov/2023011011
LC ebook record available at https://lccn.loc.gov/2023011012

British Library Cataloging-in-Publication Data is available

Editorial: Rob Tempio and Chloe Coy
Production Editorial: Sara Lerner
Text and Jacket Design: Heather Hansen
Production: Erin Suydam
Publicity: Alyssa Sanford and Carmen Jimenez

Jacket Credit: Winged death on marble plaque on church of Saint Mary.
Stephen Bisgrove / Alamy Stock Photo

This book has been composed in Arno Pro and The Fell Types

Printed on acid-free paper. ∞

Printed in the United States of America

10 9 8 7 6 5 4 3 2 1

For Grandma, Grandpa Ralph, Nan, and Grandpa Elliott.
My memories with each of you,
whether many or few, still comfort and uphold me.
I will never forget you.

CONTENTS

Foreword   ix
Introduction: A Furious Beginning   xv

PART I. PREEXISTING CONDITIONS

1	Rome's Fragile Peace	3
2	The Dry Tinder of Disease	24
3	Rumors of Death	56

PART II. OUTBREAK

4	Plague Unleashed	77
5	The Age of Angst	111
6	An Empire Exhausted	143

PART III. CASUALTIES

7	Redux?	185
8	The End of an Era	213
	Epilogue: The Spirit of Pandemic	233

Acknowledgments   241
Notes   243
Bibliography   271
Index   301

FOREWORD

In this volume in the Turning Points in Ancient History series, Colin P. Elliott writes about what was arguably history's first pandemic. The Antonine plague killed millions and was perhaps the greatest of a series of shocks in the late second century that ended the Roman Peace—the Pax Romana. Rome emerged from the era more brittle and less sure of itself. It went from being "a kingdom of gold to one of rust and iron," as an ancient writer put it. Yet despite the importance of the pandemic, it has left only elusive evidence. It takes ingenuity and assiduousness to make sense of it; fortunately, they are on offer. In *Pox Romana: The Plague That Shook the Roman World*, Elliott has written a historical detective story of the first order.

Elliott takes us through the meager data with a masterful hand. He uses both the traditional methods of a historian and the tools of social science and environmental studies. And he engages fully with both the historiographical tradition and the latest and most innovative scholarship. Historians have differed widely in their evaluation of the Antonine plague over the years, but recent evidence shows that it was a major biological event.

Direct evidence of the disease is hard to come by, but as Elliott shows, a series of "proxies"—from census records to real estate contracts to paleoclimatological evidence to amphorae finds—paints a persuasive picture of biological harm and demographic shock. That is true even if the real nature of the so-called Antonine plague remains uncertain. It was possibly smallpox, certainly not bubonic plague. Also uncertain is the extent of its impact, given the limits of the data.

Yet even a mortality rate of 1 or 2 percent might have proved devastating. One of Elliott's chief arguments is the fragility of the empire's institutions. Roman societal and governmental structures were clumsy and often ineffective. Certainly, the legions were disciplined, but the government's grasp of economics was primitive. Its response to crisis was to issue edicts that sounded authoritative but often made things worse. Elliott's description of life in an ancient metropolis—dirty, disease-ridden, and given to frequent disasters—takes a lot of the luster off the Golden Age. Rome had little margin for error.

The dislocations of the Antonine plague may have contributed to the political instability that embroiled Rome in a new era of civil war after the murder of the emperor Commodus in 192. As Elliott argues, however, perhaps the most important legacy of the disease was spiritual. It may have left in its wake a growing consciousness of catastrophe that contributed to the religious quest of the following century. That was an era in which an increasing number of Romans turned to a new religion, Christianity.

Sophisticated, complex, provocative, and readable, *Pox Romana* tells an epic tale. Our own recent experience of pandemic makes this history even more urgent and engaging.

—*Barry Strauss*

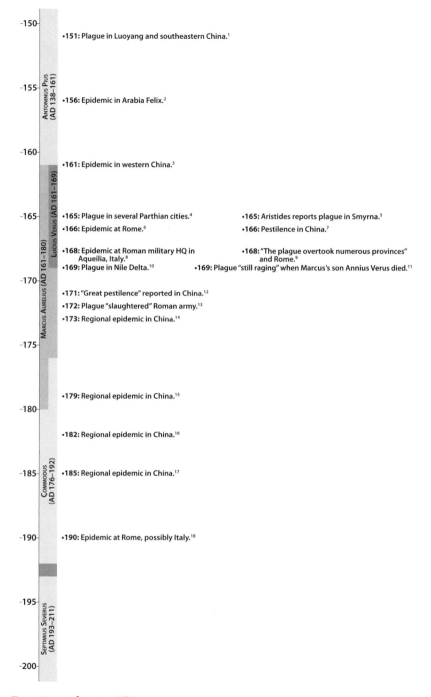

Eurasian epidemics, AD 150–200.

1. *HHS* 7.296. 2. SHA, *Anti. Pius* 9.3–5. 3. *ZZTJ* 54.1757.A. 4. Amm. Marc. 23.6.24; SHA, *Verus* 8.1–4; Luc. *Hist. Conscr.* 15. 5. Aristid. *ST* 2.38. 6. SHA *Verus* 13.1–3. 7. ZZTJ 55.1792. 8. Gal. *Lib. Prop.* 1.18. 9. Jer. *Chron.* 287f (Helm). 10. P. *Thmouis* 1, 104.9–21. 11. Gal. *De praes. ex puls.* 3.3–5. 12. *ZZTJ* 56.1826. 13. Jer. *Chron.* 288f (Helm). 14. De Crespigny 2007, 514. 15. Ibid. 16. Ibid. 17. Ibid. 18. Dio Cass. 73.14.3–4; Herodian 1.12.1–3.

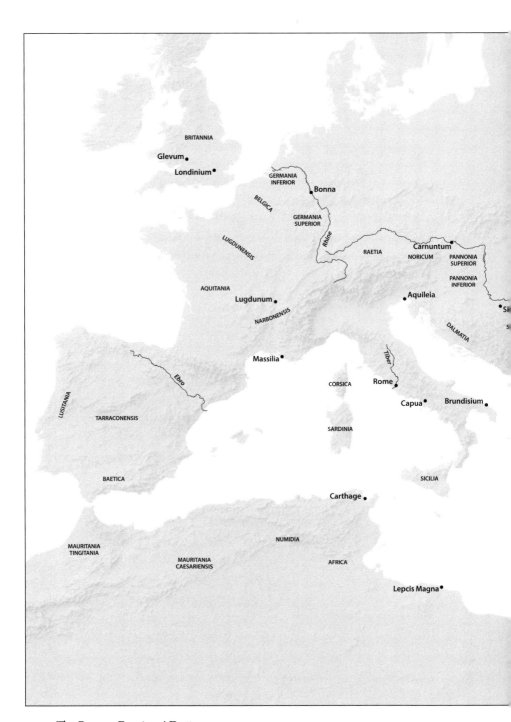

The Roman Empire, AD 165.

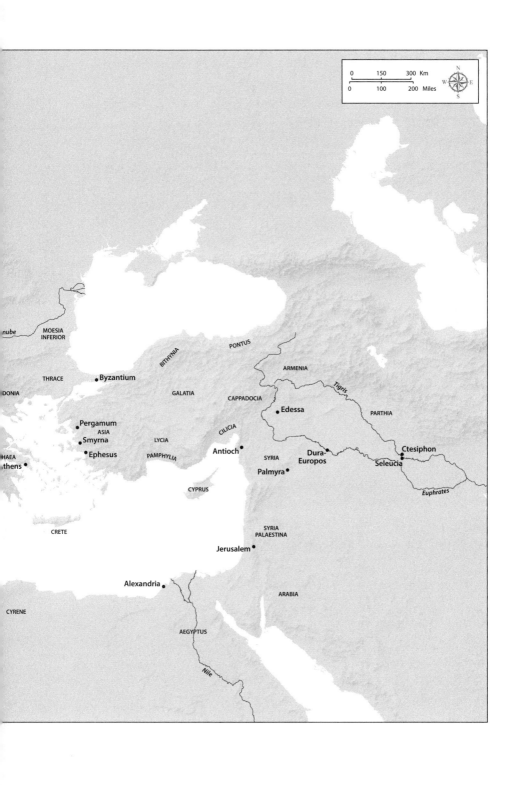

0 150 300 Km
0 100 200 Miles

N
W E
S

nube

MOESIA INFERIOR

THRACE

DONIA

•Byzantium

BITHYNIA

PONTUS

GALATIA

ARMENIA

Tigris

CAPPADOCIA

•Edessa

PARTHIA

Pergamum
ASIA
•Smyrna

CILICIA

LYCIA

•Ephesus

PAMPHYLIA

Antioch•

SYRIA

Dura-
Europos•

Ctesiphon•

HAEA
thens •

Seleucia

•Palmyra

CYPRUS

Euphrates

CRETE

SYRIA
PALAESTINA

Jerusalem•

Alexandria•

ARABIA

CYRENE

AEGYPTUS

Nile

INTRODUCTION

A FURIOUS BEGINNING

Roman soldiers surged south along the Euphrates River. After four years of indecisive battle, hostile Persia—the once unfailing bulwark against Rome's eastern ambitions—finally yielded in the autumn of AD 165. The Roman legions pummeled Parthian defenses at the Syrian border city of Dura-Europos, opening the way for a march deep into the now exposed Persian heartland. But just eighty kilometers north of Babylon, the Roman advance halted. Standing sentinel were the twin cities of Ctesiphon and Seleucia—their riches ripe for looting. Seleucia likely felt the first blows. Founded by Alexander the Great's general Seleucus in the late fourth century BC, the cosmopolis of perhaps four hundred thousand people enjoyed abundant wealth in trade due to the city's privileged position along the canal that bridged the Euphrates and Tigris. Seleucia was a melting pot of Greek, Babylonian, and Persian cultures.[1] But the city's doomed elite had no desire to endure a protracted Roman siege. Throwing open their gates, the Seleucians surrendered in the reasonable hopes of securing clemency. Forsaking mercy, however, Roman soldiers rampaged through the streets— pillaging, raping, and burning. After days, possibly weeks of impious barbarity, a jewel of the Hellenistic World was forever ruined. Rome's military machine, as many times before, reversed centuries of civilization in a matter of days. It would not be the last time.

According to ancient accounts of the sack, untamed Roman blood-lust kindled divine ire. Along some Seleucian street stood a shrine of Apollo—god of light, averter of evil, bringer of pestilence. Apollo's reputation for vengeance was as old as the classical world itself. In Greek literature's opening act—Homer's *Iliad*—Apollo inflicted a deadly plague upon an entire army because their commander, the brash Argive king Agamemnon, stole the daughter of one of Apollo's priests.[2] It was thus well-established fact that Apollo's fury was often disproportionately cataclysmic. Heedless of history's warnings, however, Roman troops broke into Apollo's holy sanctuary. Groping about for treasures, the soldiers smashed jars and pried open every nook and crevice. In their chaotic greed, the looters unsealed a nasty surprise—a deadly cloud of pestilence.[3] The soldiers breathed in the noxious air, unknowingly inaugurating a deadly plague that would decimate the entire Roman world. Furious Apollo, as always, received his vengeance in spades.

Although largely a fiction, the tale of the Romans' desecration of Apollo's Seleucian shrine survives in two separate ancient accounts. True, a disease undoubtedly infected Roman soldiers in Parthia. But other details—the violated shrine to be sure, but perhaps also even the specific legions and location—are part of a puzzling collection of sources which tell of widespread pestilence in the Roman Empire in the mid- to late second century AD. On the one hand, it seems the authors of that era wanted future readers to know that a serious disease afflicted their world. But a deeper message is embedded in what has survived. In the worldview of most Greek and Roman writers—from Homer to Procopius—disease was but a symptom of a far more corrosive and ancient malady: impiety. At the world's mythical founding, for example, Pandora disregarded the gods and cracked open a forbidden jar of curses that plagued humanity for all time.[4] Many if not most ancient descriptions of disasters reflect this connection between sacrilege and catastrophe—emphasizing the divine portents that accompanied calamities more than all other aspects.[5] The story of the sack of Seleucia fits squarely in this tradition. It seems tailor-made to connect the unprecedented disease outbreaks of that age to impieties awful enough to generate such sweeping sickness. Shrine desecration was among the most odious crimes against the gods. So too, however, was betrayal. The Roman commander at Seleucia, Avidius Cassius, would later break faith with his emperor Marcus Aurelius (AD 161–180). Cassius was, therefore, an obvious scapegoat for a pandemic which Roman writers otherwise could not explain.

The mystifying disease outbreak now known as the Antonine plague continues to puzzle to this day. Its influence on the fortunes of ancient civilizations remains one of the oldest unsolved mysteries in human history. Many nineteenth-century historians thought it a grand tragedy—an "unrecoverable blow" to the Roman Empire that left tens of millions dead.[6] But archaeological discoveries in subsequent decades yielded little proof of a calamitous empire-wide plague under Marcus Aurelius. As a result, serious doubts about the authenticity of ancient accounts emerged by the 1960s and 1970s.[7] It seemed the Antonine plague was largely a non-event in Roman history. ·

But scholarly opinion began to swing back toward plague maximalism after a physician and ancient historian revisited descriptions of the disease in ancient medical texts and diagnosed the Antonine plague pathogen as smallpox—a disease that killed around one-third of its victims.[8] Later, a pivotal article in the *Journal of Roman Archaeology* directly connected a wide range of evidence for concurrent economic and social crisis to the Antonine plague.[9] By the 1990s, the Antonine plague regained its status as one of the deadliest biological events in human history *and* became a deus ex machina to explain Rome's perplexing plummet following centuries of peace and prosperity. Now, in the wake of the SARS-CoV-2 pandemic, scholarly and popular interest in the Antonine plague has reached fever pitch.

But unlike history's other momentous scourges, even the most fundamental aspects of the Antonine plague remain unknown. To call the outbreak a "plague" is questionable. Sure, "plague" can be a generic term for "epidemic." But "plague" also implies *bubonic plague*, and historians still have no idea which pathogen (or pathogens) was responsible.[10] Many historians still favor a smallpox diagnosis, but this book will not presume such without evidence.[11] Instead "pox," like "plague," serves merely as a generic placeholder for a pustular disease that still defies historians' efforts to uncover its secrets nearly two thousand years later. When did the outbreak begin and end? How fast and how far did the disease spread? How many people died? Did some populations in the Roman Empire have preexisting immunity? And did the Antonine plague rise to the status of a pandemic? If so, it would have been the world's first.[12] Despite arriving in a period and place with a relatively high survival rate of source material, the Antonine plague left behind surprisingly little direct evidence of its deadly presence. As a result, so few of these key questions have thus far been answered with much confidence.

The meager evidence that survives, furthermore, seems confusing and even contradictory. Some ancient accounts speak of the disease "slaughtering" armies and "destroying" cities; other Roman writers are strangely silent. Why is the source material so muddled? In the pre-industrial world, disease was a normal if not chronic aspect of daily life—a constant as sure as the seasons. The social significance of epidemics was far different in the Roman world as opposed to our own. SARS-CoV-2, the defining pestilence of our era—a virus that killed millions and prompted unprecedented public health interventions throughout much of the world for years—might have gone unnoticed in the Roman world, lost in the noise of deaths from malaria, tuberculosis, influenza, and thousands of other biological maladies. Disasters of all sorts—not just diseases but famines, earthquakes, floods, and volcanic eruptions—were, as ancient historian Jeffrey Toner observes, a "structural part of Roman life."[13] So when several ancient authors speak of truly catastrophic epidemic outbreaks, we should pay attention. *Something* significant must have risen above day-to-day preindustrial misery and mortality. And the cluster of sources around the Antonine plague is obvious—even if it is ill-defined.[14] We know that ancient authors indulged in the kinds of speculation and even outright fear-mongering now common to their modern counterparts in the corporate media. In the past as in the present: fear sells. In their relentless pursuit of status—a currency more valuable than gold in the Roman world—ancient authors decorated their accounts of disease outbreaks with exaggerations meant to outdo those of their predecessors, especially the Greek father of history Thucydides's genre-defining tale of plague in Classical Athens's "Golden Age." Some Roman authors even played up plagues to cast aspersions upon political and social rivals. And so even as literary sources offer the most direct evidence of the Antonine plague's significance, such sources are also the most prone to preserve outright lies.

Worse, it is hardly obvious which sources should count as Antonine-plague evidence. Contemporary with the pandemic, for example, are vague references to sicknesses in personal letters, census records of vanishing villagers, inscriptions to gods and goddesses for health and safety, and even several mass graves. Such evidence *seems* to hint at serious disease outbreaks, while simultaneously *confirming* very little. The search for the Antonine plague's true story casts nets into the deepest parts of Roman history—material difficult to navigate, with many distracting dangers and false finds. Circumstantial evidence sings a siren song both alluring and perilous. Contemporary with the outbreak, major mining operations ceased, the output of stone quarries declined, emperors struggled to recruit soldiers, cities erupted in violence, regional officials persecuted Christians, and price inflation soared. The Antonine plague could have contributed to each and every one of these phenomena . . . or none of them. Compared to more recent and better-sourced pandemics, scholars identify the scope and scale of the Antonine plague mostly through its assumed echoes in proxies: inscriptions to Apollo, census documents, paleoclimatological data, real estate contracts, rental agreements, and fieldworker wages. If these proxies echo the effects of a pandemic, their signal is unfortunately distorted by unclear causality and muffled by time. To take just one example: Egyptian census reports show that numerous villages in the Nile Delta lost most of their inhabitants during the early years of the Antonine plague. In one village, 93 percent of citizens simply vanished.[15] We don't know if these inhabitants died of plague, or died of some other cause like starvation, or didn't even die at all but perhaps fled unpayable tax obligations or joined the revolts that proliferated in the area contemporary with the pestilence.[16] Before the disease arrived in Egypt, years of drought had forced many villagers into the Nile Delta's marshes to forage for food. Untangling the layers of crisis in just one region is challenging enough, but multiple regions of the Roman Empire leave behind evidence of chaos at the time of the Antonine plague.

The pandemic swept through the Roman Empire at the twilight of its economic and military apex—a period historians have named the Pax Romana: the "Roman Peace." The nearly two-hundred-year era lasted from the reign of Rome's first emperor, Augustus, in 31 BC through the lifetime of Marcus Aurelius, who died in AD 180. In the eyes of most commentators, both ancient and modern, the Pax Romana was a prosperous period—a golden age for Rome, of western civilization itself even. Surely it must have been? But some historians think Pax Romana a deceptive moniker—perhaps even pure propaganda.[17] For one thing, the age was hardly free from conflict. The peace of the Pax Romana was in fact quite narrowly conceived: it was the "peace" of un-questioned domination. The Roman senator Tacitus put it best: "they make a desert and they call it peace."[18] The defining characteristic of the period was hardly an absence of violence but rather an absence of any meaningful limit on Rome's ability to make violence.

Still, when Marcus was made emperor in AD 161, Roman power had been unquestioned for as long as anyone could remember. Few sus-pected they were living through the death throes of the Pax Romana. The evidence, however, as this book will detail, was all around them. Why couldn't the reigning Roman elite perceive the end of their world order? Many no doubt saw what they wanted—looking to the superfi-cial signs and symbols propagated by the Roman state. Marcus pro-moted himself as a wise and studious philosopher-king. And, for the first time in history, a second man shared the supreme power. Marcus's co-emperor was Lucius Verus (AD 161–169)—stylized as a young and charismatic military leader. The two men were bound by blood—formally adopted as brothers and united through Lucius's marriage to Marcus's daughter, Lucilla, when she was no older than fourteen. The territory Marcus and Lucius ruled was vast: roughly 7,500,000 square kilometers of land and sea—comparable to the size of the contiguous United States. And, apparently, it was not finished expanding. The Empire seemed poised to absorb lands in both Persia in Asia and Germania in Europe. Beyond those broadening horizons, Rome's wider economic influence extended from sea to shining sea, from the Atlantic to the Indian Ocean.[19]

And yet, Marcus and Lucius had barely taken power before numerous regions of the Roman Empire plunged into crisis. We still don't know exactly why. Cassius Dio—a Roman senator who lived through the tumult of the late second and early third centuries AD—later realized he had witnessed a monumental transition. On the death of Marcus, the senator grieved an age that would never return: "our history now descends from a kingdom of gold to one of iron and rust."[20] Dio's retrospective on the political events of his lifetime recounts, blow by blow, how feckless emperors, sycophantic senators, out-of-control soldiers, insurrectionists, and invaders each took turns pummeling sacred Roman institutions until, in the space of a generation, a once golden and glorious empire was mercilessly bludgeoned into a heap of slag.

Dio's report of the Pax Romana's death, however, is exaggerated. The senator had an ax to grind with Marcus's son and successor Commodus (AD 176–192).[21] Dio and other Roman writers portray Commodus as both detached and deranged—an emperor who allowed his patrimony to lapse into disorder and insurrection while he paraded in Roman arenas in the guise of a gladiator. Few modern historians fix the end of the Pax Romana on the very day Commodus ascended to the purple, but many agree that by the end of the troubled emperor's reign in the early 190s, if not before, Rome's historical path had taken a permanent turn. And there is no denying that the last quarter of the second century was transformative: key regions witnessed sustained foreign invasions, would-be emperors fought prolonged civil wars, the coinage was debased, and waves of social violence and bloody religious conflict swelled in previously peaceful cities. These disasters and more seemed to herald Rome's new normal: a Pax Romana in ruins.

The Roman Empire nevertheless plodded on for centuries following the Pax Romana's traumatic death. "Decline and fall" may offer a powerful narrative device for what followed, but the phrase is a gross oversimplification. Essential markers of a complex society endured: the Empire's sizable and socially and economically stratified population, its cultural diversity, its general unification of various heterogenic institutions into a politically if not ideologically unified construct.[22] But the Empire had nevertheless changed forever. To borrow a term from ecologist Marten Scheffer, the Roman system entered a new "stability domain" by the third century AD if not earlier.[23] This new Roman Empire—heated in the economic stresses of the mid-second century, purged in the crucible of pestilence, and hammered in the accompanying crises of the decades that followed the late AD 160s—differed from its predecessor in numerous ways. The geography of prosperity in the west, for example, shifted away from central Italy and toward places like northern Africa and Britain. In northwest Africa especially, the crises of the late second and early third centuries—including the Antonine plague—barely register in the archaeological record.[24] The crises of the age, however, devastated Italy, Gaul, the Balkans, Asia Minor, and Egypt—regions crucial to the Pax Romana's tributary economy. The patchwork Empire that survived the Antonine plague era was fundamentally less flexible, even brittle in some ways—a condition clarified in the upheavals of the tumultuous third century.

A major argument in this book is that such failures in Roman institutions channeled the course of the Antonine plague as much as the course of the plague damaged these same institutions. Dio's "age of iron and rust" witnessed a multifaceted maelstrom of disease, food shortages, war, and localized environmental changes. As with large-scale shifts in any multicultural territorial empire, the changes that occurred during and after the Antonine plague were complicated and widely varying in their causes and effects, both short and long term. Even as a new and deadly contagion punctured the Empire's porous borders, so too did foreign migrants. Disease killed Roman workers, but war and famine also stole untold lives. Nature played a key role in the chaos, but often on the regional or subregional level, and in ways tightly integrated with preindustrial political and economic realities. The Mediterranean Basin was (and still is) polka-dotted with microregions. Climate conditions in one Italian or Anatolian valley, for instance, might be vastly different than those of a hilltop just a few kilometers away.[25] Rome's roads and maritime infrastructure grafted together these diverse localities, but largely through a perplexing mixture of capricious state power, tributary demands, military might, family networks, and privileged business partnerships.[26] The Antonine plague was a crucial factor in the demise of the Pax Romana, but so too was Rome's preindustrial context.

The outbreak's direct effects—death and disease—were no doubt significant. Documented epidemic surges in Rome, Italy, and Asia Minor were sudden, severe, and disruptive. Many died—perhaps millions. But at least equally important, as the disease spread and endured—perhaps for a decade or more—the very notion of pandemic itself implanted into the collective consciousness of an entire empire. This social contagion perhaps represents the Antonine plague's most transformative power—a power derived from the disease's lingering presence as a threat both real and perceived, a disease that could strike anywhere in the known world, that killed and maimed bodies both individual and collective. The pandemic and its legacy stretched conceptual frameworks related to everything, from disease to the divine, in the minds of those who struggled to understand and cope with the rapid and comprehensive changes that took place before, during, and after the Pax Romana's curtain call.[27] Thus, as both fact and fable, the Antonine plague resonated throughout the Roman Empire and beyond.

This book, therefore, reflects the tangled evidence and ghostly legacy of what I believe was the world's first pandemic. It is an account which dwells on details, irregularities, and broader contexts of the source material—especially the preexisting stresses of the decade prior to the Antonine plague. This approach enables readers to better grasp the pandemic's true significance and meaning. The particularities and interactions among the evidence assembled here reveal some sensational surprises: the Roman Empire's connectivity was as much a liability as an asset in the face of a novel disease, the pandemic was less deadly in one place compared to another, and different causes, such as famine, war, or simply bad luck, could be just as influential on events as the pandemic itself.[28] Many of the charts in this book, for example, mark the year AD 165—the year our sources suggest the pandemic first struck Roman cities. As the charts show, sometimes that date correlates with sudden changes in key proxies, but not always. So while this book acknowledges the pandemic's significant influence, it also accounts for its variability, social context, and unique historical circumstances.

The Antonine plague's history is much like a problem known to many parents of small children. How many times have I taken out a puzzle box only to find that pieces are missing and that the box also contains a frustrating bevy of bits from other puzzles, games, and Lego sets (and a half-eaten cracker for some reason). Not only are needed pieces hopelessly lost, but not all that survives in the puzzle box is relevant. The Antonine plague is such a conundrum, only writ large. This book looks long at each piece, with frequent glances at the emerging picture. Constructing a truly thorough account requires both the historian's traditional tool kit—source analysis, contextualization, synthesis, and so forth—and methods from the social sciences and environmental studies, sorting out not only what the Antonine plague was but also what it was not. Story by story and source by source, I invite readers to collaborate with me—to follow my research, yes, but also to draw their own conclusions. Even with so much of the puzzle still missing, my hope is that what follows in this book offers readers a trustworthy depiction of one of history's most impactful biological events.

PART I

PREEXISTING CONDITIONS

Around the Mediterranean lies the continents far and wide, pouring an endless flow of goods to Rome. There is brought from every land and sea whatever is brought forth by the seasons and is produced by all countries, rivers, lakes, and the skills of Greeks and foreigners. So that anyone who wants to behold all these products must either journey through the whole world to see them or else come to this city. . . . So many merchantmen arrive here with cargoes from all over, at every season, and with each return of the harvest, that the city seems like a common warehouse of the world. One can see so many cargoes from India, or, if you wish from Arabia. . . . Clothing from Babylonia and the luxuries from the Barbarian lands beyond arrive in much greater volume. . . . Egypt, Sicily, and the civilized parts of Africa are Rome's farms. . . . All things converge here: trade, seafaring, agriculture, metallurgy, all the skills which exist and have existed, anything that is begotten and grows. Whatever cannot be seen here belongs in the category of non-existence.

—AELIUS ARISTIDES'S ORATION "TO ROME" (OR. 26.11–18),
MID-SECOND CENTURY AD

I

ROME'S FRAGILE PEACE

Rome of the Pax Romana seemed replete with the bounty of the entire known world. Eastern trade boomed. Egyptian grain poured into city storehouses each summer. Greece sent her marbles, and Dacia her silver and gold. Tens of thousands of slaves from every known land walked the city streets. Many were the fruits of conquest and hegemony—a grand harvest that inspired the orator Aelius Aristides to boast in AD 155, ten years before the Antonine plague swept through the Empire, that "all things converge here: trade, seafaring, agriculture, metallurgy, all the skills which exist and have existed, anything that is begotten and grows. Whatever cannot be seen here belongs in the category of non-existence."[1]

On the eve of the Antonine plague, the literature of the Empire's elite suggests they lived in the greatest time in not just Roman history but all human history. English historian Edward Gibbon in his *History of the Decline and Fall of the Roman Empire* famously reached this same conclusion: "If a man were called to fix the period in the history of the world, during which the condition of the human race was most happy and prosperous, he would, without hesitation, name that which elapsed from the death of Domitian [AD 96] to the accession of Commodus [AD 180]."[2] Yet in the intervening centuries since Gibbon published those quotable lines, archaeologists and historians have uncovered a trove of evidence that suggests the abundance of the Pax Romana came at tremendous cost. And although prosperity had its price, Rome's nobility—the senators and equestrians with their vast estates, moneylending networks, and control of the imperial state—rarely had to pay it.

Instead, much of the pain that produced Rome's gain was borne by those plundered and even slaughtered at the Empire's margins, both geographic and social. Universal empires in all periods promise "peace" once there are no more external enemies to fight; but inevitably, the violence previously exported merely consolidates inward in the form of oppression and control.[3] Those subject to Rome's mechanisms of compulsion were too numerous and diverse to categorize. Many lived among the various foreign peoples subject to brutal martial law, forced enslavement, or crushing expropriations. Others were indirect victims. Roman taxes, conscription, and other forms of coercion alienated farmers from ancestral lands, driving them into filthy and unwelcoming cities. Even the Empire's own soldiers paid dearly in both blood and treasure so members of the ruling class might wallow wanton in riches and repose. But at the noble heart of Rome, these costs of empire were out of sight, and therefore out of mind. Aristides's oration unwittingly captured the freeriding elite's most subtle entitlement: ignorance. "Wars . . . no longer seem real," the orator beamed, "stories about them are interpreted more as myths by the many who hear them."[4] For a precious few like Aristides, the peace of the Pax Romana seemed a gift that would continue to give into eternity.

But the Roman social order was more than just exploiters and the exploited; there were shades of gray. The hues, however, are difficult to distinguish, as elite perspectives dominate our sources. The senator Tacitus, for example, divided the commoners in the city of Rome into two distinct classes: the respectable clients and freedmen attached to noble houses, and the "dirty" plebs who were "addicted" to the circus and theater.[5] The senator generalized from his lofty position of political, social, and economic privilege. Modern historians also observe ancient Rome from a distance, but with new inscriptions, accounting tablets, and other archaeological material bringing some areas into focus. It seems that middling inhabitants—wealthy merchants, local landlords, professional artisans, and even some smallholder farmers—escaped the typical preindustrial traps of scarcity and autarky. Recent archaeological surveys of rural sites in southwest Tuscany, for example, have turned up numerous small but specialized farming and production operations. Not all non-elites were helpless victims of oppression; some used markets and other institutions to mitigate the challenges of preindustrial life in a tributary empire.[6]

Was this society capable of withstanding the world's first major pandemic? Rome was about to find out. The question demands we inspect the Empire's social and economic foundations, especially the extent to which the inhabitants of the Roman world were already teetering on the brink of poverty. Poverty on any scale—whether for individuals or whole societies—interacts with and affects many of the basic elements of human health and wellness: nutrition, labor, stress, and the environment. At the level of the general population, poverty reduces what social scientists call "resilience." In simple terms, resilience is the capacity for a society to retain its essential functions, structures, identities, and feedbacks amid or in response to disasters.[7] Massive exogenous shocks—unpredicted events that originate from outside a system—alone do not transform human societies; endogenous institutions and human choices play a crucial role in determining the significance and lasting effects of systemic crises. Resilience depends in large part on what Scheffer calls "adaptive capacity"—that is, "the degree to which a system is capable of reorganization, learning, and adaptation."[8] Resilience is, therefore, neither monolithic nor simplistic. Different shocks and different societies interact in unique and often unforeseen ways. Causality does not merely move one way—from disaster to social crisis. Widespread poverty, for instance, injects stress into the social fabric of societies before any cataclysmic acts of God. A society already struggling to adapt to endogenous stressors is more likely to undergo a transformative crisis in the face of a sudden and significant burden of parasitic microbes.

Few familiar with Roman history would pick the Pax Romana as a moment when the Roman Empire crossed the threshold of resilience.[9] The Roman Empire of the mid-second century seemingly reached the pinnacle of preindustrial prosperity and resilience—a golden age of the ancient world. Elites like Aristides propagate such perceptions plainly.

So too do the numerous victory arches, columns, and monumental buildings of the Pax Romana that still stand tall in the Eternal City. But Nobel Prize–winning Austrian economist Friedrich Hayek wisely alluded to the deceptions of imperial monumentality: "Nothing is more misleading," he said, "than the conventional formulae of historians who represent the achievement of a powerful state as the culmination of cultural evolution: it has often marked its end."[10] In fact, another Austrian— ancient historian Walter Scheidel—has gone further, arguing that only when Rome's super state ended was Europe finally free to achieve lasting prosperity.[11]

Similarly, I believe it is an open question as to whether the highest achievements of the Pax Romana sufficiently buffered the Empire's population against the novel pandemic that swept across Eurasia in the AD 160s. In fact, paradoxically, it may be in part *because* of Rome's apparent successes—its ability to wage protracted wars, its remarkable road network, its Egyptian breadbasket, its internal urban immigration, its maritime trade links with Africa, India, and East Asia—that such a large part of the preindustrial world so suddenly succumbed to global pestilence and suffered major institutional shifts in the pandemic's wake. The story of the Antonine plague therefore does not begin with the disease but with an essential exploration of its contexts—a thorough autopsy of the surprisingly weak foundations which struggled to bear the Pax Romana's glorious facade.

And so this opening chapter penetrates beneath the veneer of Roman self-aggrandizement and hubris to examine key factors of resilience on the eve of the Antonine plague. To what extent did the inhabitants of the Roman Empire, whether they lived in the cities or the countryside, experience many of the key markers of extreme poverty: high infant mortality, low life expectancy, low literacy rates, and a subsistence diet deficient in basic nutrients? Could most people obtain reliable housing, and this on a permanent basis?[12] Monumental marvels like aqueducts and bathhouses evoke awe, but did urban sanitation infrastructure make a practical difference to public health? Did elites effectively manage and redistribute resources in the face of local and regional crises? Subsequent chapters go deeper—probing the Empire's ecological context and its food supply, as well as its exposure to new pathogens via trade and military movements. The Pax Romana may have been an economic and cultural high point in the overall story of Rome and its empire, but, as we shall soon see, ancient Rome remained mired in its preindustrial limits.

The Rubbish of Empire

Even two thousand years after it was built, the house of the Vettii stands as a stunning marvel of elite opulence. Situated in northwest Pompeii, guests entering the atrium of the magnificent two-story home would have been struck by the intricate wall paintings, the refracted natural light cascading through an open rectangular skylight, and the shallow pool in the center of the atrium. If it happened to be raining, the water would have gently poured through the skylight into the pool below— perhaps catching the sunlight just right, casting vivid rainbows in the mist. Through the vapor glaze, guests caught hints of the Vettii's manicured garden in the background—its fountains and statues imposing serenity upon all who entered. The house's other rooms held similar marvels and luxuries: additional domestic pools and fountains, bright murals, gardens, statues, reception rooms, colonnades, numerous bedrooms, and even a shop to provide rental income from a local artisan.[13] And this was one of many such houses in one of many such cities in the Roman world.

But intermingled with the wealthy were the progressively less affluent. These, by necessity, left far fewer traces of their presence. Citizens of modest incomes dwelt in much smaller, moderately outfitted homes.[14] Like glue squished between the carpenter's wood, their crammed residences occupied the spaces between the larger homes of the elite. Others dwelt in tenement blocks (*insulae*) with cramped rooms, basic furniture, and without in-home access to running water or bathing facilities.[15] Multiple families might occupy a single apartment, or even a single room. But at least these people had walls and a roof. No small number of Pompeii's ten thousand or so inhabitants lacked access to permanent housing. These slept in the shadows: in alleys, sewers, tombs, and bushes.[16] Their bones are now ash and dust. But we know they were there, even if we will never know who they were.

Pompeii's homeless and transients—some of whom undoubtedly huddled against the walls of the house of the Vettii itself during the cold of winter—begged for handouts from passersby. These unfortunates could be of any age and condition—from the old and weak to the young and tough. By day, the beggars crowded the streets in search of a spare coin or two. Those young enough might earn their bread by offering their bodies for the gratification of others. Around 150 surviving graffiti in Pompeii refer to individual prostitutes, advertising prices for a range of sexual acts.[17] Adolescents sold themselves; so too did children.[18] The old, the disabled, the sick, however—those whose bodies lacked value under the cruel accounting of preindustrial poverty—simply made a nuisance of themselves at public festivals, sacrificial ceremonies, and even private weddings, demanding a small ransom to depart in peace. In fact, the very senator who first termed his age the Pax Romana— Seneca, advisor to the emperor Nero (AD 54–68)—begrudged such alms-seekers as "flocks of half-dead creatures."[19] The religiously sensitive Romans feared evil omens on otherwise cheerful days and so obligingly paid the beggars for a few hours' peace.

Unlike in many modern cities, where the middle and upper classes pay good money to thoroughly segregate themselves from the urban poor, poverty was inescapably rampant in Roman cities. Even atop Rome's famed hills—where the grandest houses of the rich cast shadows on the malarial slums below—shoddily built apartment complexes tilted in the sky, overflowing with immigrants, day laborers, and the semi-transient. But structures of stone and brick were luxuries. Both inside and outside of cities, the barely unhoused dug cave-like rooms into the sides of hills, fashioned crude wood hovels, or lay in huts of brush, reed, or even refuse. Ventilation in such dwellings was poor, and the constant intake of smoke from oil lamps and fires hung about ancient neighborhoods, accumulating in the lungs of even the wealthiest citizens. Poverty, therefore, suffocated aloof aristocrats as well as the poor. It is no wonder that Seneca claimed that his health improved dramatically after leaving Rome and its "awful odor of reeking kitchens which . . . pour forth a ruinous mess of steam and soot."[20] Under such conditions, even routine respiratory viruses must have transformed into serious killers.

But those who secured an indoor sleeping-spot—potentially in the hallway of some patron or master—endured perils invisible to the naked eye. Inside ancient dwellings, pests of all sorts left fecal matter and carcasses to taint the bodies of any who slept on floors. House owners and their families likely ate well; their servants and slaves, however, dined on kitchen scraps, including undercooked and rotten food teeming with bacteria. Household workers drank unboiled water, contaminated with colonies of parasites. Servants and slaves frequented the parts of the property where refuse of all kinds was disposed and stored. Even in luxurious houses equipped with cesspits and chamber pots, garbage and waste were frequently chucked out into the street, regardless of the quality of the neighborhood or its population density.[21] The ancient city's bustling winepress then went to work—trudging the rotten food, blood, urine, feces, vomit, insects, rodents, bacteria, and all other forms of waste into an ever-present coating of sludge that glommed onto any who ventured outside. In some quarters of Rome, for example, the bacterial muck was so thick that the poet Juvenal's legs (not merely his feet or ankles) were often "caked with mud" from the city streets.[22]

Ancient Rome was a shithole. Its roughly one million inhabitants produced around 45,000 kilograms of feces and 1.3 million liters of urine each day.[23] Where did it all end up? Graffiti in Pompeii suggests that the Empire's privileged urbanites defecated just about everywhere, and even saw fit to sign their names to mark the occasion—a way for the literate to pass the time while they vacated their bowels against some alley wall.[24] In a futile attempt to keep the streets around their establishments clean, some property owners put up signs to discourage defecators. Two bright red inscriptions in an alley between apartment buildings in Pompeii warn: "defecator, watch out for what might happen to you!"[25] But with so many people in such scarce space, piles of human and animal waste on the streets were as common as cobblestones.[26] Accepting the inevitable, some property owners merely encouraged would-be defecators to go elsewhere: "If you must defecate, pass by this place for good luck."[27] Other notices pointed out more inviting public locations: "Defecator, continue on to the wall [of the city]. If you are caught [here], you will suffer punishment. Watch out!"[28] In and around Rome, similar inscriptions warn against dumping everything from feces to bodies.[29]

In theory, Rome should have been less rife with offal compared to other ancient settlements. The Eternal City enjoyed top-of-the-line infrastructure, basic sanitation services, and legal rules aimed at regulating its million-worker feces factory.[30] Laws prohibiting the on-street disposal of human waste and corpses, however, went ignored.[31] Near Rome's Esquiline Hill, a stone's throw from surviving inscriptions prohibiting dumping corpses and sewage, excavators noted their discovery of around seventy-five pits filled with "a nauseating mixture of the corpses of the poor, animal carcasses, sewage and other garbage." The two-thousand-year-old "black, viscid, pestilent, unctuous matter" was so putrid that those digging up the site had to be granted frequent breaks.[32] Rome's public latrines—some of which still survive to the present—presumably funneled at least some waste into the sewers rather than the streets. But Rome's sewers were in fact never intended for waste disposal. Rather, they were designed to alleviate flooding and drain standing water.[33] Rome was, after all, built on a swamp. In fact, sudden or severe floods—such as the one which occurred in Rome just before the Antonine plague—backed up the sewers and vomited months-worth of sickly soup up into the city's streets.[34] Far from cleaning Rome, the sewers were a constant source of rodents, pests, and noxious gases. Clogged sewers quickly became stinking cesspits.[35] And sewers were prime dumping ground for bodies. In the drain below a bathhouse in the coastal city of Ascalon in Palestine, archaeologists found the remains of nearly one hundred newborn babies.[36] In Greek cities Athens and Messene, hundreds of infant corpses as well as dog skeletons were found dropped down wells.[37] But the sewers did not merely absorb the corpses of the unwanted or anonymous masses. Even a dead emperor or two was stuffed down the tunnels.[38] It is no wonder that most Roman homeowners refused to install in-home sewer access.[39]

Corpses occasionally clustered in Roman cities. The normal body count in mid-second-century AD Rome alone must have hit triple digits most days, with seasonal spikes in the summer.[40] While some of these cadavers received proper burial or cremation outside the city, Rome's many transient and impoverished were afforded the same respect in death as they had been given in life: none. When these died, the fortunate ones were burned on a communal pyre or simply cast into a mass grave (if one was open and nearby).[41] But many human bodies ended up in the sewers or the Tiber, or even kicked to the side of the road or in an alley to rot or be eaten by animals. Aged, sick, or disabled slaves were tossed out even before they died—left to slowly expire alone in the slimy streets. Some made it to the island in the Tiber before expiring; at least these withered away in the presence of the physician-god Asclepius. The numbers of dying slaves forsaken to a lonely and painful death became such a nuisance to the free living that emperors enacted laws to curb slave abandonment.[42]

Romans also abandoned their unwanted infants—many still alive—to refuse piles, alleys, sewers, or on the streets. The wailing of forsaken babies must have been a constant noise amid the urban background bustle. Passersby occasionally rescued these helpless ones, raising them as "foundling" slaves and selling them later for profit—often into prostitution. But many infants died cold, hungry, alone, and in searing agony—crying for days until their breath failed, and they simply expired. But there were worse fates. The Jewish philosopher Philo of Alexandria leaves little to the imagination:

> [Some parents] do the deed with their own hands; with monstrous cruelty and barbarity they stifle and throttle the first breath which the infants draw or throw them into a river or into the depths of the sea, after attaching some heavy substance to make them sink more quickly under its weight. Others take them to be exposed in some desert place, hoping, they themselves say, that they may be saved, but leaving them in actual truth to suffer the most distressing fate. For all the beasts that feed on human flesh visit the spot and feast unhindered on the infants, a fine banquet provided by their sole guardians, those who

above all others should keep them safe, their fathers and mothers. Carnivorous birds, too, come flying down and gobble up the fragments, that is, if they have not discovered them earlier, for, if they have, they get ready to fight the beasts of the field for the whole carcass.[43]

The Empire's cities were impossible to cleanse. The Roman government employed slaves to perform the grim work of body removal. Additional help was provided by roving animals—dogs, carrion, and pigs; these feasted on the decaying flesh before it putrefied.[44] The poet Martial terrified his readers with such a fate. He wrote of a destitute man on the edge of death "hearing around him the howling of dogs for his body, and driving away birds of prey by shaking his rags."[45] Human remains could turn up just about any time or any place. Even the emperor Vespasian (AD 69–79) sat down to breakfast one day, only to have his meal interrupted by a dog carrying a human hand in its mouth.[46] Routine body removal was probably manageable; corpses hardly rotted on every corner. But the numerous anecdotes in literary sources about bodies on the street only work in an environment where death was not only highly visible but could at times inject its gruesome presence in the daily routines of the living.

Aqueduct water flushed out some of Rome's inexhaustible filth. In the age of the Antonine plague, ten working aqueducts supplied Rome with millions of liters of fresh water from rural Italy each day. The famous Pergamese doctor Galen—our most reliable eyewitness to the Antonine plague—was certainly impressed: "In Rome . . . there is the goodness and abundance of fountains and the water of none of them is smelly, toxic, muddy, or hard."[47] And as Scheidel says: "a counter-factual Roman world without aqueducts would have been (even) worse."[48] But Rome's aqueducts, like its sewers, served more as monuments to elite vanity than as a practical means of sanitizing the city. Aqueducts exemplified Roman self-presentation of political power; only the lords of an expansive and wealthy empire could construct such wonders.[49] These practical, applied works of engineering, according to the Roman water specialist Frontinus, were superior compared to the "idle Pyramids or the useless, although famous, works of the Greeks."[50]

In aggregate terms, Rome's aqueducts may have brought more than one hundred liters of water per person per day. Undoubtedly many Romans relied upon aqueduct water. However, drinking such water was not without risks. Unbeknownst to the Romans, their groundwater contained excessive fluorine due to local volcanoes. Also, while Romans understood the dangers of lead, their use of lead for pipes, tools, weapons, jewelry, makeup, and even food seasonings exposed them to hemolytic anemia and lead poisoning.[51] Galen observed that the Aqua Alsientina, an aqueduct that brought water to Rome from several freshwater lakes, caused diarrhea if drunk.[52] Rome appointed officials to nominally oversee the provision of drinking water, but maintaining clean water seems to have been beyond Roman capacities.[53] And around 40 percent of the water that came into the city via aqueduct was not drunk at all; instead, it went to various public and ornamental uses in meeting places, baths, barracks, arenas, display fountains, and so on.[54] Another 20 percent of the flow was reserved for the personal enjoyment of the emperor. Emperors doled out the remaining 40 percent of waters to those wealthy enough to pay a hefty "water tax," and who carried enough political and social clout to earn the emperor's favor.[55] So while Roman aqueducts were indeed a marvel to behold, such marveling was in fact their raison d'être—to evoke awe. Aqueducts' improvements to overall health and sanitation—and of course there would be some benefits— are contested at best.[56]

Similar could be said of the Empire's many public baths. While bathing may indeed have washed some contaminants and parasites off Roman bodies, it is nevertheless an open question as to whether a trip to the bathhouse made one more or less clean on net.[57] The emperor Marcus Aurelius used ancient Rome's most pristine bathing facilities, and yet, even he quipped: "What is bathing when you think of it? Oil, sweat, filth, greasy water, everything revolting."[58] The bathwater in ancient bathhouses contained no sterilizing chemicals. It was never disinfected or cleaned. Rather, bath patrons marinated in tepid, stagnant water infused with the dirt, grease, and bacteria added hour by hour, day by day, by hundreds of other bodies—not all of them human. No evidence survives to suggest any rules for changing out bathwater, and scholars believe that the water cycled through a slow process of over-flow.[59] Ancient peoples also engaged in the timeless tradition of urinat-ing in their own bathwater.[60] Contemporary writers discuss how bath-ers washed the fluids, excrement, and feces off their private parts in the baths.[61] Doctors like Galen and Celsus sent many sick people to the public baths for a lengthy soak. People with sores and illnesses were such a common sight among bathers that the emperor Hadrian (AD 117–138) mandated that the sick be given exclusive rights to bathe in the first half of the day.[62] We know that people with open wounds used the baths because medical sources observe cases of gangrene following pub-lic bathing.[63] Prostitutes of all kinds, and their patrons—all presumably rife with cocktails of untreated sexually transmitted diseases—not only bathed but conducted their most intimate business dealings in and around the foul waters.[64] Of course, the prostitutes and clients most likely to fornicate in the public baths were those who lacked more per-manent premises.[65] Non-human residents also copulated near bathwa-ter. In his *Natural History*, Pliny the Elder observed that the main breed-ing ground for Rome's cockroaches was "in the damp warmth of bathhouses."[66] Even invisible vermin—parasites such as roundworms and whipworms—found the baths replete with hosts.[67]

Rome's sanitation infrastructure, therefore, not only failed to mitigate disease and infection, it actively aided and abetted the dispersion and evolution of the parasites and pathogens brought to the cosmopolis from all corners of the known world—like pilgrims to a microbial mecca. A recent comprehensive study of fecal remains from sites across the Roman Empire shows that despite (or maybe because of) the aque-ducts and bathhouses, human parasites thrived in the Roman Empire at similar if not greater levels than in previous eras.[68] Disease was every-where, but especially in Rome. Galen, for example, guessed that ten thousand Romans suffered daily from jaundice and another ten thou-sand from dropsy—invented numbers, but still suggestive of wide-spread poor health.[69] The most persistent killer in Rome and several other ancient cities, however, seems to have been malarial parasites. Several species, but especially *Plasmodium falciparum* and *Plasmodium vivax*, seem to have been endemic in Rome.[70] Ancient sources are replete with malarial symptoms: fevers, chills, impaired brain function, seizures, and faints.[71] Those who survived a bout with malaria, however, were then prone to additional maladies such as pulmonary tuberculosis and gastroenteric infections.[72] Those with *P. falciparum* often died. Malaria was especially bad in the low-lying areas of cities. Much of Rome had been marshland. The poet Horace jibed that spending time in the Roman forum would bring on "fevers and opened wills."[73] Living near the top of Rome's hills may have allowed some relief from the malarial mosquitoes of the lowlands, but unchlorinated baths and pools, street refuse, vermin, and lead poisoning all did their part to make life miserable for even wealthy Romans. Simply living and working away from malarial lowlands could have conceivably added years to one's life expectancy.[74]

Even as Roman cities attained their highest levels of population, prosperity, and wealth during the Pax Romana, the inhabitants of those cities suffered increased biological stress. A recent study of more than ten thousand skeletons from throughout the Roman world shows a serious dip in stature—an indicator of poor physical health—from the first century BC through the end of the fourth century AD.[75] Romans were a good ten centimeters shorter than their Classical and Hellenistic Greek counterparts, Iron Age Celts, and even early medieval Italians.[76] Despite the varied urban diet and higher standard of living relative to the countryside, Roman bones testify that prosperity required a biological price.[77] Who exacted the toll? According to researchers, the microbes that thrived in the high-density low-sanitation cities—viruses, bacteria, parasites—wracked those well-fed Roman bodies.[78] Isotope signatures also show an urban Roman diet low in animal proteins. Romans were simply ill-equipped for the adverse biological jungle that surrounded them. Still, Roman skeletal evidence tends to come from cities; we don't know whether rural Romans enjoyed statures more comparable to those of their ancestors and descendants.[79]

Grinding poverty, poor sanitation, malnutrition, and disease ensured that a person born in the city of Rome could expect to live around twenty-five or thirty years at most. Even elites suffered from the low life expectancy common throughout the preindustrial world.[80] Infant mortality tips the statistics, however. If a person was fortunate enough to live past age five, they likely reached their forties or fifties. Results varied, of course, based on several factors—some of them ecological, some behavioral. Seasonal water quality, for example, was a primary factor in infant mortality, as water supplies blossomed with deadly pathogens in the warm weather.[81] For most Romans, including the elite, the grim prospects for life expectancy placed extreme pressures on young women to reproduce early and often to maintain the population.[82] The math seems insurmountable. Each Roman woman needed to birth at least three daughters and three sons to keep the population stable.[83] Obviously, such birth rates were unrealistic on the aggregate— so how did Pax Romana Rome and other ancient cities preserve and even grow their populations? A steady stream of immigrants and refugees swarmed in from the surrounding countryside. Scholars rightly call ancient Rome a "population sink."[84] Genetic analysis of bodies buried near Rome shows that the city received net immigration from the Near East, Europe, and North Africa.[85] But immigrants' immune systems were unprepared for the biological onslaught that awaited them. No doubt many new arrivals to Rome and other ancient cities succumbed to the pathogens and parasites teeming in their midst.

Above the routine din of death resounding throughout ancient urban streets, the Antonine plague would rise into preeminence in the mid-160s. This epidemic was clearly more than a sudden surge of one of the Empire's familiar pathogens.[86] It was something new, and this is why the disaster caught the attention of elites, city officials, soldiers, and medical professionals. Once the disease took hold, elites and commoners alike suffered similar fates. In a sense, the disease was a perfect match for the ancient city of Rome: it was no respecter of persons.

Disaster Unpreparedness

Before the Antonine plague struck, Rome was home to around one million people—the most populous European city in all of human history prior to the industrial revolution. The wider Empire was also flush with people. Of the global human population in the era of the Pax

Romana, perhaps as many as one out of every four souls—fifty-five to seventy million people—resided in territory directly administered by Rome.[87] Such high population numbers represented a powerful resource, but these were also a tremendous responsibility, especially when disaster struck. To what extent did the governing structures of the Pax Romana protect populations before, during, and after disasters like plagues and food shortages? The answer to this question hints at how the epidemics associated with the Antonine plague would have been handled on the local level. Anecdotal evidence suggests many governing officials were passive, corrupt, and even predatory during calamities. What roused them to pro-social action in challenging times? Mass violence.

The administration of the Roman Empire was simultaneously simple and yet sophisticated. On the one hand, one man—the emperor— enjoyed absolute and even at times capricious authority. He was the paterfamilias—the patriarch and patron—of a household of millions. Emperors, therefore, usually focused on grand matters of state: warfare, diplomacy, major infrastructure projects, founding new cities and colonies. Surviving imperial rescripts of the Pax Romana—direct edicts from the emperor given in response to petitions—nevertheless record imperial interventions in even the most tedious local disputes.[88] Emperors often used their dictatorial power to alleviate disasters. When a plague struck Rome under the emperor Titus (AD 79–81), for example, the imperial biographer Suetonius tells us that "there was no aid, human or divine, which [Titus] did not employ, searching for every kind of sacrifice, and all kinds of medicines for curing the plague and reducing the epidemic's force."[89] But some imperial interventions exacerbated calamities. Nero allegedly used the Great Fire of Rome (AD 64) as a pretext for expropriating "vast sums from private citizens as well as from whole communities," even "depriving the Romans of the free dole of grain."[90]

Roman officials—emperors included—lacked a vision for public health. Practical aid during plagues was instead narrowly focused: mobilizing corpse removal, distributing food, freezing prices, or even issuing direct payments to citizens.[91] Emperors may have also adopted measures like those taken by authorities in Republican Rome during epidemics: suspending festivals, markets, political meetings, and even elections. Such measures were not aimed at mitigating disease transmission; rather, people were just too sick to carry on with business.[92] Shutdowns simply gave official recognition to existing behavior.

Prior to the Antonine plague, the Roman Empire had never encountered a pandemic. Or at least no previous pandemic spread so rapidly and widely as to be identified as such in the sources. In the pre-pandemic age, pestilences were perceived as local phenomena, usually limited to individual cities or regions. Somewhere between 10 and 20 percent of the population of the Empire lived in urban environments.[93] These cities were probably not all as filthy as Rome, but they were nevertheless crowded and, during disasters, chaotic. Local nobility ruled these cities, although always answerable to imperial governors. These elites were duty-bound to care for the crowds—especially in times of plague and famine. But the source material is rife with examples of local rulers exploiting their people more often than not, even when calamities struck. Routine and otherwise "official" exploitation—through taxing citizens' meager surpluses, and thus keeping living standards low—was augmented by the mismanagement and wastage of such surpluses, often on self-aggrandizing status enhancement. Even Roman euergetism—elite gift-giving to communities—was not motivated for public welfare nor did it often accomplish such in practical terms.

The Empire featured several "aqueducts to nowhere," for example. Sometime around AD 110, the emperor Trajan sent his friend Pliny (nephew of the elder Pliny) to the city of Nicomedia as governor of the province of Bithynia in northern Asia Minor. The town council of Nicomedia had dropped millions of sesterces on several aqueducts with no serious plan for completion. Fiscally, the province was a shambles. Pliny did not mince words about the thriftless Nicomedians—tattling to Trajan in a letter that local elites were "throwing away money."[94] In his reply, Trajan was furious, and expected Pliny as governor to solve the problem. The emperor fumed: "I swear that it is also part of your diligent duty to find out who is to blame for the waste of such sums of money."[95] But governors like Pliny were sent out with few if any staff or specialists to accomplish their tasks. Instead, they were granted *imperium*—the right to command and expect automatic compliance.[96] It came down to the governor's *auctoritas* to put this theoretical power into practice and co-opt locals in the business of governance. Local officials could and did passively resist. Councillors of the town of Apamea, for instance, kept their accounting logs back from Pliny despite his official station and (theoretically) grave powers.[97] Rome may have had an expansive territorial empire, a strong military, and a dominant culture, but the Pax Romana was administered more like a household than a modern government bureau.

Pliny's financial problems in Bithynia were soon profligate throughout the Empire. By the mid-second century AD, civic treasuries—meant to be filled by contributions from wealthy local elites (sometimes voluntary, sometimes coerced)—were in a state of chronic insolvency.[98] The emperor Hadrian toured the Empire with money pouring from his pockets—revitalizing declining towns and cities with new public buildings and grants-in-aid.[99] His successor, Antoninus Pius (AD 138–161), granted even small towns rights to levy additional taxes to fund their shortfalls.[100] Of course, more taxes did not solve the systemic problems of mismanagement and outright corruption; if anything, giving corrupt and wasteful officials more money only encouraged them. The Roman Empire, like many predatory systems, was both wealthy and impoverished at the same time. By this, I mean that resources abounded, but they did not consistently reach the multitudes at the margins—a terrible position for a society to be in just prior to a pandemic.

What then kept Roman cities from descending into chaos when disaster struck? A volatile combination of ad hoc elite benefaction and mob violence.[101] Food crises elicited the most extreme reactions. Emergency aid in Roman cities was fairly simple: elites collected in-kind taxes in cereals, some of which they held in reserve for redistribution in key times: for celebrations, holidays, and festivals but also during shortages. Whether as emergency relief or regular entitlements, such redistributions were a matter of basic morality to ancient peoples: the produce of the land was for everyone; landowners were caretakers of community supply, and thus obligated to keep prices low and grain flowing to the general population.[102]

Such social and moral pressures can be powerful regulators, but greed is often more powerful still. Many of the same elites responsible for distributing grain also owned significant patrimonial estates that produced cereals as cash crops. If elites had grain in the storehouse, then famine was good for their bottom line. Shortages brought price spikes, and high prices meant high profits. High profits funded elites' conspicuous consumption and enhanced their social status against their elite peers. It was a thin line to walk, and famines strained the system by disrupting the flow of entitlements. Rioters may have lacked food, but they were full of moral outrage. So it is unsurprising to see scenes like those during a famine in the city of Aspendus in Pamphylia (southern Asia Minor) where, according to the third-century AD Greek sophist Philostratus:

> People lived off anything that gave sustenance, as the upper classes were keeping the grain stored up to create a shortage in the territory. People of every age were infuriated with the chief magistrate, and had begun to light torches to burn him alive, even though he clung to the statues of the emperor.[103]

Fortunately, as the crisis was about to boil over, a wandering philosopher named Apollonius intervened. He shamed and threatened grain-holders in public until they relented and "flooded the market with grain, and the city revived." Sometimes the coercion of the masses was enough to prick elite consciences.

Ammianus Marcellinus, a soldier and historian writing in the fourth century AD, called rioting "a thing which constantly happens in Rome."[104] Earlier under the Pax Romana, mass violence was also endemic.[105] Emperors were especially mindful of the threat. Riots might blossom into insurrection. Ironically, the terror of insurrection competed with emperors' duty to mitigate crises. Hence Pliny, after a massive fire destroyed parts of Nicomedia, sought Trajan's approval to draft a three-hundred-man fire brigade—a moderate and practical proposal. But the emperor offered this paranoid reply:

Societies of this sort have greatly disturbed the peace of the province in general, and of those cities in particular. Whatever name we give them, and for whatever purposes they may be founded, they will not fail to form themselves into factious assemblies, however short their meetings may be.[106]

Fear of out-of-control street violence was so strong that officials even sacrificed their elite peers to appease mobs. The emperor Gallus in the mid-fourth century AD looted grain stores in the city of Antioch (in modern southeast Turkey) to feed his army on the way to Persia. The resulting food shortage, exacerbated by a local drought, spawned a furious rabble. As the violence threatened to overwhelm the city, the emperor blamed the shortage on the provincial governor, telling the unruly crowd: "no one could lack food if the governor did not wish it." It was not only classic blame-shifting but an unveiled authorization for targeted violence. According to a contemporary account, the mob assailed the governor "with kicks and blows, and trampling him under foot when he was half-dead, with awful mutilation tore him to pieces."[107] Why do the difficult work of dealing with the disaster itself when scapegoating is so much easier?

Crises created crowds, and crowds sustained and spread diseases. The Antonine plague was looming on the horizon, and the festering disorder in cities in the mid-second century was a menacing omen. But the situation was even worse. Recall from earlier in the chapter: where did many of the crowds in Rome, Antioch, Ephesus, and other large cities come from in the first place? They were not born in the cities.[108] Rather, they were refugees and migrants from the countryside. In the hinterlands of the Empire, when food shortages degraded into famines, peasant farmers had to make terrible choices: take flight or starve to death. For some, relocation might be only temporary, but the truly desperate sold their possessions and land and moved elsewhere. Severe famines would depress land values in affected regions; some victims no doubt had to practically give away their land and family heirlooms. Anything that could not be carried was let go at bargain prices. The patrimonial rich, however, not only could weather the bad years but often prospered during short-term crises. Elite landowners bought up the lands of the poor, and might even employ the former owners as tenant farmers. This drop in status for the dispossessed—which was usually permanent—was not always a desirable outcome for peasants. Besides, some tenant farmers could expect to be treated worse than the slaves working in the fields with them.[109] Slaves represented long-term investments for their owners; tenant farmers were expendable. And so to avoid such a fate, migrants flocked to the cities—seeking patronage or occasional labor.

The refugees entering the cities, therefore, were often not the strong but the weak, the hungry, the malnourished. Having few if any contacts in their new city, they would have concentrated in the worst areas and in the most filthy and unhealthy conditions in the already unsanitary context of the preindustrial urban environment. Their naive and fragile immune systems would have suddenly faced the onslaught of novel diseases and microbes battle-hardened in the urban arena.[110] For the pathogens endemic to the Empire's cities, such migrants were fresh meat.

During the Pax Romana, immigrants from the countryside drowned the cities. The numbers are unknown, but population estimates suggest immigration was high enough to sustain or even grow urban populations despite infant mortality and the horrid conditions of ancient cities.[111] As Antioch faced famine in the fourth century AD, for example, one contemporary observed "crowds of squatters everywhere," noting that "the governors resent the migrations, but in the uncertainty about the future, they cannot stop them."[112] In fact, elite spending, seasonal or ad hoc job opportunities, and public grain distributions offered migrants good reason to move.[113] But as the hungry flooded the cities, already limited urban supplies were put under increased strain. And hopeful *perceptions* of life in an ancient city may have far outstripped the harsh reality migrants discovered once they arrived.[114] Rome, for example, clamped down on handouts to non-citizens and migrants. Other cities likely imposed similar barriers. And yet many perceived that it was better to go hungry and even homeless in the cities than to face certain death when famine struck the countryside.

Some migrants turned their transience into an advantage. They worked different jobs in different places at different times. The populations of ancient cities thus ebbed and flowed with the seasons. Spring and summer brought artisans who worked in the open air, dockworkers who arrived into ports with the opening of safe sailing around late March or early April, construction works, shipbuilders, brick makers, and others. At the same time, fieldworkers and farmers exited cities in preparation for the harvest.[115] In the hottest months, the wealthy escaped the city swelter for cooler country villas. Those who worked for these elites—directly and indirectly—may have followed in their train.[116] In the autumn and winter, the reverse occurred. The urban centers of the Empire—especially Rome, the Empire's heart—pumped hundreds of thousands of people in and out each year.

When it finally arrived in Roman territory, the Antonine plague pathogen attached itself to these circulating mass movements of migrants. Moreover, as the following chapter shows, the stresses of the mid-second century swelled these movements at exactly the wrong time. According to numerous proxies, food shortages in key localities ramped up in the decades prior to the Antoine plague. It is reasonable to assume internal migrations increased in response, reducing resilience, especially in urban areas. The Empire's once vibrant and dynamic cities—islands of Roman civilization—suddenly transformed into an archipelago of infection. Elite writers took notice, and the old era of local pestilence gave way to something new: an age of pandemics.

2

THE DRY TINDER
OF DISEASE

With his co-emperor and adoptive brother Lucius Verus waging war against Parthia in the east, Marcus Aurelius settled into a life of scholarship at Rome. Cloistered in the imperial palace, reprieved of the vile city streets, the emperor read the speeches and treatises of Republican heroes—Cato, Cicero, Sallust, Gracchus.[1] He attended lectures given by philosophers and rhetoricians.[2] But Marcus found himself most drawn to the Stoics. These philosophers attempted to live reflectively in the present moment—neither fearing pain nor pursuing pleasure. In those early days, Marcus probably had no idea how much he would come to rely on Stoic principles during the crisis that was coming—a crisis that would consume the remainder of his life, and define his legacy.

Marcus's Roman holiday was brief. According to the emperor's private letters, "pressing anxieties" came upon him within two years of taking the purple.[3] The first of these was a major natural disaster in Rome itself. In the spring of AD 162, the River Tiber breached its banks and flooded the lower city.[4] Roman records occasionally note such once-in-a-generation floods—preserving for posterity both the immediate effects and the lingering devastation.[5] Under Rome's first emperor Augustus (31 BC–AD 14), for example, the Tiber flooded to such an extent that many city streets were only navigable by boat.[6] Typically, the sewers backed up, pouring refuse of all sorts into the streets of Rome. New corpses augmented the old, as the flood killed rodents, livestock, and people—their bodies swelling the already horrific flotsam. The deluge of death greedily consumed buildings made of unfired clay or bricks. One eyewitness account of such a flood describes the raging Tiber carrying away whole herds of cattle and entire groves of trees.[7] These were powerful waters indeed.

But the flood itself was only the beginning. The nasty waters slowly contaminated everything they touched, soaking furniture, carpets, bedding, utensils, food, and water supplies. Few Romans could afford to part with any possessions or food stocks that survived the initial deluge—including those contaminated by invisible yet deadly microbes. And so the days and weeks after the waters receded were more deadly than the flood itself. Pestilence spread throughout Rome following the Augustan flood, for example. Disease then diffused into greater Italy.[8] In the wake of floods, whether in Rome or elsewhere, fecal-oral bacterial diseases and parasites, such as shigellosis, typhoid fever, and a whole zoo of parasitic worms, would have continued the carnage long after the floodwaters vanished. Mass outbreaks of dysentery, diarrhea, and vomiting further fouled cities. The slowly receding waters drew mosquitoes in abundance, spreading malaria. Exposed corpses attracted flies and rats, which in turn brought typhoid and leptospirosis ("rat fever"). No wonder Marcus became such a well-studied philosopher; who would venture out in such conditions?

The flood under Marcus, however, also illustrates a key link explored throughout this book. The Antonine plague occurred in a context. Factors like food supply systems and climate were "dry tinder" that could exacerbate and even establish epidemics. Major Tiber floods, for example, aided local and regional outbreaks of disease, but scholars also believe that hemispheric and global ecological forces—such as volcanic forcing or changes in solar irradiance—prompted the rise of epidemics.[9] A massive eruption of Alaska's Okmok volcano in 43 BC, for instance, coincides with reports of famine, disease, and political unrest in the Roman world in the aftermath of Julius Caesar's assassination.[10] The Justinianic plague that began in the AD 540s—the world's first bubonic plague pandemic—was directly preceded by a period of extreme volcanic activity with major global environmental effects.[11] But smoking

volcanoes are not always smoking guns. Large eruptions in AD 163 and
170 show up in paleoclimatological records, but these eruptions—the
locations of which are yet to be confirmed—did not eject sunlight-
blocking sulfates into the atmosphere at comparable levels to Okmok
and mid-sixth-century AD eruptions.[12] It is not immediately obvious
whether volcanic eruptions were key events or mere background noise
in the Antonine plague's shrouded story.[13]

But some links between Roman history and environmental history
are clearer. On the grand scale, the political rise and fall of the Roman
Empire coincides with a period of warm and mild weather in Eurasia
from around the third century BC to around the third century AD, a
period many refer to as the Roman Climate Optimum.[14] Regional and
even microregional details, however, reveal a far more complicated and
dynamic situation.[15] It is true that many parts of the Roman Empire
became drier and colder after the mid-second century AD, but several
localities bucked the general trend.[16] Measurements of tree rings from
central Western Europe, for example, show that temperatures in that region dropped a full degree Celsius in the second century AD compared
to the previous century.[17] At the same time, mineral deposits in caves
from both Spain and the Austrian Alps do not always show the anomaly.[18] Then again, cave deposits (speleothems) don't offer the kind of
resolution other proxies do.[19] A rapidly growing body of ever more precise paleoclimatological evidence—tree rings, ice cores, lake sediments,
and other proxies—bring a once opaque picture into vivid detail: for the
past eleven thousand years, the Mediterranean has been on a "climate
see-saw" with various regions swapping dry conditions in some centuries for wet ones in the next few centuries, and then back again.[20]

To properly understand the dry tinder of the Antonine plague, therefore, we must think *locally* before we think globally. We must also consider *causes* over correlations. On the one hand, yes, the pandemic occurred at or just after the peak of the Roman Climate Optimum. But
there were important regional ecological shifts and variations in local
climate patterns. Although not part of a uniform environmental decline
and fall, it is possible to show that these anomalies were well-placed and
timed to expose the economic and administrative fragility highlighted

in the previous chapter—inflicting food shortages amid the Empire's culture of ever-present risk.[21] And no region was more central to Roman food supplies than Egypt.

The Pax Romana in fact began with Egypt, and this was no accident. In 31 BC, Augustus conquered and looted Egypt. He then made it a special "dominion" (not a mere province) of his newly inaugurated empire, solidifying Roman control over the most bountiful grain-producing region in the history of the preindustrial world.[22] Previously under the republic, Rome drew grain primarily from Sicily and North Africa—excellent breadbaskets to be sure, but nothing like Egypt. With Egypt now in hand, subsequent emperors reoriented grain production and distribution systems on the assumption that Egyptian grain would flow forever.

Egypt was so alluring precisely because of its distinct climate mechanisms compared to the rest of the Mediterranean. Instead of the sometimes fickle western Mediterranean rains, the rhythmic flooding of the Nile watered Egyptian crops—creating what seemed like an inexhaustible supply fit to meet the unending demands of Rome's hungry mob. When Nile waters in Egypt overflowed, so too did Roman granaries—leading to a healthier, more resilient Roman population.

By the middle of the second century AD, much of the wheat that fed Rome's more than one million inhabitants came from Egypt, and this not through the invisible hand of markets but the visible hand of state power.[23] The state accumulated more and more Egyptian fields. From field to port, Egyptian grain moved along state-maintained infrastructure. State-regulated "fleets" of state-underwritten ships sailed grain from Alexandria to Rome. Once there, state officials supervised, scheduled, and regulated how and when Egyptian grain was unloaded. The grain was then distributed by a state-run process and at state-subsidized prices.[24] In setting up such an apparatus, Roman officials took a gamble and placed the fate of the Eternal City into the hands of the gods that kept Egypt's Nile floods flowing.[25] What could possibly go wrong?

Unfortunately for Rome, the risk-reward ratio in the Empire's most crucial breadbasket flipped just ahead of the Antonine plague. A growing body of evidence suggests the bad years began to outnumber the good in Egypt around the AD 150s. The causes of the change, however, are unclear. Temperature anomalies hit the Pacific and Indian oceans. Mediterranean storms may have increased. Volcanic clouds of sulfate in the 160s may have reduced sunlight and precipitation.[26] Roman officials were unaware that gradual environmental changes were slowly manifesting. Necessary adaptations in their food production and distribution systems were delayed or simply not pursued at all; and the state sunk more and more resources into an increasingly shaky operation. So even before the pandemic hit, the Roman state's seemingly wise investments in Egypt began to backfire.

The Storm Cometh

Rome's half-millennium hold over the Mediterranean was a remarkable exception in a history of otherwise revolving regional powers. One of the few polities to surpass Rome's impressive longevity was Pharaonic Egypt, which—despite several intermittent civil wars and revolutions—retained much of its social and political identity over millennia. As with the Romans, climate may have been a significant factor for the endurance of the Egyptian regime. Despite Egypt's proximity to the Mediterranean, the pharaohs fed their populations independent of the often chaotic Mediterranean weather patterns. Instead of Mediterranean springtime rains, the Nile and its annual late summer flood seeded Egypt's healthy harvests with water and nitrates from the heart of Africa thousands of kilometers south. Egypt was merely the final destination for the rich, silty waters that initially fell in the summer monsoons over the highlands of equatorial east Africa. As the monsoons doused the highlands, the runoff drained into Lake Tana. The 3,000-square-kilometer lake then filled to the brim, sending a mud-brown surge down the Blue Nile on its 4,500-kilometer journey to flood the grain fields of Egypt. And so, like clockwork, surging waters burst the Nile's banks in Egypt in the late summer months. Unlike the floods of the Tiber, which ushered destruction and disease in Rome, the rising Nile waters brought emerald-green life to the arid Egyptian desert and, consequently, to those who controlled Egypt.

Even still, the monsoons over equatorial east Africa were hardly perfect. Climate scientists have identified a few multidecade "megadroughts" over the last five thousand years. Interestingly, such periods coincided with social and political disruptions to the otherwise stable Egyptian civilization.[27] However, the exceptions prove the rule: the Nile has otherwise been fairly consistent at providing Egypt with an abundant source of grain production year in and year out. As a result, the river was, as papyrologist Roger Bagnall observed, "not only worshipped as a divinity but also monitored like a patient in intensive care."[28] Each year, as the floodwaters began to rise, Egyptians looked to nilometers—columns, wells, or even small buildings that marked the flood levels at key locations along the Nile. "The watchers," the Roman geographer Strabo called them, "give out word to the rest of the people" on the expected flood level.[29] Seneca ridiculed Egyptian farmers: "not one of them looks at the sky!"[30] The arrogant senator seems to have been utterly oblivious to the fact that his own peace and prosperity depended upon the labor of those ground-gazing farmers. His descendants in the late second century found out the hard way.

During the Pax Romana, the nilometers had a sweet spot. A water height of between 14 and 16 cubits (6.3–7.2 meters) brought maximum grain production. Whenever floods flowed outside that critical range, however—whether too high or too low—the Egyptian harvest suffered. At 18 or 20 cubits, for example, the surging waters wrecked agricultural infrastructure, destroyed villages, and even killed fieldworkers. And, yet, as we are told by Pliny the Elder: "when the water rises to only 12 cubits, Egypt experiences the horrors of famine; when the flood attains 13 cubits, hunger is still the result."[31] In very rare years, the floods failed entirely. Pliny tells us that the Nile rose to a mere 5 cubits in 48 BC—the year Julius Caesar won control of the Roman Empire in a civil war against Pompey the Great and his senatorial collaborators.[32] Perhaps not coincidentally, Egypt was also embroiled in civil war that year, and Caesar personally ventured to Alexandria and threw his lot in with Cleopatra. Two decades later, after that same Cleopatra and her Roman lover Mark Antony committed suicide, Caesar's adopted son, who became known as Augustus, made Egypt the crown jewel of the Roman Empire.

Historians tend to focus on Augustus's political acumen and his impressive ability to generate ideology and inspire loyalty. But Rome's first emperor was unquestionably a product of his environment. By securing the riches of Egypt—both the grain produced by the Nile floods and the gold and silver accumulated by the pharaohs—Augustus wiped away the nightmare years of famine, starvation, and civil war that accompanied his tyrannical rule in Rome during the previous decade. The Roman senator Cassius Dio said that the wealth Augustus brought back from conquered Egypt was so vast that "the Romans forgot all their unpleasant experiences" of the past.[33] The regularity of Egyptian harvests made it seem as though even nature itself bowed to the new emperor. The etched vines, tendrils, and reeds that surround his famous altar of Augustan Peace reinforce this dominance. Rather than growing organically and chaotically, the vines form rigid, ordered shapes. "Every bud and leaf," notes the archaeologist Paul Zanker, "has its prescribed place . . . a model of perfect order."[34] Such subtle but relentless propaganda undoubtedly rang true as Egyptian grain ships filled Roman storehouses year after year. The new territory was so crucial to the fortunes of the Empire that Augustus banned any Roman senator from even visiting Egypt, let alone serving as governor.[35] Augustus's conquest grafted the fate of Rome to the fortunes of Egypt, for better or worse.

The Nile floods and the province's plethora of crops were blessings the Romans could not refuse. No wonder the emperors who followed Augustus—especially Claudius (AD 41–54) and Trajan—invested in expanding the flow of grain from Egypt to Rome. Mob violence was a major catalyst for change. During a food shortage in the winter of AD 51, an angry crowd accosted Claudius in Rome.[36] The capital was down to a mere fifteen days' worth of food, but the grain ships from Egypt were still months from arriving. Claudius's predecessor, Caligula (AD 37–41), had tried to hide similar shortages from the public to avoid exactly the kind of outcry now threatening Claudius.[37] Caligula, however, became so hated that his own bodyguards assassinated him. Claudius wished to avoid such a grisly end. So, at tremendous risk, he sent ships on a perilous journey to acquire grain in North Africa in the middle of the winter storm season. The move betrays the desperation of the moment. But just before chaos erupted in Rome, the city was resupplied in what seemed like a miracle. Tacitus attributed Rome's salvation to "the grace of the gods and the mildness of the winter."[38] To avoid tempting fate again, Claudius splurged on port facilities and crafted incentives for those who shipped grain to the capital. The emperor guaranteed compensation for any losses contractors endured in shipping grain to Rome.[39] Claudius extended legal privileges and even conferred full Roman citizenship on those who constructed ships large enough to carry at least 10,000 *modii* of grain (around 70,000 kilograms) to Rome and contracted them for this purpose for at least six years.[40] It seems the measures were initially successful. In a flamboyant act of propaganda, Claudius's successor Nero ordered heaps of the city's grain dumped into the Tiber.[41]

Ties between Egypt and Rome became stronger in the second century AD. By the reigns of Trajan, Hadrian, and Antoninus Pius, images of Egypt and the Nile proliferated on gold and silver coins produced not only in the east but also in Rome. On many of these coins, a divine personification of the Nile points to the number "16"—the number of cubits that guaranteed an optimal harvest.

In the first century AD, Seneca mocked Egyptians for not looking to the sky, but only a few decades later even the Romans obsessed over reports from Egypt's nilometers. The news was usually wonderful. For much of the late first and early second centuries, Egypt brought Rome bumper crops. Romans interpreted Egypt's bounty as a sign of divine benevolence and their own wise political leadership. Pliny the Younger boasted that the Nile "has never flowed more generously for our glory."[42] His arrogance even led him to claim that Rome had "no need of Egypt, but Egypt must always need us."[43] In fact, the opposite was true. Without Egypt, the Roman Empire might well have failed to outlive its first emperor.[44]

As the Pax Romana persisted, Roman hubris rose to new heights. The Nile's floodwaters, however, soon moved in the opposite direction. The plunge was gradual, but more frequent failed floods—sometimes for multiple years in a row—began occurring from around the middle of

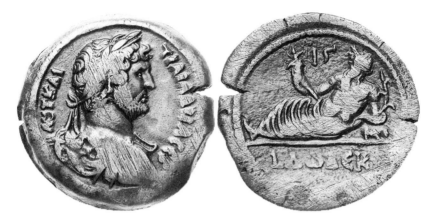

FIG. 2.1. Bronze drachm of Alexandria minted under Hadrian (AD 127/8) showing Nilus reclining near a hippopotamus (at left elbow), holding a reed and cornucopia. Nilus points toward "IS." Milne 1267. Used with permission of Wildwinds (https://www.wildwinds.com).

the second century AD.[45] And even when high waters returned, they were more often *too strong*—destructive even. Historians first came to suspect the change by surveying Roman tax records from Egypt that preserve farmers' pleas for tax relief. In years when floods failed to inundate their crops, Egyptian residents had little grain to hand over to government officials. Their reports thus enable historians to guess at flood levels in Egypt and, hence, better date and understand food shortages. According to this evidence, the 150s saw a sustained drop in flood levels, which then carried on through the worst years of the Antonine plague.

Following the terrible flood of AD 151, Egyptians could not pay their allotted tribute in grain. As a result, the tax collectors fled; after all, they were personally liable to the government for the taxes owed by the people. Recovery evidently stalled, and the starving and overtaxed Egyptians rioted, taking the extraordinary step of killing the Egyptian prefect—the de facto governor of the entire province, and the emperor's personal representative. Under normal circumstances, we would expect Rome to butcher Egyptians in response. The new governor, however, recognized the dire agricultural situation and offered an am-

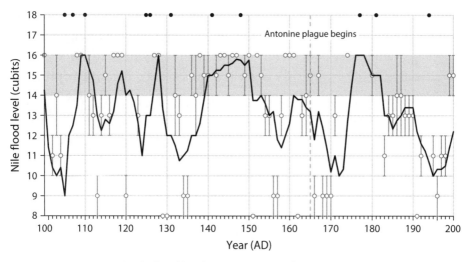

FIG. 2.2. Reported Nile flood levels, AD 100–200. Black circles represent "destructive" floods of 18 or more cubits. Ideal flood levels of between 14 and 16 cubits are shaded.

Values derived from Bonneau 1971, 239–52. In some cases, Bonneau makes an educated guess about flood levels; the error bars represent this uncertainty. The trend line represents a 5-point moving average (not a 5-year moving average, due to gaps in the data) beginning from data from AD 95. Destructive floods are omitted from the moving average to avoid skewing the trendline. The 170s are particularly unreliable, as six of these years have no data. Another caveat: government tax incentives—namely a 50 percent tax break for those who farmed land on the edges of floodplains—may distort these data, as some of these reports come from such marginal lands. Marginal lands may have failed to flood even when flood levels were otherwise favorable for much of Egypt; see *P. Giss* 1.4.19–12, 5.13–14, and 6.14–1; comments in Blouin 2014, 159, 169; Bonneau 1971, 176–79.

nesty. "Let them return . . . without fear," his official announcement proclaims in a preserved papyrus.[46] At the same time, the governor refused to reduce grain taxes.[47] Why would he? In the past, bountiful floods had always returned in short order. But that's not what happened this time.

Floods appear noticeably bad in the AD 150s through 180s compared to periods both before and after. In the first century AD, for example, floods dropped below 12 cubits—the level of severe drought—only fifteen times, and destructive floods occurred in a mere six years.

Third-century AD numbers are similar: fifteen poor floods and four destructive floods. But the second century was terrible, with a whopping twenty-three poor floods, and another twenty-three that were destructive. In other words, for nearly half the second century, flood problems plagued Egypt.[48] But historians must be careful with these flood reports.[49] Fragmentary records like these are prone to error and can only tell us so much anyway. Some years (the AD 170s most crucially) provide little data. We must also wonder whether survival bias skews the picture. The reports thus give clues, but not confirmation. For that, we need better evidence.

Fortunately, due to ongoing interest in modern anthropogenic climate change, new and more robust data are coming in faster than ever. A whole host of new long-term climatological proxies make it clear: there truly was a food crisis brewing on the eve of the Antonine plague, but its causes were complicated, varied, and distant. Unlike the prelude to the Justinianic plague—where most every climate proxy points in the same direction—climate proxies for the decades prior to the Antonine plague offer subtle, even strange signals. Unraveling the layers of ecological causes and effects necessitates a journey down a paleoclimatological rabbit hole.

It begins with the oceans. The Romans had little if any knowledge of the eastern equatorial Pacific Ocean, but changes in its surface temperature—even by just a few degrees—affect weather patterns all over the globe to this day. The phenomenon known as the El Niño–Southern Oscillation (ENSO) features a warming phase (El Niño) and a cooling phase (La Niña). The effects of these temperature changes are not always the same in each locality, yet many regions are strongly linked, even across hemispheres. So when ENSO-related droughts hit equatorial east Africa, parts of the North American Southwest and Southeast also tend to dry out.[50] The La Niña episode that developed in late 2010, for example, unleashed a drought that killed several hundred thousand people across southern Ethiopia, Kenya, and Somalia. By 2012, a multiyear drought afflicted parts of California, Arizona, New Mexico, and southern Colorado. The drought endured for so long because the eastern equatorial Pacific remained cool well after the se-

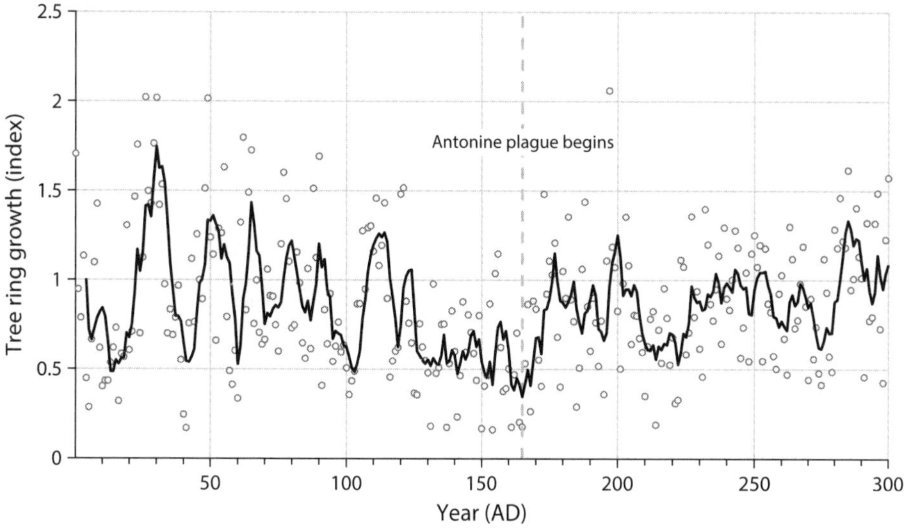

FIG. 2.3. Tree ring growth in American Southwest bristlecone pines, AD 1–300. Routson, Woodhouse, and Overpeck 2011. Line is a 5-point moving average.

vere La Niña episode itself diminished. Even the record-setting El Niño of 2015 failed to turn the tide and end the drought in the American Southwest.[51] But even worse, the 2015 El Niño triggered a new drought in the northern highlands of Ethiopia—the region that produced the annual Nile floods. ENSO indicators in the second century AD thus bear watching.

Remarkably, ENSO-induced droughts correlate with Egyptian flood records. In the San Juan Mountains near the headwaters of the Rio Grande, ancient bristlecone pines dot the landscape. Some of these trees are more than two thousand years old—accumulating rings each year.[52] Thin rings are a telltale sign of drought. Samples from several of these trees show sustained low ring growth in the mid-second century AD, with the most severe period occurring between the years 148 and 173.[53]

The drought in the American Southwest need not automatically correspond to an identical drought over northern Ethiopia—where the Nile floods originate. Again, global climatological relationships are complex. In fact, researchers studying the Nile flood in recent years have determined that "extreme" floods are most likely when weather patterns suddenly flip—for instance, when a La Niña event follows on the heels of an El Niño event.[54] Some east African climate proxies show such variability during the Pax Romana, but some do not.[55] Seasonality also matters, as late spring and early summer El Niño events provoke the most severe droughts. The local problems in Ethiopia created by the ENSO are not always predictable, but it is merely one example of a large-scale climate mechanism that locks together otherwise disparate regions across the globe—and undoubtedly had some negative impact on Egyptian harvests.[56]

The ENSO is just one piece of the climatological puzzle that contextualized the Antonine plague. Regional weather patterns in the Gulf of Guinea also generate east African rains, as does weather in the Red Sea. The Indian Ocean is even more crucial.[57] Changing temperatures in the Pacific due to the ENSO influence the monsoons in the Indian Ocean—usually referred to as the Indian Ocean Dipole (IOD).[58] These monsoons are a significant source of the summer rainfall in northern Ethiopia and, subsequently, the overflow that pours out of Lake Tana and down the Nile.[59] When sea surface temperatures in the Eastern Pacific drop, the summer Indian Ocean monsoon tends to be stronger in the east but weaker in the west (over Ethiopia).[60] Summer sea surface temperatures in the region have averaged around 29 degrees Celsius during the last 11,000 years. In the decades just prior to the Antonine plague, however, the waters cooled by about one degree in the South China Sea and stayed that way through much of the remainder of the second century.[61] Waters in the region also became less salty—suggesting that monsoon rains poured into the eastern Indian Ocean.[62] Such cooling and increased salinity were hardly catastrophic in and of themselves; the shift, however, signals that over Ethiopia, a lengthy drier period probably set in from the late 140s through early 170s AD.

The Romans could not conceive of these complex global relationships and how they affected harvests in Egypt, their main breadbasket in the mid-second century. For modern researchers, however, the climate data bolster the evidence from traditional sources. While additional and more precise data is still needed, it now seems plausible that

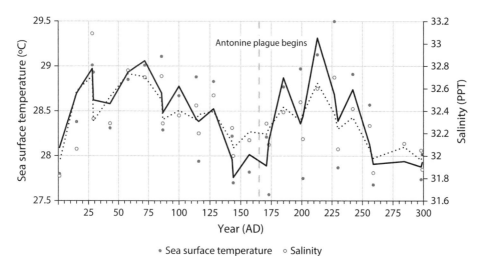

FIG. 2.4. Salinity and sea surface temperature in the South China Sea, AD 1–300. Woodson 2014. Data are combined from two cores (D45, D42). Trendlines are smoothed at a 2-point moving average. Intervals between data points in D45 are roughly 20 years, while D42 has a higher resolution at roughly 15-year intervals. Combined, however, the two cores offer a more robust data set.

Nile floods became less consistent around a decade before the Antonine plague pathogen reached the Roman Empire.

But Egypt was not the only Roman region that experienced climate troubles on the eve of the Antonine plague. Recent data also suggest that some central and northern European regions endured short-term climate anomalies from the early 150s. Although Egypt supplied much if not most of Rome's grain for state redistribution, a good deal of the city's privately sold grain came from Sicily and North Africa. Smaller amounts came from elsewhere, including Gaul.[63] We know, for example, that during grain shortages under Commodus near the end of the traditional Antonine plague chronology, the emperor set up an African grain fleet to ferry emergency grain from Carthage to Rome.[64] Tree ring data from several parts of Europe clearly show a prolonged period of colder temperatures in the second half of the second century.

It is unclear how much reduced temperatures in these regions affected food supplies in Rome and other Mediterranean cities. Wheat farmers in Italy, Sicily, and North Africa would have planted in autumn

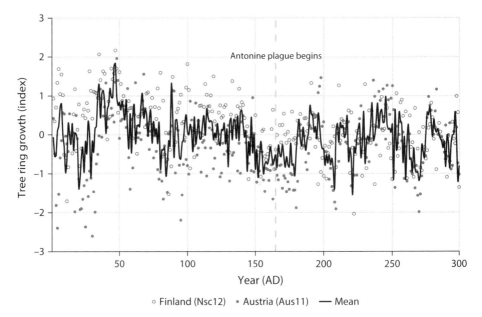

FIG. 2.5. Tree ring growth in Europe, AD 1–300.
McKay and Kaufman 2014.

and winter to take advantage of the wet season as well as the reliably cool but not cold temperatures. Wheat matures more slowly in colder temperatures.[65] Harvest followed late in the spring—the most volatile time in the agricultural cycle. Sudden frosts or hot dry winds could strike, causing crops to yield fewer kernels.[66] The summer droughts in Europe suggested by these tree rings would have augmented existing regional grain shortages in parts of the Mediterranean. The droughts also drove nomadic tribal populations south—directly into Roman lands—in search of better foraging and hunting. So even if the droughts did not affect Mediterranean grain supply, they may have indirectly increased pressure on demand.

Aside from grain production, the ramifications of cold European and Mediterranean weather for grain *distribution* are also coming into focus through new environmental proxies. Roman sources record that even when grain was available, famines occurred when ships were blown off course or could not land.[67] Severe storm activity, especially in the western part of the Mediterranean, tends to correlate with colder tempera-

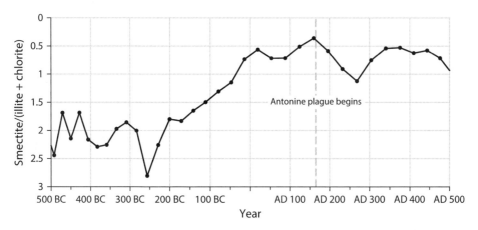

FIG. 2.6. Ratio of smectite to illite and chlorite—a proxy for storm activity—in the Gulf of Lions, 500 BC–AD 500.
Sabatier et al. 2012. The y-axis is inverted to display more intense storm activity as higher on the axis.

tures. An impressionistic data set seems to confirm high levels of storm activity in the mid-second-century AD western Mediterranean. Researchers recently pulled sediment cores from the coast of southern France to examine changes in the size and makeup of sand grains over time. Lower ratios of smectite to other minerals, for example, indicate increased deposits from the ocean—a sign of intense western Mediterranean storms (top of y-axis in figure 2.6).

These data lack the high-resolution year-by-year detail of other data sets in this chapter. The apparent pinnacle of storm activity in 160 AD is one of only three data points in the second century. More studies are needed. But the long-term trends are unmissable: the mid-second century AD witnessed the most significant storm activity not only throughout the Classical Era but for the last ten thousand years of the Holocene Epoch. And while we cannot know exactly how these storms affected grain distribution, it is reasonable to suspect increased instability in maritime transport in the western Roman provinces in the mid-second century.

Various environmental factors were crucial to food production and distribution in the Pax Romana. These proxies are, of course, selected from many. Some regions would not have experienced any changes, even as others dealt with serious ecological challenges. There was no total environmental calamity. But it is worth asking: did local environmental changes in places like Egypt and parts of the north and western Empire stress food production and distribution systems?[68] As with epidemics, the relationship between human societies and their environmental context is two-way. Human institutions can either mitigate or exacerbate the forces of nature. We also need to consider the crops themselves, as different species and subspecies responded to climate changes in different ways. To gain a better perspective on the state of food supply and nutrition on the eve of the Antonine plague, we must now turn to human systems and institutions.

Food Supply on the Eve of the Pandemic

"You are what you eat" was no Roman adage; French and German writers crafted the famous saying in the nineteenth century. In that period, food supply and distribution were rapidly modernizing, allowing many to access types and quantities of food their ancestors could hardly imagine. Capitalism had cracked the once hard ceiling on preindustrial prosperity, although not everywhere or at the same pace. The cities of France, Britain, and the United States—even as they became connected to food-producing colonies and trade partners—suffered mortality rates more than double those in the countryside. Overcrowding, poor sanitation, adulterated food, pollution, and disease were all contributors, but so too was a lack of variety in diet and access to nutritional foods.[69] Roman cities dealt with many of these same challenges, even during the Pax Romana. Yet in some ways the Roman Empire should have been better-off. Large ships carrying food crisscrossed the Mediterranean. At the heart of most cities, a forum or agora, often with permanent market stalls for retailers, offered inhabitants with enough money the right to buy the produce of distant hinterlands. City governments also furnished citizens free or cheap staples—cereals, wine, oil, and even pork. Rome's agricultural economy could withstand normal stresses.

It is true that the Empire's food production and distribution systems were impressive—but in the same way that a juggler riding a unicycle on a tightrope is impressive. As we've seen, one destabilizing force was regional climate change. But there were also inbuilt flaws in the system just waiting to fail. The economies of scale that moved heaps of Egyptian grain to Rome, for example, siphoned resources and distorted market signals. As gradual changes in the climate induced stress, especially in the capital, officials reacted in line with their imperialistic frame of reference—expanding coercive measures in the vain hope of solving a complex set of problems that they didn't truly understand. As we will see, negative knock-on effects—like ticking time bombs—were gradually implanted in the system. Many of these embedded disturbances exploded at the worst possible time: in the midst of the Antonine plague pandemic.

We begin with cereals, the central staple in many diets across the Roman world. From east to west, in cities and on rural farms, ancient peoples from every walk of life ate a wide range of wheat, barley, and millet types, among other cereals.[70] The diversity of cereals was perhaps the strongest attribute of the Roman food supply. Many cereal types endured environmental changes—droughts, rises in soil salinity, even frosts—better than others. Ancient farmers thus avoided specializing in just one crop type. Instead, often in the same fields, they planted a variety of cereal species and subspecies. Within the normal range of environmental variability, this diversification strategy ensured that at least some crops made it to harvest each year. But the gradual changes that began in some agricultural regions in the second century AD, as well as the short-term variance of the 150s–180s, may have overcome the strengths of crop diversity. And, of course, the reduced specialization in ancient farming practices came with a trade-off: in years where conditions were right for certain varieties to thrive, and to thus recover from the shortages of previous years, farmers as well as the food system as a whole missed out on higher overall yields.[71]

Quantity of food, therefore, rather than quality was the main driver of malnutrition in the Roman world. In turn, malnutrition was a key factor in the severity of epidemics, and vice versa. We can see the relationship on the regional scale through a vignette captured at the start of the sixth century AD. In spring of AD 500, the prosperous but landlocked city of Edessa (in Syria) succumbed to both a local drought and a plague of locusts in the vicinity of the city. Hundreds of thousands of people were subsequently plunged into a sea of famine. A disease outbreak soon followed. A contemporary account chronicles the timeline of devastation:

> In the month of [April], there began to be a dearth of grain . . . in the months of [June and July] the inhabitants of those areas . . . sowed millet for their own use, but it was not enough . . . before the year came to an end, misery from hunger had reduced the people to beggary, so that they sold their property for half its worth. . . . many forsook their native places . . . and the sick who were in the villages, as well as the old men and boys and women and infants, and those who were tortured by hunger, being unable to walk far and go to distant places, entered into the cities to get a livelihood by begging . . . the pestilence came upon them in the places to which they went.[72]

As pestilential crowds formed in the cities, the region's governor finally acted—handing out cash and bread—but the situation deteriorated as winter set in:

> The pestilence became worse . . . when there began to be frost and ice . . . children and babies were crying in every street. Of some the mothers were dead; others their mothers had left, and had run away from them when they asked for something to eat, because they had nothing to give them. Dead bodies were lying exposed in every street, and the citizens were not able to bury them, because, while they were carrying out the first that had died, the moment they returned they found others.[73]

One city at the eastern edge of the Empire suffered a single poor harvest. But crowded, famine-wrought Edessa then spawned a regional plague that spread throughout Syria, from Antioch to Nisibis. The waves of immigrants into Syrian cities triggered the epidemic spread of a disease with some apparent similarities to smallpox.[74] Our source tells of bodies "full of boils or pustules, down even to the palms of their hands and the soles of their feet."[75]

The story highlights a well-known tendency: disease and malnutrition often work in concert.[76] Poor population health—especially in urban settings—increased vulnerability to pathogens which, in turn, depressed nutrient intake even further.[77] In 1968, the World Health Organization published a major study linking malnutrition with more severe outcomes from infectious disease.[78] As a result, previously established disease history continues to be rewritten. Many people still believe, for example, that Native Americans succumbed to smallpox primarily because they lacked immunity. In fact, preexisting and then ongoing malnutrition exacerbated disease outbreaks among Native American populations, as European settlers expropriated Native lands, disrupted hunting and foraging patterns, and reduced Native populations through war and extermination.[79] Even Roman-era writers noted connections between disease and malnourishment. Galen himself observed during the years just prior to the Antonine plague that desperate people forced to eat uncooked, rotten, indigestible, or even poisonous "food" were fodder for local epidemics.[80] And the ancient Greek word for starvation (*limos*) is nearly identical to the word for epidemic disease (*loimos*). The connection between malnutrition and disease seemingly predates the classical world itself.

But was the Pax Romana—with its impressive food redistribution programs and access to markets—really "a world on the edge of starvation," as one eminent ancient historian claims?[81] Still others conclude ancient peoples suffered from "endemic" malnutrition—a systemic deficiency of the nutrients and energy necessary to maintain physiological health.[82] On the one hand, we should be careful of such rhetoric. Yes, Romans struggled to obtain sufficient quantities of cereals, but the cereals they ate were more nutritious than modern varieties. In the 1960s, scientists developed high-yield, disease-resistant genetically modified wheat that could be grown in places where it was not grown before.[83] While this wheat type has kept billions from starving, it lacks in micronutrients compared to older cultivars. The fact is that ancient people were able to survive on less grain than their modern counterparts because

Roman grain contained higher quantities of micronutrients that supported basic body functions and macronutrients that provided energy.[84]

But Roman grain also contained less desirable additives. The heat of the Vesuvius eruption in autumn of AD 79 carbonized wheat stored in a granary at nearby Herculaneum. That grain, as it turns out, was laced with vetch, rye, straw, and gravel and full of insects and their larvae; it would have made even Charles Dickens squirm.[85] Galen claimed ancient wheat was often mixed with darnel (also called tare or "poisonous rye")—a grass that grew noxious fungus.[86] A common darnel-borne fungus—*Claviceps purpurea*—wreaks havoc on the central nervous system, leading to a loss of the use of fingers, hands, feet, or even entire limbs. Even the bread of the elites contained poisonous plants, bacteria, parasites, insects, and larvae.

Rome's insatiable appetite for tax also drove grain contamination. With so much of their produce stolen by the state, farmers struggled to survive the long periods between harvests. When the taxman came round, farmers got creative. They surrendered the worst-quality wheat to the state—that was a given. Many also purposefully adulterated tax grain—mixing in just enough water to add bulk without being too obvious. Such watered wheat could, according to Galen, pass immediate inspection.[87] But not long after reaching the storehouse, the moisture in the grain fueled fungus and rot. Vermin and bacteria then fed on the soaked seeds. Entire storehouses of cereals could become corrupted. And when fed to urban populations, such grain brought mass sickness and even death.

Herculaneum left behind more than just contaminated grain. The eruption of Vesuvius killed many, and some of the bones of those who ate that grain have since been analyzed. Nearly half of all female and a third of all male skeletons bore clear signs of iron deficiency, as well as related conditions like porotic hyperostosis and enamel hypoplasia.[88] One large cemetery in the Roman suburbs yielded an 80 percent enamel hypoplasia rate and a 70 percent rate of cribra orbitalia.[89] Mineral analysis of the bones also showed zinc deficiency, even while suggesting higher levels of vegetable consumption than even modern Americans enjoy.[90] Despite their varied plant- and seafood-based diet, urban Romans' lack of animal protein reduced their stature and perhaps their overall health relative to those who came before and after them.[91] Skeletal stature is influenced by a variety of factors. Diet was partly responsible, but so too was disease.[92] But there is no overlooking it: at the Pax Romana's height, Romans themselves were short.[93]

Malnutrition is not the same as starvation. Urban Romans did not lack basic staples like cereals, and proteins from fish sauce and pork.[94] Rather, the cause of their malnutrition was food insecurity and disease. The record in the literary sources suggests that food shortages occurred every three to four years in the ancient Mediterranean.[95] The causes varied. Usually, either declines in food production or problems with food distribution were responsible.[96] Nature both gave and took away: droughts, flooding, heat waves, and cold spells often reduced production. Times of warfare also placed serious strains on food supplies, especially at the local level. Even in years of abundant harvests, storms sunk ships brimming with grain. Other factors were entirely human. Failures of markets or state redistribution schemes kept food out of the hands of tens of thousands even when it was otherwise available. The weather was impossible to predict. Years of plenty and years of dearth came at random and varied from region to region. Even those areas which enjoyed bountiful harvests most years felt the strain on their resources when nearby cities were in want.

Connectivity mattered most in securing adequate food, whatever the scale. At the level of the individual or family, those with reliable employment or patronage ate better than those lacking such connections.[97] Citizens received the grain dole; non-citizens did not. For about twice the cost of grain, one could access milling technology and ovens for baking.[98] Those without means might use crude stone instruments to crush grain to mix with cold water to make gruel. During those apparent meager decades prior to the Antonine plague, Galen traveled Asia Minor with his teenage friends and saw "quite a lot of peasants" eat boiled grain seasoned with salt.[99] Galen tried the concoction but soon felt as if "mud was lying in the bottom of the stomach." He became "unable to eat anything, suffering from flatulent bloating, headaches and blurred vision."[100] Galen was just a well-fed, rich tourist trying the food of the local poor; his system could handle one bad meal. The malnourished rural locals on the other hand probably suffered far worse fates.

Settlements and cities with access to navigable water enjoyed a wider range of food types. Most foodstuffs, especially cereals, were expensive to move across land. Landlocked communities (like Edessa above) especially struggled in times of shortage.[101] And outright famines plunged ancient populations—in both city and countryside—into hellish oscillations between starvation and sickness. We might say that such outcomes were baked into Rome's tribute-based economy. Food, even nutritious food, was available—just not always where and when it was needed most.

Food production and distribution was so precarious in the Roman Empire that minor food shortages easily transformed into famines—levels of food shortage that caused mass starvation. Toner aptly called famine "an inbuilt, albeit terrifying, part of normality" of life in the Roman world.[102] If "normality" in the Roman world was food insecurity, outright famines must have been truly terrible. Once the grain ran out, humans turned to animal fodder. The Greek physician Oribasius tells us that starving people ate "food for beasts of burden"—oats boiled in water or millet boiled in milk.[103] And after that was gone, undercooked, raw, rotten, or even poisonous plants became fit for fare. Starving peoples ate acorns, grass, tree bark, roots, and wild mushrooms, some of which were poisonous.[104] The Christian historian Eusebius recounts how famine drove the hungry to chew "on tiny scraps of animal feed and . . . poisonous plants, which wasted their bodies."[105]

Such horrific conditions seem inconceivable under modern capitalism. Hobbled and rigged as they are, today's markets nevertheless spontaneously provide inexpensive and high-quality bread for billions. At the equivalent value of merely a few minutes' work, people in many nations can purchase a loaf of clean, standardized, presliced bread on demand at a well-stocked store within minutes of wherever they live. This modern miracle is an inescapable result not of political planning but of voluntary trade, technology, and market integration.[106] The absence of such postindustrial economic wonders helps explain why the majority of those who lived under the shadow of Rome had such trouble securing daily bread. And, in turn, it becomes possible to see why a pandemic pathogen found the Empire's undernourished inhabitants so palatable.

There is no question that Roman agriculture—from large estates to small peasant farms—generated surpluses. So did Soviet farms. The Roman state's obsessive focus on feeding the city of Rome and its hundreds of thousands of soldiers, however, either consumed or wasted this surplus.[107] The economic system of the Pax Romana was no communist command economy—so it could have been much worse—but state interventions nevertheless distorted markets and compounded supply-chain problems. By robbing the peasantry to feed the cities, for example, redistribution schemes exacerbated the threat of starvation in the countryside—weakening rural populations and driving the newly destitute into already crowded cities to beg and scavenge from privileged urbanites.[108] Galen, who toured Rome's exploited periphery, grasped the perverse consequences of urban predation at the expense of grain-producing hinterlands:

> People living in towns . . . by taking from the countryside all the wheat along with the barley and the beans and lentils, left for the countrymen all the other grains, which they call pulses and legumes, after taking not a few of these too to the city. So these foods that were left to them the country people use up during the winter, and are forced to use foods productive of bad humor for the whole of the spring. They eat twigs and shoots of the trees and bushes, and bulbs and roots of plants with bad juices and consume the so called wild greens, whichever happens to be in good supply, without sparing until they are satisfied, just as they boiled and ate whole green grasses which they had never tasted, even to try them.[109]

Roman cities siphoned surpluses from the countryside in the zero-sum game of state expropriation and redistribution.[110] Nowhere was this ghastly trade-off more apparent than at Rome, which consumed vast quantities of grain taken from numerous regions, but especially Egypt. Only after hundreds of thousands of Rome's entitled citizens had their share would other cities taste the scraps.[111]

Still, we would expect grain redistribution schemes in the cities to have reduced endemic malnutrition and mitigated food crises. But general welfare was never the aim of food handouts. Food redistribution schemes—including Rome's model *annona*—were pure political bribery and elite aggrandizement. Rome's *annona* began with the populist politician Gaius Gracchus trying to curry votes for his reelection campaign, almost a century before the Roman Republic died its slow, violent death. By Gaius's heyday in 123 BC, Rome's population had grown exponentially; conquering and enslaving many of the peoples of the Mediterranean will do that. Rome's masses were hungry—for food, yes, but also for sweeping political change. Gaius's grain program provided both. The Roman Senate, however, would have none of it. After a wave of violence in increasingly volatile Rome—a premonition of things to come as the Republic began to disintegrate—the charismatic Gaius lay dead. Afterward, the Senate weakened Gaius's grain redistribution scheme to the point where no one qualified for cheap grain from 81 to 73 BC. But the buried program soon sprouted once again as opportunistic politicians demagogued power by reviving the subsidy. By 73 BC, 40,000 citizens received grain at subsidized prices. Just a decade later, the number had more than tripled. In 58 BC, subsidies gave way to outright free grain. By the time of Julius Caesar's dictatorship in 46 BC, 320,000 Roman men ate grain at state expense. Once Caesar secured uncontested absolute rule, however, he cut the number of recipients down to 160,000 by purging non-citizens from the list of recipients.[112]

Two centuries later, at the height of the Pax Romana, around 200,000 Roman men relied upon direct government handouts for their grain. The *annona* provided 5 *modii* (about 32 kg) of free grain to each recipient each month. It was enough to feed an adult male and maybe one additional dependent. Thus, in reality, the *annona* served some 300,000–400,000 Romans.[113] Receiving such aid bore no stigma. Quite the contrary; it was a privilege—one made hereditary and only available to new recipients by imperial benefaction or lottery. Slaves and non-citizens were prohibited from *annona* grain. So too were immigrants. In the Roman world, the right to feed off the labor of others was a prized mark of status, even for the poor.

In order to fulfill obligations to entitled *annona* recipients, the Roman state expropriated and then stored tonnes of grain, most of it obtained from Egypt. At the southern end of the city near the Tiber, around 21,000 square meters of warehouses made up the Horrea Galbae—the main storage for public grain and other goods for public distribution.[114] In times of dearth, officials could draw upon such stores to alleviate the worst excesses of food crises in the city. But redistribution schemes then as now were not mechanistic; rather, human beings, with all their faults and prejudices, ran them. Even when officials' motives were not self-serving or corrupt, their knowledge was incomplete. The wisdom found in Hayek's 1974 Nobel Prize lecture was true in ancient Rome too: "If man is not to do more harm than good in his efforts to improve the social order, he will have to learn that . . . where essential complexity of an organized kind prevails, he cannot acquire the full knowledge which would make mastery of the events possible."[115] In other words: even if Rome's wisest and most well-meaning experts ran their system of grain redistribution, these individuals lacked the economic knowledge necessary to keep the scheme running smoothly. Indeed, legal writings and literary sources from the Roman period show that elites had no clue as to how markets worked; they often assumed that sudden outpourings of private greed dictated market phenomena.[116] Even as Roman monetary standards rapidly degraded in the third and early fourth centuries AD, for example, the emperor Diocletian confidently blamed the "raging and boundless avarice" of merchants rather than his own profligate spending and the decades of coin debasement that ultimately destroyed the previous Roman monetary system and shot inflation into the stratosphere.[117] In reality, while landed elites and speculators undoubtedly profited from shortages, they lacked the coercive monopolistic power to control the entire grain market.[118] There is little evidence that Romans succeeded in grasping the fundamental workings of their own economy.

It is hard to fault Roman ignorance, or their cynical worldview. Inequality was hard-wired into Roman society, in large part on purpose. It was not merely a matter of unequal distribution of resources, although epidemics and food shortages highlighted such disparities.

Eusebius, for example, describes a combined plague and famine in the third century AD in which beggars overwhelmed the cities, but the "harsh and hard-hearted" wealthy refused to provide more than basic relief to the suffering.[119] But Roman patronage—even in the midst of calamity—was designed to protect class divisions. Free grain was a civic ritual meant to reinforce elite dominance and superior status. In Rome's patronage-driven culture, those who gave were better than those who received. Roman elites did not aim to fight poverty but to keep the impoverished in their proper social tier. The dependence and passivity incentivized among handout recipients were not bugs in the system but features. In an economy dominated by reciprocity and re-distribution as both pragmatic and moral, the well-known Victorian adage could very well have been reversed: give a man a fish so that he owes you future services; but never teach a man to fish, lest you lose your power over him.

In some years, the overall food needs of the cities, and especially Rome, must have outstripped supply and distribution capacity. The mathematics were simply too brutal. At one million inhabitants in Rome—each requiring around 3 *modii* (~21 kg) of grain per month on average (with children requiring less and some adults requiring more)—the city may have consumed around 36 million *modii* (~250 million kg) of grain per year.[120] While Roman sources imply that ships with capaci-ties as high as 1,000 tonnes (1,000,000 kg) sailed the ancient Mediter-ranean, a lack of archaeological evidence has made some suspect the veracity of such claims. Still, there were ships that could carry between 65 and 300 tonnes (65,000–300,000 kg) of grain.[121] Rome's normal grain needs would have demanded something like two full 300-tonne ships or ten 65-tonne ships be unloaded each day of the year. But Medi-terranean grain transporters could not operate year-round even if they wanted to. From November to March, the sea was too stormy for sailing, and the entire Mediterranean was effectively closed (*mare clausum*).[122] Sailing even a month or two outside these dates was deemed risky, al-though many ships would sail in April and October. However, a period of a mere 111 days—between May 27 and September 14—was the extent of what was considered the Mediterranean's safe season for sailing.[123] This limited window left little time for grain ships, especially those that traveled over long distances, say from Egypt to Italy. Once the stormy weather subsided in spring, crewmen in Alexandria loaded ship holds with grain harvested the previous year. After leaving the Egyptian capital, contrary winds forced ships in the grain fleet along a circuitous two- to three-month-long route along the northern Mediterranean coastline in the hopes of arriving at Italian ports around July.[124]

Ecological limits on the food systems of the Pax Romana coincided with the maleffects of state intervention. We know from a letter sent by a ship crewman that the Alexandrian grain fleet was controlled, and could be delayed because ships were required to wait together in port for official permission to travel.[125] In the letter, the crewman explains that his ship arrived at the port of Ostia on June 30 but was still awaiting permission to return to Alexandria over a month later. This ship was not part of a random collection of "entrepreneurial" merchant ships responding to supply and demand. Instead, all ships, despite their variable speeds, seem to have traveled in a "convoy" at the speed of the slowest ship in the fleet.[126] Such throttling of grain shipments may have been "fair" in a sense, but it also necessarily meant that less grain could be transferred to and from Egypt over the course of each sailing season, compared to a situation in which some ships were allowed to travel at a faster pace. We do not know if the Alexandrian ships endured the same rigid rules that governed later fleets. Ships in the African fleet set up in the AD 180s, for instance, had to leave and arrive in the same order they departed.[127]

Mandates, rules, and other interventions even restricted how ships were unloaded. It was common practice in Rome, but also elsewhere, for officials to grant monopolies to dockworkers. Hadrian gave a single company transport rights along the Tiber between the port at Ostia and Rome.[128] Later imperial edicts show a similar pattern of market capture in port facilities.[129] Such conditions weakened market-based incentives, making the unloading process slower and more expensive. From harvest to consumption, state interventions constrained grain production, transport, and distribution in the years prior to the Antonine plague's first waves.

There were market alternatives to state redistributed grain, but these were limited by the same preindustrial context that stifled the *annona* system. Overland transport, for example, provided little grain for markets. The Empire's famous roads may have allowed animal-drawn carts to move fast, but beasts of burden still needed constant food along the journey. Even using well-maintained roads, a loaded cart pulled by oxen or donkeys could travel a mere fifteen kilometers a day.[130] The journey by land from the port at Puteoli (near Naples) to Rome, for example, would have taken about three weeks.[131] Those who drove the carts also required lodging each night and food each day. Land transport was too cumbersome to make a dent in the food requirements of Rome.[132] So once the sea closed in autumn, Romans had to hope their stores would last until the following summer. Often by spring, however—the season of hunger—tensions in the city rose, and the population eagerly awaited the arrival of the Alexandrian fleet. Adequately feeding all of Rome's one million plus inhabitants must have been challenging even in years of plenty; in times of dearth, it was impossible.

On the one hand, Rome's *annona* program was a monumental preindustrial achievement. *Annona* grain traveled more than 1,800 kilometers by sea from Egypt. Roman emperors and administrators, moreover, deployed a combination of laws and incentives to secure a proper fleet of contracted ships to transport the hundreds of millions of kilograms of grain annually required to feed those entitled to free grain.[133] Pliny the Younger praised imperial control of the grain market:

> We are blessed with a prince who could switch earth's bounty here and there, as occasion and necessity require, bringing aid and nourishment to a nation cut off by the sea as if its people were numbered among the humbler citizens of Rome! . . . He can so join East and West by convoys that those peoples who offer and those who need supplies can learn and appreciate in their turn, after experiencing license and discord, how much they gain from having one master to serve. Divide a common property, and each individual must bear his

own losses; but where everything is jointly held, no one suffers personal loss and all share in the common wealth.[134]

And yet, the superficial grandeur of the *annona* obscures its inherent inefficiencies, limitations, and tremendous costs to the Empire's periphery. On the eve of the Antonine plague, these costs were clearly catching up even to those at the top of Roman society. The generous incentives provided by Claudius and Trajan were curtailed. By the reign of Marcus and Lucius, privileges were only extended to the largest shipping operations—those shipowners with at least one 50,000 *modii*–capacity ship (around 350,000 kg), at least five 10,000 *modii*–capacity ships, or shippers and traders who had "the greater portion of their property invested in maritime business and commodities."[135] To the extent that middling and small-scale shippers provided grain to Rome, they were now at a major competitive disadvantage compared to the state-privileged larger enterprises. It is also far more likely that these smaller merchants supplied grain for markets rather than state redistribution. The Roman state picked winners and losers—undermining the overall health of the food system.[136] State-led attempts to secure more grain for the capital unwittingly stifled the more dynamic, responsive, and resilient elements in food supply systems. Thus officials fell into the kind of short-term thinking that so often entangles societies in times of insecurity. These problems would come to haunt the Romans once the Antonine plague sharpened and strengthened the unfolding stresses already at work prior to its arrival.

From Stress to Crisis

Stresses multiplied in the mid-second-century Roman Empire. Still, the essential functions and identities in Roman society persisted; stress need not have inevitably led to crisis. The system's capacity to adapt, however, was undergoing a major test. Increasing energy and resources were needed to prevent a variety of challenges—food insecurity, endemic diseases, urban migrations, climatic changes in key locations, and so forth—from coalescing into a full-blown crisis. The changing ecosystem that surrounded the Roman Empire was not helping matters either. And Roman institutions were changing too—and not simply in reaction to exogenous stimuli, or even uniformly in the direction of decline. Roman trade networks and military power, for example, punctured through geographic and political boundaries. But this expansion carried its own risks and consequences, and in some ways augmented existing strains on the system. It was a moment of fragility in an already fragile pre-industrial system.

As fate would have it, Rome's luck ran out. We do not know how the Antonine plague pathogen entered at this crucial moment, but it did. Historian William McNeill's *Plagues and Peoples*—among the most influential books on the history of disease—offers one theory: "in the first Christian centuries . . . Europe and China, the two least disease-experienced civilizations of the Old World, were in an epidemiological position analogous to that of Amerindians in the later age: vulnerable to socially disruptive attack by new infectious diseases."[137] But studying the Roman Empire's vulnerabilities belies a more dynamic situation than McNeill assumed. The Roman Empire (and especially its capital) was in the middle of naturogenic and anthropogenic challenges to its food supplies in key regions, prompting movements and migrations. Internally, droughts and other climatic disturbances hit certain regions at exactly the wrong times, sending the rural malnourished into nearby cities. There, the already limited mechanisms for relief such as we saw in the previous chapter were stretched to breaking. External climate refugees too—Celtic, German, and Sarmatian peoples from the far north and the Eurasian Steppe—pressed hard against the Empire's European borders, inaugurating territorial clashes that would last centuries.[138] The migrations highlighted differences in immunities—among urban and rural populations but also among the Empire's insiders and outsiders. With urban squalor, malnutrition, and regional climate shifts wedging open the widening cracks of the Pax Romana, the changing immunity profiles in the Empire's various populations evidently offered the incoming pandemic exactly what it needed to thrive.

The next chapter shows how long-distance trade as well as large mobile armies breached the geographic and social buffers on the eastern Mediterranean. Romans thought their attempts to engage and subdue this wider geography a sign of their power and might. To the evolving pathogens of the preindustrial world, however, the Pax Romana created new opportunities for transfer and conquest. So even while the institutions of the Roman Empire shook under their still expanding weight and bulk, the era of premodern pandemics commenced its historic rise.

3

RUMORS OF
DEATH

Late in the year AD 161, the Parthian king Vologases IV invaded the Roman protectorate of Armenia. With impressive speed, Vologases deposed Armenia's client king and installed his own ruler on the throne. Dutifully but foolishly, the Roman governor of the neighboring province of Cappadocia launched a counterinvasion with but a few thousand solders. After mere days of marching in the Armenian highlands, the Persians destroyed the overmatched Roman force. Humiliated, the Roman governor promptly committed suicide. The antagonistic Parthians obviously required a stern rebuke. Marcus's co-emperor Lucius Verus would deliver the punishment personally. His instrument? An army of around thirty thousand Roman soldiers. After decades of retrenchment and stagnation under the emperors Hadrian and Antoninus Pius, the Roman military roared back to life.

Responding to Lucius's call to arms, massive numbers of troops and officers poured eastward from all over the Empire. These gradually coalesced into a human flood that surged into Parthian territory. Lucius himself, however, never ventured past the eastern capital of Antioch. Instead, the emperor dallied with women and drank himself into stupors. Lucius's co-dependent generals and governors took up the slack, prosecuting a five-year war that culminated in the sack of the Parthian cities of Ctesiphon and Seleucia in Mesopotamia. When the war ended in early 166, the generals and their legions withdrew back into the

Empire, only now they carried a deadly disease. Rome had secured its eastern border only to have it breached by an invisible enemy. For Roman writers, the Parthian War's closing scene was also the Antonine plague's opening act.

Yet despite Roman claims of an eastern origin, we don't know where the Antonine plague pathogen came from. The pandemic's entrance into the Empire seems to have been a tragic historical coincidence— the result of a contagious, deadly, and likely novel disease reaching the eastern edges of the Mediterranean Basin just as mass movements of soldiers, as well as traders and refugees, were most active in the area. The contagion's most likely routes probably followed Red Sea trade networks and Roman military movements along the Empire's eastern boundaries. Perhaps Roman authors—despite their anti-eastern prejudices, superstitions, and misunderstandings about how diseases spread—got something fundamentally right about the disease's transmission? Maybe the clash between Roman soldiers and their Parthian neighbors in the mid-160s was the breach that sent plague surging into the Mediterranean? But there need not have been just one entrance. *Both* Lucius's returning soldiers and, for example, large caravans transporting goods from the Red Sea port of Berenike to Coptos along the Nile could have carried the disease. Ecological historian Robert Sallares pithily observes: "the appearance of pandemics was a side-effect of the general increase in inter-regional trade and movements of people in classical times."[1] So even if we lack practical information, at least one principle seems certain: Rome's economic and military power was a crucial precondition for the pandemic.

Oceans Together

Less than a decade before the first epidemics associated with the Antonine plague, strange rumors of a looming disease emerge from just beyond the eastern ends of Roman territory. A fourth-century AD biography of Antoninus Pius notes a local pestilence in Arabia during his reign. The mysterious throwaway comment appears among a list of outlandish "misfortunes and prodigies" that supposedly occurred in the AD 140s and 150s:

> A comet was seen, a two-headed child was born, and a woman gave birth to quintuplets . . . in Arabia, a crested serpent larger than the usual size . . . ate itself from the tail to the middle; and also in Arabia there was a pestilence, while in Moesia barley sprouted from the tops of trees. And besides all this, in Arabia four lions grew tame and of their own accord yielded themselves to capture.[2]

Historians typically dismiss such obvious sensationalism. Why would an undated and vague claim of pestilence in Arabia be any different? However, in the 1990s an inscription was found in the highlands of Yemen, a country that falls well within the area the Romans designated as Arabia. The inscription tells of a regional plague in AD 156. According to the text, the outbreak afflicted "the whole country"—presumably the Qaran region from which the inscription originated.[3] It is plausible, however, that "the whole country" included the entire southern Arabian Peninsula. Qaran was an often contested territorial mesh point for three kingdoms in southern Yemen—and any or indeed all of these kingdoms may have suffered the pestilence. Amazingly, the frequently dismissed biography of Antoninus Pius had its story straight in this one instance; it seems a sustained bout of disease indeed struck southern Arabia on the eve of the Antonine plague.

But was that mysterious pestilence the same disease associated with the Antonine plague? It is impossible to know. The chronology is suggestive, but historians need more detail to even begin to connect the dots.[4] The inscription itself hints at a few characteristics. First, it tells us that the disease was durable: it had lasted at least four years by the time the inscription was erected, and the pestilence was still ongoing. The inscription also notes that "there was infection in all the wells of the valley"—information that may point not to the water in the wells but to the wells' function as semi-settled gathering places for the otherwise rural and nomadic populations in the area. This disease surged where populations were most dense. In the more remote countryside, however, it lingered at a slow burn. The disease behind the Antonine plague too, as we shall soon see, hit Roman cities in epidemic bursts while, at the same time, meandered slowly through Roman hinterlands for years on end. So there is a connection here, albeit one clouded by the vagaries of ancient evidence.

How did the disease, whatever it was, find its way to the rural hinterlands of the southern Arabian Peninsula in the first place? A likely answer is trade. The people of southern Yemen—a region the Romans called Arabia Felix ("Fortunate Arabia")—were a crucial local link in the wider long-distance luxury trade networks of the Red Sea and Indian Ocean. Frankincense, myrrh, and other high-value goods moved overland through the kingdoms of southern Yemen and then up through the Nabataean Kingdom into an area the Romans called Arabia Petraea ("Stony Arabia") before reaching the city of Petra (in modern Jordan) itself. From there, goods made the short journey to the Mediterranean via the port at Gaza. But those in the Yemeni highlands also had contact with their southern and eastern neighbors along the coast—paying tax and providing soldiers. By the middle of the second century AD, luxury goods increasingly moved via maritime trade in the Red Sea and through major Arabian ports of Aden, Qanī', and Mocha.

The trade links between Rome and Arabia Felix were strong and well-established in the second century AD. Recent underwater excavations along the southern coast of Yemen confirm the presence of wine, oil, and other products from as far away as Gaul, North Africa, and Spain.[5] The southern Arabian kingdom of Saba even produced imitation Roman silver coins inscribed with portraits of Rome's first emperor, Augustus. The coins' silver content made them roughly equivalent to the Roman silver denarius—suggesting frequent and regular two-way trade.[6] As a pivot point in the larger Indian Ocean trade matrix, the southern Arabian Peninsula was, therefore, a natural point of contact for travelers (and their microbes) from India, Sub-Saharan Africa, the Middle East, and the Mediterranean. It is not surprising that the mid-second-century plague inscription was just one of several such inscriptions dating from between the first and sixth centuries AD.[7] The epidemic outbreak described in the mid-second-century Qaran inscription is therefore at least a plausible candidate, whatever pathogen became the infamous Antonine plague.

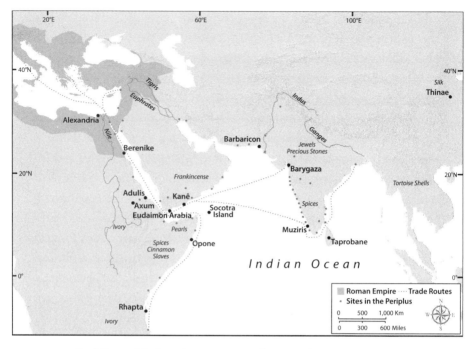

FIG. 3.1. Red Sea and Indian Ocean ports in the second century AD. Kyle Harper, *The Fate of Rome: Climate, Disease, and the End of an Empire* (Princeton: Princeton University Press, 2017), map 9: Romans and the Indian Ocean.

Still, hopping geographic barriers was no easy task for antiquity's microorganisms. But the Red Sea was like a funnel. Into it poured merchant ships carrying goods and people from all over the Afro-Eurasian world.[8] A first-century AD Greek logbook, the *Periplus of the Erythraean Sea*, describes a wide array of peoples, goods, ports, and routes around and beyond the Horn of Africa, Arabian Sea, and Indian Ocean.

The *Periplus* confirms that regional traders moved goods not only via *cabotage*—short-distance coastal trade routes linked together into a long-distance chain—but also via long-haul voyages across empty ocean, such as the established route from Qanī' in eastern Arabia Felix to Limyrike on the southwestern coast of India.[9] The author of the *Periplus* tells us that traders "used to make [this voyage] in small vessels, sailing close around the shores of the gulfs" until the first century BC. Around that time, the Greek navigator Hippalus discovered something

that changed Roman-Indian trade for good: it was possible for east-
bound ships to ride the monsoon winds on a direct route across the
open Indian Ocean, bypassing the smaller ports to the north.[10]

Many of the Roman ships that took advantage of the monsoon-aided
route were massive—perhaps fifty meters in length.[11] With lead-lined
hulls, these ships easily fit in the deep-water port of Berenike, the last
Roman-controlled outpost along the western coast of the Red Sea.
From there, barges rode in convoys—each ship staffed by dozens of
traders, workers, and soldiers (to deal with pirates)—across the warm
Indian Ocean waters to distant locations thousands of kilometers away,
from the southeast African emporium of Rhapta (likely off the Tanza-
nian coast) to Sri Lanka.[12] They made few stops—perhaps offloading
Roman goods at a port or two along the southern Arabian Peninsula.
The luxury goods brought back on these trips were desired by Roman
elites, for both consumption and profit; they therefore invested heavily
in such ventures.[13] By the second century AD, Roman sources—such
as the writings of the geographer and mathematician Claudius
Ptolemy—demonstrate much expanded and more precise knowledge
of the areas far to the east of the Roman Empire, including East Asia.[14]
Romans themselves, and in larger numbers, saw with their own eyes
lands that their grandparents might have once thought mythical.

The reach of Pax Romana traders was astonishing. In AD 166, a
group of Alexandrian merchants even managed to set foot in the Han
capital of Luoyang. The merchants claimed to be an official envoy of
Marcus Aurelius, but even the Chinese doubted their story.[15] A Chinese source from the Han emperor's court, the Hou Hanshu ("Book of
the Later Han"), records one of preindustrial history's most remarkable first contacts:

> The king of this country [the Roman Empire] always wanted to
> send envoys to the Han, but Anxi [Parthia], wishing to control the
> trade in multi-coloured Chinese silks, blocked the route to prevent
> [the Romans] getting through [to China]. In the ninth yanxi year
> [AD 166], during the reign of Emperor Huan, the king of Da Qin
> [the Roman Empire], Andun [Marcus Aurelius], sent envoys from

beyond the frontiers through Rinan [on the central-eastern Vietnam-
ese coast] to offer elephant tusks, rhinoceros horn, and turtle shell.
This was the very first time there was [direct] communication [be-
tween the two countries]. The tribute brought was neither precious
nor rare, raising suspicion that the accounts [of the "envoys"] might
be exaggerated.[16]

The Parthians had evidently kept the Romans and the Chinese from
connecting.[17] Their medial position between the two empires gave the
Parthians a trade advantage, both by land and sea, against their neighbors. Roman victories against Parthia, however, opened up new business for Rome. Roman goods reached previously unknown destina-
tions. Expanded Indian Ocean trade made exotic foreign goods available
to wealthy Romans at cheaper prices. But increased connectivity also
exposed the inhabitants of both empires to novel pathogens.

Trade connections between the four largest empires of Eurasia—the
Roman, Parthian, Kushan, and Han empires—reached their zenith.
Maritime routes across the Indian Ocean and overland highways via the
Silk Roads were replete with travelers.[18] We know that diseases hitched
rides along these routes, even the lonely paths across empty wilderness
and desolate plains. The proof is in the poop. Analysis of two-thousand-
year-old human feces found in a latrine along one Silk Road waypoint
confirms that travelers carried parasites with them over thousands of
kilometers.[19] Could traders have also carried the Antonine plague
pathogen? Many historians believe so, but the case is speculative, resting
primarily upon the chronology of vague records of epidemics across
Eurasia.[20] The earliest show up in Han China in AD 151.[21] Then westward in the Kushan Empire, sculptures of Hariti—goddess and plague
demon—appear in high numbers from AD 156 through 165. By the seventh century AD, she was associated with pox-like diseases as both protector and destroyer.[22] Does her sudden and frequent presence in the
mid-second century hint at the Antonine plague in the Kushan Empire?
The aforementioned Arabia Felix inscription (AD 156) then follows, as
do Roman references to plague in the Parthian Empire (AD 165). It may
well be that slow but steady trade moved the pandemic westward across

Eurasian empires, from China, through Kushan territory, then to Parthian cities, and finally into the Roman Empire. Alternatively, unrelated local epidemics may have struck these regions, and historians who see a larger pandemic at work are fitting the evidence into preexisting assumptions. Historians must do more than note instances of disease among sources with varied geographic origins; they must also identify the vectors that bridged social, economic, and geographic buffers between populations, as well as their potential paths.

The threshold between Indian Ocean and Mediterranean networks was Egypt—the narrowest segment of the Red Sea funnel. In the second century AD, the flow of goods into and out of the eastern Roman Empire ran through Egyptian ports along the Red Sea. Arriving from further east, traders unloaded cargoes at Red Sea ports, such as Berenike. Getting these goods to the Nile then required a two-week journey, usually taken by night, across Egypt's desolate eastern desert. This part of the journey was the most cumbersome and expensive of the entire trip—requiring the service of not only pack animals but also armed guards.[23] Desert travelers then arrived at Coptos on the Nile, where river barges carried cargoes on a three-week voyage downriver to the capital city of Alexandria—which Strabo called "the greatest emporium in the habitable world."[24]

During the Pax Romana, the city founded by Alexander the Great in 331 BC had become the dominant mediator between huge trade networks—a gateway between empires. By Strabo's day, Alexandria had "a monopoly of trade, and is almost the only receptacle for [luxury] merchandise and place of supply for foreigners." High-value goods, foreign wealth, and merchants from far beyond Roman frontiers flooded the eastern cosmopolis. Alexandria's ethnic diversity struck the Greek orator Dio Chrysostom, who met on the streets or in the temples not only Mediterranean peoples—Greeks, Italians, and Near Eastern peoples—but also "Ethiopians and Arabs from more distant regions" and "even Bactrians, Scythians, Persians and a few Indians."[25] A large Jewish population also inhabited the city. And watching over all who walked the gridded streets was the great Lighthouse—the Pharos of Alexandria. The ancient wonder stood over one hundred meters tall—an ever-present reminder of the abundant trade that animated the Egyptian capital.[26]

Wondrous Alexandria was nevertheless wracked with sickness. Due to its status as a high-volume entrepôt for both Mediterranean and Indian Ocean goods, the populations of Roman Alexandria and other parts of Egypt along the Nile trade routes probably encountered more diseases than just about any peoples in all of preindustrial human history. The inhospitable desert surrounding the reliable Nile River channeled goods and the people and animals who carried them into a narrow "artery of communication" through highly urbanized and dense populations.[27] Around 30 percent of Egyptians dwelt in cities, where diseases spread quickly and widely.[28] Consequently, Egyptian cities were among humanity's oldest and most resilient reservoirs for antiquity's deadliest pathogens.[29] Malaria, for example, was a common malady in Alexandria due to the marshes and mosquitoes in the Nile Delta. As an endemic disease, malaria cases rhythmically swelled in the fall and winter before declining again in spring and summer.[30] Some of the earliest medical papyri from Egypt are in fact wards against "the pestilence of the year"—presumably a reference to the annual surge of endemic diseases.[31] Pliny the Elder called Egypt "the fruitful parent of diseases" for good reason.[32]

Such routine encounters with an emporium of ancient diseases must have awarded many urban, if not rural, Egyptian populations increased immunity to some diseases. In an era without vaccines, population immunity—acquired when large numbers of people survived infection—offered the best resistance to the spread of many different diseases. This form of immunity, however, rarely quenched outbreaks, in both the past and present. Instead, endemic diseases settled into predictable patterns that ebbed and flowed with seasonal weather, migration patterns, and demography. Children (due to a lack of preexisting immunity) and the elderly (due to comorbidities) were often most at risk to endemic diseases. But when novel pathogens latched on to high-density Egyptian populations, the corresponding flare-ups would have been devastating.[33]

It is true that Egypt was not the only point of connection between the Indian Ocean and Mediterranean Sea, but it was by far the most convenient—and therefore the most well traveled. Although increasing maritime trade crowded out its overland counterpart during the Pax Romana, caravans and other land-based transport continued. Persian texts describe working supply stations and towns along the Silk Roads to Roman territory.[34] The major commercial city of Palmyra took goods from the Silk Roads and Persian Gulf. Riverine transport along the Tigris and Euphrates made Mesopotamia a vital connection as well. Spice and incense traders still moved goods through Arabia Felix. The dusty path between the Red Sea port of Aela (modern Aqaba, Jordan) and the port of Gaza in Judea took a mere two weeks to walk, but hostile wildlife ("an abundance of snakes" according to Strabo) made the journey perilous.[35] The road-building emperor Trajan constructed a paved path from Aela to Bostra in southern Syria, but the route seems to have been intended to serve Bostra's legionary base.[36]

Egypt outcompeted these land-based alternatives with help from Rome's emperors, who were incentivized to limit eastern entrances to their territory. Trade in luxury goods was a sizable source of tax revenue. It made sense to funnel trade through as few routes as possible; it was easier that way to collect the 25 percent tax on both imports and exports. Merchants seem to have taken the high costs of Roman infrastructure in stride. They may not have liked the taxes, but at least for their troubles they received some modicum of security, infrastructure, convenience, and predictability. One critical reappraisal of the Pax Romana put it this way: "the imperial peace . . . may well have benefited trade; but traders were also made to pay."[37]

While several trade arteries penetrated the Roman Empire, Egypt offered the pandemic a well-trafficked and densely populated pathway. But as Parthia and Rome grappled for control over Mesopotamia, catalytic communities of soldiers marched at a pace suitable to collect pathogens in one area and carry them into naive populations while transmissibility remained high. So while land and sea traders undoubtedly transmitted the Antonine plague pathogen at a slow pace through

eastern Roman cities, Rome's legions delivered the disease a direct
route toward the Mediterranean's millions of waiting victims.

Plague's Human Highways

On the eve of the Antonine plague, Marcus and Lucius commanded an
army just shy of half a million men. Roman citizens alone made up
thirty legions—or about 180,000 soldiers in total, give or take a few
thousand. More than 200,000 auxiliary troops—infantry, cavalry, and
sailors from across the Roman Empire—accompanied the regular legions.[38] Roman military camps were larger and more cosmopolitan
than many Roman cities. They contained not only thousands of soldiers
from diverse parts of the Empire but also equal if not greater numbers
of dependent women, children, and servants.[39] Excavations at the fort
at Vindolanda on the Roman side of Hadrian's Wall in Britain, for example, turned up shoes for women and children.[40] Similarly, at the
other end of the Empire at Dura-Europos in Syria, archaeologists found
high numbers of women's hairpins and bracelets inside the military base
there.[41] Wherever Roman soldiers were, whether lingering in garrisons
or marching across thousands of kilometers, merchants, suppliers, mes-
sengers, and many others latched on. And when soldiers moved, especially in large numbers to fight in Rome's wars, they formed mobile
cities—excellent breeding grounds for all sorts of microbes. For the
Antonine plague pathogen, there could be no better strategic conquest
than Rome's legions.

Historians would like to know more about the military movements
that preceded the Antonine plague outbreak in the mid AD 160s. Still,
the available evidence—circumstantial though it may be—suggests that
the pandemic entered the Roman Empire via the movements of Roman
soldiers and those who followed in their camps. Contemporary Roman
writers, inscriptions, and sources from well outside the Roman Empire
record several important contacts between Roman troops and the Red
Sea and Indian Ocean societies that carried novel diseases poised to run
rampant in the Roman Empire, should an army of sufficient size ever
carry them there.

Political and economic expansion during the Pax Romana dispersed Roman troops well beyond the Empire's boundaries. In fact, when history records Roman soldiers crossing into foreign territories, tales of encounters with new and deadly diseases often follow. Such stories were as old as the Pax Romana itself. In the mid- to late 20s BC, Augustus sent the Egyptian governor Aelius Gallus, along with 10,000 legionaries from Egypt, as well as a detachment of 500 Jewish troops borrowed from King Herod in Judea, into the deserts of Arabia Felix.[42] In his report to the geographer Strabo, Gallus complained of an expedition fraught with "sickness, fatigue, hunger and bad roads." The Roman army was unprepared for the novel diseases that awaited them in Arabia Felix, as well as the dangers of a lengthy campaign in the desert.[43] The outbreak was so lethal and lasted so long that Gallus's army was forced to halt for several months through winter "for the recovery of the sick" before carrying on with the expedition.[44] In the end, Gallus abandoned Arabia Felix with as many excuses as surviving troops, retreating to Egypt with the beleaguered remnants of his once proud army.

After Gallus's failure, the Romans never again sent a large force to the southern Arabian Peninsula. Instead, the strategy shifted toward the use of naval forces accompanied by detachments of soldiers to control and tax both land and seaborne imports from beyond the Empire's eastern and southern boundaries.[45] Key to this strategy was Trajan's annexation of the Nabataean Kingdom of northwest Arabia and its ports along the northern tip of the Red Sea. The Nabataeans were crucial middlemen in the overland trade between southern Arabia and the Romans.[46] After the annexation, Trajan accomplished what no previous emperor had: he conquered Parthia. Trajan's invasion brought Mesopotamia briefly into the Roman Empire. The emperor then took his army to the Persian Gulf. There he grieved that he was too old to follow further east in the footsteps of his hero, Alexander the Great.

Ironically, however, Trajan did follow Alexander—by dying from a disease caught in the east. According to Cassius Dio, Trajan first fell ill shortly after an unsuccessful siege of Hatra (in northern Iraq) in the winter of AD 117. Then Trajan's newly conquered territories erupted in revolt. The health of the *optimus princeps* declined rapidly. Trajan was dead by summer, along with his expansionary vision of a Roman-controlled Persia. Unfortunately, sources reveal little of the emperor's symptoms or whether his army also became infected with whatever disease flared up that winter.[47] But as luck would have it, no epidemic followed Trajan's solders back home.

The rapid pace of conquest under Trajan came to a screeching halt under his successors Hadrian and Antoninus Pius. Mass military movements correspondingly slowed down.[48] Instead, money poured into infrastructure projects along the Red Sea. Emperors constructed fortifications, canals, and roads to better control and tax trade from Arabia Felix, India, Ethiopia, and beyond.[49] It was in these areas that smaller clusters of soldiers from the eastern legions—especially those normally stationed in Egypt, Arabia, and Syria—traveled hundreds of kilometers beyond the last outposts within Roman lands to monitor and administer these lucrative rents for the Roman state. In Hegra (in modern northwest Saudi Arabia), for example, an inscription dated to the mid AD 170s records a military dedication to Marcus Aurelius set up under the supervision of centurions from Legio III Cyrenaica—normally resident some eight hundred kilometers away in Bostra.[50] These troops were almost certainly in Hegra to control and tax the overland spice trade that moved through the prosperous Arabian city.[51] Much further south, the name and title of one Publius Cornelius, an equestrian, appear on a puzzling and difficult-to-date inscription found in the Al-Jawf region of inland western Yemen—an area within a day's walk of the aforementioned Yemeni plague inscription from the mid-second century AD.[52] On the eve of the Antonine plague, Roman soldiers once again traveled back and forth between distant lands.

But these troops fanned out farther than ever before. Remarkably, two inscriptions found on the largest of the Farasan Islands off the west coast of Yemen—almost one thousand kilometers beyond Rome's last southern port at Berenike—confirm that detachments from Rome's eastern legions, as well as a fleet of ships, patrolled the area.[53] In AD 120, just three years after Trajan's death, soldiers from Legio VI Ferrata out of Bostra were stationed on the island. A second inscription from AD 143/4 provides even more detail and testifies to a serious and sustained Roman presence. A new detachment, this one a full *vexillatio* of about one thousand soldiers from Legio II Traiana, normally based in Egypt, as well as axillary troops plus some additional support units, had taken over duties at the distant outpost.[54] These detachments may have discouraged pirates—Rome's main competitors in the expropriation of commerce. According to contemporary sources, piracy was rampant in the region.[55] The 143/4 inscription even refers to a *praefectus Ferresani portus et Ponti Herculis*—a Roman prefecture of "the harbor of Farasan and of the Herculean Sea" (probably the straits of Bab el Mandeb)—a sign of long-term Roman governance in the region.[56] *Vexillationes* themselves, however, rarely served long-term stints. These ad hoc detachments occupied frontier areas on limited and specific assignments; upon completion, they rejoined their parent legions. The inscriptions, therefore, suggest that service on the Farasan Islands was not the responsibility of one group of soldiers, or even a single legion. Instead, Roman troops rotated to and from the island on a semi-regular basis.

Buoyed by more frequent and far-flung movements of the Roman military, conditions in the mid-second century AD may have finally aligned for a novel disease to travel into Roman territory. Instead of sending infrequent invasion forces, the Romans blanketed their eastern legions across thousands of kilometers along and beyond their borders. In addition to traders, groups of Roman soldiers now regularly moved back and forth and in the midst of Indian Ocean trade networks. Even the most distant detachments were concentrated into ships, forts, and island garrisons in proximity to areas with confirmed outbreaks of diseases for which the Romans likely had little if any preexisting immunity. Such movements may explain how Roman sources even came to know about a mid-second-century plague in Arabia in the first place. Did a detachment of soldiers witness it firsthand, and then return to their commanding officers in Bostra or Alexandria to tell the tale? Did some of these soldiers catch the disease themselves, and subsequently spread it among their comrades in the eastern Empire? The aforementioned Arabia Felix inscription records an active plague for at least four years— plenty of time for it to spread among nearby Roman troops.

Then there was the Parthian War. The invasion collected (and afterward dispersed) the outstretched eastern legions, as well as soldiers and
commanders from across the Empire. Seven legions occupied the provinces of Egypt, Arabia, Syria Palaestina, and Syria. It was standard practice to muster these soldiers together and then deploy them in eastern
campaigns.[57] If, as expected, Lucius's invading army borrowed heavily
from these legions, he would have left behind auxiliary regiments of
several hundred men to provide minimum order in the eastern provinces.[58] After all, no one wanted a repeat of the eastern revolts that undermined Trajan's Parthian War some fifty years prior.

Surviving sources confirm troop movements from even farther afield
just prior to the Antonine plague. Upon the suicide of the Cappadocian
governor in AD 161, for example, the senator Marcus Statius Priscus—
an experienced military commander and governor—traveled all the
way from Britain across nearly the entire Empire to take over the now
vacant post. We know from inscriptions that he commanded two legions in the Parthian War: Legio I Minervia and Legio V Macedonica.[59]
Both of these legions marched over from Europe—the former from
Bonna (modern Bonn, Germany) while the latter left behind a fort at
the Danube Delta (in modern southeast Romania). Additional legions
from Aquincum (modern Budapest) and Vindobona (modern Vienna)
along with several detachments from other European legions also made
the trip east. The list of commanding officers and members of the imperial retinue was long, and these arrived from posts across the Empire,
including Britain, Africa, Italy, Gaul, Egypt, and the Balkans.[60] In all,
Lucius's campaign amassed people from various parts of Europe, Asia
Minor, the Near East, and beyond, mixed them together, and then concentrated them in groups on and off again for the duration of the war.
Even if the Romans managed to escape contamination via trade, the
movements of the Empire's eastern legions almost certainly exposed
them and those nearby to new diseases, if not the Antonine plague
pathogen itself.

Finally, there is still the conventional account to reckon with—that
superstitious story of Apollo's wrath when Lucius's subordinate Avidius
Cassius sacked Seleucia. Could Roman soldiers have (also?) picked up

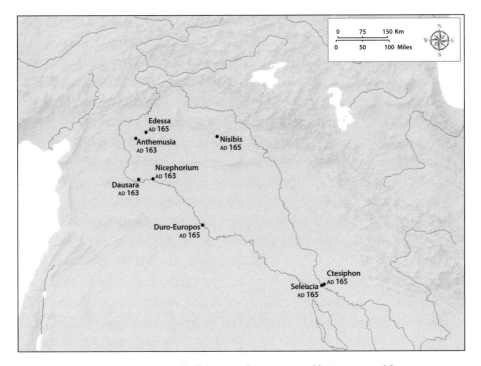

FIG. 3.2. Parthian cities attacked, besieged, or occupied by Roman soldiers during the Roman offensive against Parthia, AD 163–165.

the disease at the end of the Parthian War? Although tales of divine vengeance following the desecration of Apollo's shrine were later inventions, it remains possible that the disease that spawned the Antonine plague spread among the Roman legions during their winter marches through Mesopotamia. Hints in the evidence implicate at least four Parthian cities in the spread of disease during the Parthian War: Seleucia, Ctesiphon, Nisibis, and Dura-Europos.

Roman soldiers ravaged densely populated Seleucia and Ctesiphon in the winter of AD 165/6. Each city's population, but especially that of Ctesiphon, was in dire straits. Whereas Seleucia had opened its gates, the citizens of Ctesiphon—perhaps after hearing what happened to their neighbors—hunkered down for a siege. While the city probably had some supplies, the poor masses in Ctesiphon—if they were not already malnourished because of the war—would have been the first to suffer under the blockade. When Ctesiphon finally capitulated, many in the city were likely starved and diseased. During the murder, rapine, looting, and burning that followed, the rampaging Roman soldiers unwittingly offered their own bodies as hosts and vectors, adding to the existing mass of starving, sick, and potentially contagious citizens.

But this was not the only violent, potentially sickness-spreading intermingling of Romans and Persians that year. In the summer of 165, the northern wing of the Roman force occupied the strategic city of Edessa, the capital of the small Roman client-kingdom of Osrhoene. With Edessa under Roman control, Legio V Macedonica pursued the Parthians east. The Parthians dug in at Nisibis and prepared for a siege. Details about this phase of the war are hard to come by. A history of the conflict, penned by one Crepereius Calpurnianus, is lost. We only know of it from a scathing review written by one of antiquity's most spicy satirists. Lucian of Samosata relentlessly mocked Calpurnianus for plagiarizing Thucydides to embellish portions of his account of the siege of Nisibis.[61] A plague struck the city during the siege, tempting Calpurnianus to draw motifs from antiquity's most famous pestilential disaster in Classical Athens. And yet, buried in the hyperbole must have been a kernel of truth. Thousands of Romans besieged and then perhaps occupied the city while it suffered an epidemic.[62]

Last is the puzzle of Dura-Europos—the minor cosmopolis on the banks of the Euphrates at the boundary of the two great empires. Although not as populous as Seleucia and Ctesiphon, Dura-Europos was both the terminus for upriver trade from the Persian Gulf and the starting point of a major land route to the Roman Empire's eastern cities of Antioch, Palmyra, and Damascus.[63] Archaeological excavations in the city's ancient ruins have uncovered a vast diversity of temples and other religious and cultural buildings, implying a population of many cultural and ethnic backgrounds.[64] Avidius Cassius attacked the city on his southern march in late AD 165. The literary sources tell us little about what happened over the winter, but archaeological evidence suggests that Cassius kept a detachment of soldiers within the city walls during the winter of 165/6—exposing the soldiers to the seasonal spike of the city's endemic diseases. First, the city was not sacked—a merciful fate that normally preceded Roman occupation. A Roman garrison may also explain the construction of an underground temple to the god Mithras, a deity of special significance to Roman soldiers.[65] Someone also repaired the city walls.[66] The Roman garrison would have included the twentieth auxiliary cohort in Syria. Indeed, a unit called the Cohors XX Palmyrenorum seems to have originated at this time.[67] The most interesting evidence for occupation, however, is the base of a statue dedicated to the emperor Lucius Verus in, of all places, the temple of Artemis.[68] Artemis, like Apollo, was capable of curing disease, and the goddess's powers were sought out numerous times during the Antonine plague in the eastern Empire. Did a plague outbreak flare up in the city during the winter of 165/6, infecting a garrison of Roman troops? Was the disease still viable among these soldiers when the Roman legions returned to their bases the following year? A statue on its own does not make a pandemic, but it does suggest Roman occupation in the midst of a pestilential moment.

Many historians, both ancient and modern, seem confident that the pestilence associated with the Antonine plague latched on to Roman soldiers in Parthia. And while the explicit evidence for such a pathway is thin, the circumstantial links are strong enough to make a case for transmission—especially in the cities. So there may be some grains of truth mixed in with Roman writers' otherwise dismissible anti-eastern prejudices. Perhaps we should give more credence to writers such as Ammianus Marcellinus—one of the Empire's last great historians—who described the Antonine plague as an "incurable disease . . . which corrupted everything with contagion and death from the boundaries of Persia all the way to the Rhine and to Gaul."[69]

And yet, there remains some evidence that the conventional date for the start of the Antonine plague—AD 165—could be dead wrong.[70] A statue to Apollo "Averter of Evil" was erected in Hierapolis in southwestern Asia Minor in AD 164.[71] While this statue alone hardly confirms that a novel pathogen spread in the eastern Empire, neither should historians dismiss its presence as mere general concern for health.[72] Apollo "Averter of Evil" was *the* god to petition as a ward against serious epidemic disease.[73] As far back as the Peloponnesian War (431–404 BC), the Athenians placated this fearful iteration of Apollo with statuary during their famous plague.[74] And a dream journal written by the Roman orator Aelius Aristides contains a curious account of a deadly plague in nearby Smyrna in the summer of AD 165.[75] An undated mid-second-century AD inscription also praises the god of the river Meles near Smyrna for "deliverance from the pestilence and evil."[76] So an epidemic hit parts of western Asia Minor in 164—a year *before* Roman troops in Persia supposedly first caught the disease that would soon be thought of as the Antonine plague.

Unfortunately, we will never know whether the outbreak in Asia Minor was just a curiously timed local epidemic or the same scourge responsible for the Antonine plague. Roman authors probably would never admit their side got the disease first. Anti-Persian rhetoric was rampant, as was Roman association of disease with impiety. Facts could easily be changed to suit a preferred narrative. A wrathful Apollo suddenly striking sacrilegious soldiers in the distant east fits several pieces of propaganda at once. But, in fact, instead of the Parthians infecting the Romans, the Roman army could have brought the disease from Asia Minor, Syria, or Egypt into the cities of Mesopotamia. But even if Lucius's legions were not the Empire's first victims, or even its main vectors, the returning legions undoubtedly gave the Antonine plague pathogen purchase in Roman territory.[77] So however and whenever the Roman army became infected, the dramatic movements of large bodies of soldiers in the 160s would have planted seeds of plague wherever they went. By the Parthian War's victorious end, if not earlier, Rome's defenders became unwitting agents of disease and death. The pandemic had arrived.

PART II

OUTBREAK

Woe! Woe! A powerful disaster leaps onto the plain—a pestilence inescapable. It wields a sword of vengeance in one hand. In the other, it lifts up the deeply mournful images of newly blighted mortals. In every way, it harangues the newborn ground donated to death, and hastily torments and ravages men.

Every generation perishes!

—APOLLO'S ORACLE TO CAESAREA TROCETTA (*IGRR* 4.1498), SECOND CENTURY AD

4

PLAGUE
UNLEASHED

Rome's doctors were in an uproar. A twenty-one-year-old noblewoman was dead of an unknown disease. Her initial symptoms were quite mild: chronic cough, shortness of breath, reddened face, and light menstruation. The family's physicians, led by one of Rome's most experienced and respected anatomists, Martianus, decided against bleeding the woman. A young, hot-headed, and probably uninvited physician from Pergamum, however, injected himself into the discussion—arguing that the patient would quickly deteriorate unless she was bled. No one listened. But then the woman's health took a nasty turn. She coughed up so much blood that she suffocated to death. It was agonizing to watch. Furious that no one heeded his advice, the Pergamese doctor lambasted the older men, calling Martianus "malicious and contentious." And yet, it was the young doctor who put up his fists and needed to be physically restrained, lest he brawl with his elders. Galen of Pergamum, the doctor whose name would go on to become legendary not only in ancient Rome but in all of medical history, began his combative career in Rome with a near knockout.

The imperial capital during the Pax Romana seemed tailor-made for innovative and ambitious physicians.[1] In normal times, Rome was rife with disease of all sorts, offering fledgling doctors challenges fit to launch famed medical careers. Galen arrived in Rome around the time of the great Tiber flood under Marcus Aurelius—a bumper year for diseases. As the waters receded, the finest medical minds, many arriving from the Greek east, flooded the city. But demand for health care far outstripped supply. Greek doctors could therefore charge exorbitant fees, and Rome's wealthy elite begrudgingly ponied up.[2] And as medical costs rose higher and higher, the complaints followed. Pliny the Elder gives us a flavor for the love-hate relationship between Roman elites and their medical experts:

> Doctors learn by exposing us to risks, and conduct experiments at the expense of our lives. Only a doctor can kill a man with impunity. . . . Let us not indict the greed of doctors, their financial rapacity in dealing with patients whose life is in the balance, the fees charged for curing ailments, the payments on account that lead to death, and the secret instructions to ease aside a cataract rather than remove it completely. In the final analysis, the large number of sharks using medical practice to prey on people seems to be the best thing about the situation, in that competition between rivals—rather than any sense of decency—reduces fees.[3]

Galen quickly figured out how to exploit the latent distrust that hounded many Roman physicians. Like a populist politician who, without any hint of irony, denounces establishment incumbents even while desperately seeking membership in their ranks, Galen aggressively lambasted Rome's most illustrious doctors, often naming names. By the mid-160s, the thirty-seven-year-old doctor had become a persistent thorn in the side of his older, more established colleagues. At his most audacious, Galen anointed himself the medical field's Trajan—a doctor *optimus maximus* ("best and greatest"). Galen said that his improvements over Hippocrates—the fifth-century BC Greek father of medicine and originator of the Hippocratic Oath—were akin to Trajan's civilizing of the countryside through the construction or repair of hundreds of kilometers of roads.[4] There may not be a word in the English language sufficient to capture such unbridled arrogance. Yet Galen's antics earned him a passionate following, as well as the attention of emperors.

But perhaps more than any intrinsic talent, Galen benefitted from circumstance. He found himself in the right place at the right time. His meteoric rise to fame commenced just as the Antonine plague first settled into its multiyear residency. Galen's career arc aligned perfectly with the pandemic. Through serious study and treatment of numerous plague victims, including perhaps the emperors and their family members, Galen obtained expert knowledge of what he called "the great pestilence." In fact, the Antonine plague is so associated with the doctor that some still refer to it as "the Galenic plague." Although Galen never wrote a proper treatise on the disease, several passing references in his massive corpus survive to the present day, offering historians captivating clues to the pandemic that shook mighty Rome at its height. The proud doctor, of course, focused his prose on his own clever treatments; he said far less about the disease itself. Most of Galen's plague patients probably died, and thus the boastful doctor would not have preserved details of their final days.[5] Still, especially in those that lived, Galen described several symptoms of the malady, although with frustrating brevity. Galen most wanted to memorialize his cures, not the disease that inspired them. Ironically, Galen criticized Thucydides for describing the Athenian plague of the late fifth century BC like a historian rather than a doctor; but Galen, in describing the pestilence of his own day like a doctor, left historians with a puzzle they cannot quite complete.[6]

Historians do not know exactly which pathogen promulgated the Antonine plague. Galen's notes on the outbreak are tantalizingly brief; he provides enough clues to suggest several diagnoses—a *poxviridae* family infection being the most favored. But pinning down the exact pathogen has proven impossible. It's a real shame. Solving this ancient medical mystery would allow historians to deploy epidemiological models to better estimate how quickly the disease spread and how many it killed and even draw firmer conclusions about its economic and social effects.[7] At the moment, historians can merely offer retrospective diagnoses. Such efforts, however, are challenging at best, and likely to mislead. Absent genetic evidence, the descriptions of ancient authors are tricky to turn into robust diagnoses. Even without a definitive identification of disease responsible for the Antonine plague, however, some of the disease's main characteristics are discernable in the sources.

First, the disease survived and spread in large groups of human beings in regular close contact with one another. Our sources consistently tell us the cities and the soldiers were hardest hit. Galen himself compares the pestilence to an insatiable beast which "does not just kill a handful, but spreads over entire cities and destroys them horribly."[8] We know far less about what happened in the sparsely populated countryside. It is unfortunate that we cannot know the exact mechanism by which the pandemic moved from person to person, otherwise we could better model the densities, behaviors, and population dynamics required to sustain it. Some of the most transmissible diseases spread via droplets, aerosol particles suspended in liquid or gas and on objects or surfaces (fomites).[9] Measles, for example—among the most contagious viruses in existence—diffuses rapidly as infected persons cough or sneeze both aerosols and droplets.[10] Other pathogens survive in clothes, in bedding, or on food—allowing transmission without direct human-to-human contact. In some cases, rodents or insects act as disease reservoirs. Humans can pick up bubonic plague, for example, from infected fleas or through direct contact with the tissue of human victims. If the Antonine plague pathogen lacked an animal reservoir, however, the spread of the disease would have slowed considerably in the countryside due to the limited number and frequency of human-to-human contacts.

Second, we know the epidemic was deadly. Sources claim not only that many people died but that they died in groups or households. This is a mark of a true epidemic scourge. When SARS-CoV-2 ripped through the world in 2020 and 2021, total mortality was high for a modern outbreak, but seroprevalence studies show its pre-vaccination global infection fatality rate for those under age sixty was a mere .03 percent.[11] Compare SARS-CoV-2's historically benign mortality with that of, say, bubonic plague, which some scholars believe killed around 50 to 60 percent of its urban victims during its preindustrial pandemic phases.[12] Of the two modern smallpox strains, *Variola major* killed as many as 30 percent of those infected in some cases. The far-less-deadly variant *Variola minor*, which emerged in the late nineteenth century, killed less than 1 percent.[13] Historical context matters. In the modern era, several hundred people catch bubonic plague each year, but access to modern medicine ensures that almost all victims survive. Modern populations understand how diseases spread and take preventative measures. In sixth-century AD Constantinople, however, bubonic plague preyed upon underfed, unhealthy, and unwashed urban populations. The resulting body count was too massive for proper burial. The same would have been true of the Antonine plague; the prevailing conditions of poverty and malnutrition in the ancient world would have only fed the appetite of an already deadly disease.

Finally, the seasonality of the disease is complicated but also intriguing. Galen and the senator Cassius Dio both link outbreaks with colder weather.[14] Sources for the Parthian War likewise suggest fall and winter transmission. But Aelius Aristides claims to have witnessed a summer pestilence in Smyrna. It seems likely that lower temperature and humidity facilitated the spread of the Antonine plague pathogen, but other factors—population density, migration patterns, preexisting immunity, and others—could clearly overcome seasonal forcing. In this one respect, the disease was not unlike modern smallpox—a disease with a similar relationship to climate.[15] In many early modern smallpox epidemics—eighteenth-century London, Paris, and New Mexico, and twentieth-century India—smallpox surges often correlated with colder and drier conditions.[16] Smallpox historically spread best when temperatures dropped below 26 degrees Celsius (78.8 degrees Fahrenheit) and when humidity fell under 85 percent.[17] Diseases are dynamic, however; and so are human populations. As smallpox ravaged early modern England over three centuries, for example, its seasonality and peak mortality gradually shifted from early fall to late winter.[18] Seasonality also seems to have influenced epidemics during the Antonine plague, but the novelty of the disease probably allowed it to spread even when seasonal factors were unfavorable.

But when temperature, humidity, and population dynamics all aligned, epidemic bursts must have been devastating. The winter of AD 165/6 was a deadly one for Roman soldiers in Parthian territory. Both famine and disease decimated the legions before they made it back to

Antioch.[19] We have what seems like corroborating evidence in a Spartan monument, which records the fate of a potential plague victim: "Hail to thee Dioscoras, who lived 26 years. He had gone to the successful campaign against the Persians, and on his way back he died in Hierapolis [in Syria]."[20] Soldiers such as Dioscoras returned from the northern prong of the invasion force that deadly winter. These were the soldiers that conquered the cities of Edessa and Nisibis in August or September of 165. Their victories earned Lucius the title *Parthicus Maximus* ("Greatest Conqueror of Parthia")—a title which appeared on his coinage before the year was over.[21] Some of these soldiers undoubtedly lingered in Nisibis and became caught in (or perhaps caused!) the outbreak there. But no later than spring of AD 166, most were back in Antioch to make the journey home. Because of both the reference to plague in Nisibis from Lucian's writings and the expectation of a spring rather than summer return, this army may have been the force to spread the disease deep into Roman territory. The population of Antioch may also have become infected that year. But if plague-carrying soldiers arrived late enough in the spring, the city may have been spared a major flare-up, at least until the following winter.

The southern wing of Lucius's army, however—the soldiers led by Avidius Cassius—remained in Parthian territory over the winter. Perhaps as a reward for his devastating blitz down the Euphrates in late 165, Cassius was made consul—the highest magistracy open to a Roman aristocrat. But Cassius did not rest on his laurels. Seeking additional glory and spoils, he burst east out of Ctesiphon and Seleucia in spring of 166 and into Media, the territory of the once mighty empire of the Medes. This excursion, short-lived though it was, earned Cassius's boss Lucius the title of "Medicus" or "Conqueror of the Medes."[22] It was this army that sources claim brought plague back to Rome. But if Cassius's soldiers had indeed suffered a horrific high-mortality epidemic over the previous winter, would they have been in sufficient shape to press on into Media? It was, in fact, the other army that hastened back to Antioch, not Cassius's soldiers.

Rome's earliest potential exposure from the eastern soldiers came in late spring of AD 166. A young junior officer of the Syrian Legio III Gallica named Junius Maximus was appointed as the lucky messenger to deliver news of the victory to the Roman nobility. In order to give the announcement personally in the Senate House—where only members were allowed to speak—Junius was given a battlefield promotion to quaestor, a financial magistracy that included automatic Senate membership.[23] He and his party must have arrived in Rome in May or June of 166, where he sang the praises of Cassius to both Marcus and the senators.[24] The bulk of Cassius's army, however, remained in Persia just beyond midsummer.[25] Cassius himself never returned to Rome. He stayed in the east administering ever larger segments of the Empire until his life met a tragic end, as this book will soon relate. But all roads lead to Rome, and the contagion quickly found a route into the Empire's unprotected heart.

The First Wave

The summer of AD 166 saw a slew of soldiers stream into Asia Minor from the now subdued Parthian Empire. These travelers, who would have numbered in the tens of thousands, did not return to their European camps and forts in one large mass. But cellular collections of soldiers marched along familiar roads and arterials, stopping off in many of the same cities and waypoints. We know from an inscription found at Ephesus, for example, that many legionaries passed that way on their return. In Ephesus, the men were fed at the expense of the wealthy sophist Falavius Damianus. Damianus outlaid enough grain to feed around forty thousand soldiers for a period of five months.[26] There is no question that crowds of soldiers moved through Asia Minor.

From southwestern Asia Minor, the veterans of the Parthian War fanned out to find their legionary bases.[27] We know where some of these soldiers went. The majority traveled north along the western coast of Asia Minor and then overland through the province of Thracia. Members of Legio V Macedonica were reassigned from Moesia Inferior to a fort at Potaissa, a dangerous outpost north of the Danube in the center of Dacian territory. Legio II Adiutrix returned to Aquincum (modern Budapest). The longest known journey, however, belonged to Legio I

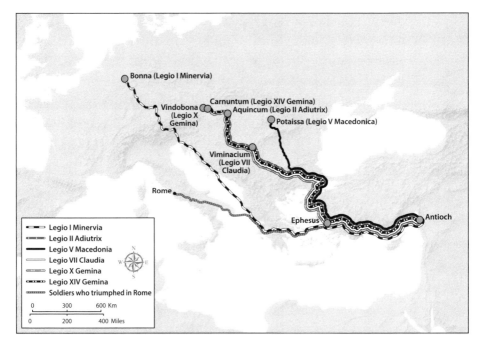

FIG. 4.1. Probable routes of soldiers from Antioch to their legionary camps following the Parthian War of AD 161–166.
Constructed from the ORBIS network model road map (https://orbis.stanford.edu/) with the following settings: season: summer; priority: shortest; network modes: road, river, coastal sea; mode: foot, military, and daylight. Based on *AE* 1913.170, all routes pass through Ephesus.

Minervia. These men likely sailed around Greece before making landfall in Illyricum and passing through Aquileia in Italy on their way back to Bonna (modern Bonn) along the Rhine. A portion of the soldiers triumphed in Rome. We cannot know the route these soldiers took, but it seems unlikely that they returned all the way back to their bases only to suddenly have to make another long journey to Rome; they probably took a direct route to the capital from either Antioch or Ephesus.

How contagious were the returning troops if they carried the Antonine plague pathogen back with them? The hot, dry Mediterranean climate may have kept the disease at a low simmer among the soldiers and cities in which they stayed. Perhaps the disease remained at most a lingering threat, trickling from the traveling soldiers at each populated rest stop? But winter was coming.

No doubt some of these soldiers unknowingly passed a legendary physician as he sauntered in the opposite direction. Galen had left Rome in a huff in the summer of 166. He told his friends that he was heading back east on a short country holiday, but the doctor ended up spending several years away from Rome.[28] The first epidemic wave in Rome explains his prolonged absence, but does it also explain his sudden departure? Galen portrays himself in early writings as a young genius fighting against older, better-connected but nevertheless ignorant competition in Rome. A threatened medical establishment hounded him out of the city after he showed them up in his writing and public dissections.[29] In a letter he wrote decades later, however—when Galen had himself become a paragon of the medical establishment—the doctor changed his story dramatically. He claimed to have had a premonition that a deadly plague would soon strike the city, and so the doctor fled in advance.[30] Galen's earlier explanation for his departure, although likely exaggerated, seems easier to believe. After all, if Galen truly fled because he knew plague was on its way, why set course eastward directly into the pestilential tidal wave?[31] No, Galen at best may have heard rumors that Lucius's army was swarmed by plague in Parthian territory.[32] Neither Galen nor anyone else in Rome was prepared for the contagion quietly but quickly creeping across the Empire.

Galen was not alone in vacating Rome that summer. Elites often left the sweltering city midyear. The hot months ushered in disproportionate degrees of death according to epitaphs and inscribed cinerary urns.[33] Poor hygiene, flies, rodents, incoming seasonal workers, multiplying bacteria, and higher levels of human and animal excrement created an environment rife with killer dysenteries, diarrheas, bacterial infections, and other stomach and intestinal maladies. These were the most deadly of the routine afflictions to strike Rome.[34] For the elderly, however, their most dangerous days were in winter, when low temperatures brought respiratory viruses out of their summer dormancy. The Antonine plague contagion also awaited the coming cold.

As autumn arrived in AD 166, many of Lucius's veterans coagulated in the Eternal City. It was their privilege to join the emperor's public triumphal parade—a spectacular celebration of the eastern conquests credited to Lucius. Thousands marched along crowded city streets on October 12, 166.[35] Tens of thousands more individuals—citizens and slaves alike—packed into the fora, the temples, and the amphitheaters for days on end. Rome's street traders, hawkers, and peddlers swarmed throughout the swollen throng, offering souvenirs and street food out of baskets or trays or from mats on the ground.[36] It was a super-spreader event on the grandest scale. The weather turned. And all hell broke loose in the city of Rome.

The entry in Lucius's biography is jarring. Even as the festivities wound down, the emperors began quiet preparations for a new war against the Germanic tribes; then, suddenly, heaps of bodies over-whelmed the city.[37] There was evidently no warning. Only by using wagons and carts could victims be removed. We know from ancient accounts of other plagues that urban epidemics quickly overwhelmed the limited capacity of body collectors.[38] The sight of rotting corpses in the streets, the dogs and rats fighting over the macabre morsels, the unrelenting rancid stench, the pustular flesh and fluids being crushed into the grime of the city streets—it would have been unendurable.[39] The bodies were enough of a problem that the Romans, normally care-ful about burial rituals and funerary rites, bypassed their protocols—prompting the emperors to enact "stringent laws on burials and tombs" according to one account.[40] Surviving Roman legal records confirm new burial laws under Marcus and Lucius, although none specify plague as their cause.[41] Accounts from other ancient urban plagues, however, tell of survivors sneaking corpses into the tombs of other families.[42] If the body count in Rome was as high as the sources suggest, civility may have been abandoned.

Rome had little capacity for dealing with mass death. In the cata-combs of Saint Peter and Marcellinus just outside Rome, archaeologists in 2002 cleared away the debris blocking a series of ancient chambers.[43] To their surprise, they discovered several tombs containing bodies un-ceremoniously dumped from above and doused in lime or covered with shrouds—well over a hundred adults and a few children. None of the bones showed signs of trauma. Some appear to have been victims of an epidemic (or even *epidemics*). With much of the catacombs still to be excavated, several thousand more bodies may be entombed. Typically, the bodies in catacombs are delicately laid to rest either in individual places or as carefully organized group burials. Indeed, such care is seen in the layers of remains both above and below the tangled bodies. The burial patterns in these tombs seem consistent with an epidemic that initially killed at a manageable pace before cresting into a wave that overwhelmed the site with bodies.[44] Threads of gold, amber resin, and traces of silver were intermingled in the tangle of human remains. One woman bore a pair of gold earrings. At least some of these people were wealthy. Many of the dead were of above-average height, suggesting a better diet than their contemporaries.[45] Artefacts found among the burials in the best excavated rooms include coins of Titus and Marcus Aurelius—indicating burial contemporary with epidemics at or near the reigns of those emperors.[46] These rushed mass burials suggest that waves of disease pummeled Rome even in its era of prosperity.[47]

Apart from the fatalities, social norms also may have suffered in the Antonine plague's first wave in Rome. With the death of elites, for example, Rome lost not only leadership but also some of the accompanying grain, oil, and wine that those elites would have typically redistributed during and following the crisis. Plague upended the complex social hierarchy of patrons and clients in the city. Amid the chaos, Marcus took the lead. In an act which must have inspired confidence in the face of social fragility, the emperor dipped into state funds to pay for memorial services for myriad plague victims. Rome's nobles were given memorial statues, the non-elite mass funerals.[48] The emperor's actions not only helped rid the city of bodies but reminded the Romans of their dignity in the middle of the chaos.

Economic conditions may have also deteriorated. Comparative sources from future urban epidemics suggest that market activity would have shut down. When the Justinianic plague first pummeled Constantinople, one witness tells us that "work of every description ceased, and all the trades were abandoned by the artisans, and all other work as well."[49] Economic shutdowns then as now compounded the death toll from epidemics. During an early fourth-century plague in the cities of the eastern Empire, Eusebius claims that "through every alley, agora, and forum there was nothing to see but lamentation and the customary dirges and clamor that come with it." City streets were crammed with beggars. Even noblewomen begged for food. Others lacking sustenance ate hay or poisonous herbs.[50] In Rome, the Antonine plague's initial wave may have only lasted a month or two, but death and sickness would have left few available to provision the survivors with daily food, oil, and other goods.

For the best evidence of plague's socioeconomic impact, we follow the money. The 81,044 denarii contained in the single largest hoard of Roman silver coins ever found—the Reka Devnia hoard uncovered in northeastern Bulgaria—serve as a reliable year-by-year catalogue of Roman coin production from AD 64 to 251. The hoard shows in vivid detail the effects of the Antonine plague's first wave in Rome. From the hoard, it seems the production of coins minted in Rome from December 166 through the last few weeks of 167 took a massive nosedive—dropping to around a third of the reign's previous average. It is unlikely that metal shortages were responsible—those were to come later in the pandemic, ushering in even more prolonged and profound consequences. Rather, this isolated one-year drop in coin production in Rome was almost certainly a local problem. Mint-workers may have become badly ill or may have even died in the winter of 166/7. Depending on the severity of the disruption, it could have taken the better part of a year before replacement workers were trained or brought from elsewhere.[51]

Personal stories of loss from the first wave are almost unknown. Perhaps the emergency was so grave that it defied efforts to memorialize it until later. The emperors Marcus and Lucius seemingly suffered the loss of their old tutor and mentor, Marcus Fronto.[52] A surviving cache of personal letters shows that the three men were in regular correspondence until the contagion hit. For Marcus, Fronto provided ongoing instruction in rhetoric, logic, and virtue as the emperor managed affairs in Rome.[53] For Lucius, Fronto was writing up a history of the emperor's

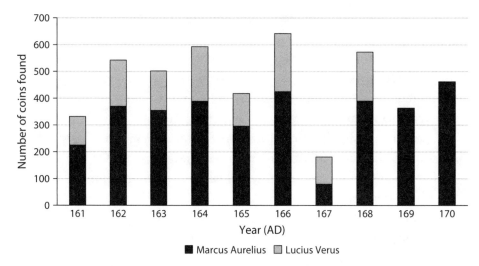

FIG. 4.2. Numbers of datable silver denarii found in the Reka Devnia hoard per regnal year, AD 161–170.

After Duncan-Jones 1996, 130–31. Coins are catalogued in *Coin Hoards of the Roman Empire* (https://chre.ashmus.ox.ac.uk/). Coins of Marcus and Lucius are dated by annual renewal of tribunician power, which took place for both emperors on December 10 of each year. To avoid using split years to account for a few weeks in December, the chart treats those few remaining weeks in December as belonging to the following year's coin production (a practical likelihood anyway, as coin production probably did not commence immediately upon the renewal of tribunician power). Coins of Faustina II (produced between 161 and 175) and Lucilla (produced between 164 and 180) and the posthumous coins of Lucius Verus cannot be securely dated to particular years and are therefore excluded from the graph. There is a noticeable drop in numbers of coins of Marcus from 174, and it seems likely that the coins of Lucilla and posthumous coins of Faustina II (produced between 176 and 180) filled the gap.

recently won war against Parthia. Lucius expected the account to "dwell at length on the causes and early stages of the war, and especially our ill success in my absence. Do not be in a hurry to come to my share. . . . make quite clear the great superiority of the Parthians before my arrival, that the magnitude of my achievements may be manifest."[54] This from the man who set not one of his imperial feet in Parthian territory. But Fronto did not survive to write Lucius's war stories. In his final letters, Fronto was both ill and in the throes of grief—having lost both his wife and three-year-old grandson to causes unnamed. Then, in 166, Fronto's letters abruptly end. Among the statues Marcus erected to the noble plague victims, Fronto's image too may have stood.[55]

Galen likewise, although he saved his own skin by fleeing the capital, suffered a personal tragedy. Teuthras, the doctor's old schoolmate from Pergamum, elected to stay behind with the other physicians in Rome. Galen laments that "the first visitation of the plague" snatched away the life of his old friend.[56] Galen also mourned the loss of an entire houseful of slaves to plague. He does not tell us whether these unfortunates perished in the first epidemic wave or a subsequent outbreak. But did it really matter? Plague now raged in the heart of the Empire, and no one could stop it. Its indiscriminate attacks afflicted nobles and commoners, physicians and slaves. Rome—the largest consumer city in all of pre-industrial human history—had managed to draw in death itself. The same economic and social gravity that siphoned goods and people from three continents now absorbed a pandemic into its core that would poison the city and its peripheral territories for a generation.

A Disease without a Diagnosis

The disease behind the Antonine plague was, and still is, a mystery. Without knowing the exact pathogen, it will never be possible to fully understand transmission and mortality. Scholars have so far been unable to isolate genetic samples from victims—the surest way to identify the malady. If the Antonine plague pathogen was a virus, its genetic material was either DNA or RNA. DNA viruses like smallpox and herpes contain large genomes and tend to replicate accurately. Their genetic material withstands time and environmental hazards fairly well. RNA viruses—influenza, measles, Ebola, SARS, and so forth—have a high mutation rate, making them unstable, error-prone during replication, and far more difficult to recover over time, at least with current technology. If a form of measles caused the Antonine plague, for example, historians will probably never have the genetic evidence needed for confirmation. If an ancient orthopoxvirus, however, it is probably just a matter of time until scholars obtain a sound diagnosis.[57]

The most severe orthopoxvirus is modern smallpox (*Variola major*), a nightmarish disease. During outbreaks in the early modern period, smallpox killed around a third of those who contracted it. Children and infants were especially susceptible; death occurred in roughly half of all cases when the victim was under a year old. Smallpox survivors often carried the scars of their encounter for the rest of their lives. Around a third of these also permanently lost their eyesight. The fight against this scourge took centuries, but victory finally arrived in the 1970s when vaccination efforts eradicated the disease. In the scholarship of the past few decades, smallpox (even *Variola major*) emerged as a preferred candidate for the Antonine plague.[58] One of the lone cautious voices during this time was my Indiana University colleague Ann Carmichael, who saw no evidence of the severe disease associated with *Variola major* in Europe before AD 1600.[59] Recent genetic evidence proved Carmichael correct. In 2017, a team of researchers sequenced smallpox DNA from seventeenth-century mummified human remains found in Lithuania.[60] Strangely, these old smallpox samples were nearly identical to samples collected in the 1970s—pointing to an emergence of modern *Variola major* in the 1500s at the earliest, more than a millennium after the Antonine plague.[61] Subsequent studies have since pounded the final nails in an Antonine plague diagnosis of modern smallpox.[62] The Antonine plague was not modern *Variola major*, but past human populations have nevertheless suffered orthopoxviruses many times.[63] And the evolutionary history of disease signals a foreboding future: human populations are by no means beyond the death grip of some future pox.[64]

In the meantime, historians return again and again to the tantalizing hints of the Antonine plague's main symptoms scattered in Galen's notes.[65] Fever seems to have been the earliest and most common sign of infection. From there, the condition of victims worsened significantly over the course of the following week. Some developed diarrhea with a blood-blackened stool (the sure sign of a deadly case, according to Galen). In other victims, their breath became foul and they soon coughed up blood and the scabs of ulcers. Unsurprisingly, many had trouble sleeping.

But the most striking and distinct symptom in Galen's description is the presence of a dry, black pustular rash between days nine and twelve. The sores scabbed over, then fell away "like husks."[66] Galen's language is precise. He avoids the Greek word for buboes in his descriptions of the Antonine plague.[67] Therefore, it seems safe to rule out *Yersinia pestis*—the bacteria responsible for all three major bubonic plague pandemics, including the infamous Black Death of the Late Middle Ages, and perhaps over one hundred million total deaths.[68] The rash Galen describes covered victims' entire bodies. Bubonic plague buboes tend to emerge at the groin, armpits, or neck.[69]

Even more astounding, Galen alludes to scarring of the pustular sores. Galen only discusses scarring in the instance of one patient, and this in a strange way. Ever seeking to take credit, Galen claims he "helped the wound become a scar" or "cicatrize" through applying drying medicines.[70] Disease historians tend to jump at such language, as scarring pustules are telltale signs of smallpox.[71] But Galen's comment requires caution. He says nothing of how long the scarring lasted nor whether any other survivors bore scars. And Roman writers, Galen included, were obsessed with physical disfigurements; why did he (or anyone else for that matter?) say nothing more if the scars were widespread and permanent?[72] If millions of pandemic survivors were left with permanent scarring, we should expect more in the sources than just Galen's cagey observation.[73] So while Galen's references to pustules and scarring suggest some kind of pox, caution is warranted. Historians eagerly await some future genetic discovery that may one day confirm the Antonine plague's true diagnosis.

That evidence may arrive sooner than we think. In 2020, researchers screened genetic material from Viking Age human remains from Europe and found something shocking: "ancient smallpox."[74] The DNA was not *Variola major* precisely but an ancestral relative (aVARV) that has since become extinct. Evolutionary modeling offers no definitive date of emergence, but it is no leap to postulate that aVARV was active during the time of the Antonine plague. Were these Viking Age peoples some of the final victims of an ancient orthopoxvirus that earlier ravaged the world as the Antonine plague?[75] The notion is tempting, but still premature.

The mystery of the Antonine plague thus continues to perplex, but new evidence is ever emerging. Genetic confirmation of the pathogen could be imminent. And yet, a confirmed diagnosis will only make historians' work all the more essential. Myriad contextual conditions—population dynamics, ecology, the resilience of political institutions, health regimes, and so on—factored into the disease's overall impact. Confirmation of the Justinianic plague pathogen as *Yersinia pestis* in 2011, for example, blew open new debates over how far the disease spread, how many it killed, and the extent to which it generated historical change; scholars continue to fight it out to this day.[76] With or without a diagnosis, the same questions surround the Antonine plague, especially the big one: how many of the Empire's tens of millions succumbed to the disease?

Counting the Bodies

In 2020 alone, around 2 million people died of or, to be more precise, *with* SARS-CoV-2—a frighteningly high figure. Nearly 3.5 million more died in 2021, despite the administration of more than 8 billion doses of mRNA vaccine. How should such inconceivably large numbers be framed? When compared to one of the most memorable tragedies of the 2000s—the September 11, 2001, attacks on the World Trade Center in New York City which killed 2,977 people—SARS-CoV-2 deaths seem astronomical. Victims of SARS-CoV-2, however, represent a minuscule .025 percent of the global population. By contrast, the estimated 70–80 million casualties of World War II represent a full 3 percent of the estimated 1940 global population. For truly grotesque figures, we look to the pandemics of the distant past. The Black Death swept through mid-fourteenth century Europe, killing tens of millions. Was the disease behind the Antonine plague a true scourge like the bubonic plague or was the pandemic's death toll overhyped by ancient authors?

We lack an accurate body count for the Antonine plague. But we know the disease killed in large numbers, especially in cities. How deadly was it? Historians have made several educated guesses over the years. Unsurprisingly, their mortality figures have been all over the map.

Minimalist historians in the 1960s and 1970s offered low estimates of between 1 and 10 percent total mortality.[77] The lack of evidence for widespread plague did not allow for any other interpretation. By the 1990s, however, the number of estimated dead ballooned upwards of 25 percent, with more recent estimates as high as 30 or 35 percent. Why the dramatic shift? Advances in epidemiology, climate science, and social-scientific modeling, as well as new evidence—fragmentary wage and price data from Roman Egypt and comparative evidence from medieval Europe—offered historians new perspectives and tools to better quantify and estimate the impact of the Antonine plague. In just the past few decades, scholars have elevated the pandemic's dead from less than one million to closer to ten or twenty million.[78] Such a dramatic demographic shock—if the new estimates are correct—must have shaken if not toppled the foundations of the Pax Romana's political and economic systems.

All the models in the world, however, cannot avoid a harsh empirical reality: we do not have reliable mortality figures to plug into our models, simulations, and equations. What few numbers we have are either speculative or symbolic.[79] Did anyone count the corpses? In major cities perhaps. Cassius Dio claimed that an epidemic wave in Rome in AD 190 killed 2,000 people a day.[80] But where did the senator get his figure? Comparative evidence offers a few possibilities. Ottoman officials tracked plague deaths in Istanbul in the late fifteenth century.[81] A thousand years earlier in the same city, the Byzantine emperor Justinian stationed men at the harbors, straits, and city gates to tally the numbers of bubonic plague victims.[82] The numbers became so overwhelming, however, that the counters soon gave up. So it could be the case that Dio had an accurate count; but it is equally possible that he just made the figure up. Ancient authors were notorious for their hyperbole and exaggeration; after all, then as now, death sells.[83] It may be that Dio just picked a large number to accentuate his claim that the outbreak was the greatest he had ever seen. The Christian writer Jerome similarly claimed that a novel disease killed five times Dio's amount (10,000) each day in Rome under the emperor Titus in AD 79/80.[84] In reality, the first wave in Rome in 166—when presumably none of Rome's million or more inhabitants possessed immunity—was likely the deadliest event by far during the entirety of the pandemic.

Even then, there are hints that most people survived the worst of that deadly surge. A small group of aged senatorial priests tasked with worshipping the divine Antoninus Pius—the *sodales Antoniniani*—were named and numbered just before the outbreak in AD 166.[85] These were men of consular rank at the time of their appointment, which means they were in their fifties or sixties at minimum when the contagion struck Rome. Because of their fame, their fates are almost all known. Only one perished following the initial epidemic, and he could have died of any cause. A full ten of the fourteen elderly men are known to have still been alive after AD 170. The sample size here is small, to be sure, but it is nevertheless significant. Of those most likely to die in an outbreak of novel disease in Rome, the elderly must have been especially vulnerable—and yet these men survived.

There were inbuilt limits on the disease's ability to kill. Like many diseases, it conferred upon survivors some degree of immunity. Few deadly diseases strike the same person twice, or do so with the same severity. Measles reinfections, for example, are very rare and are typically asymptomatic. Reinfection never occurs in smallpox survivors—a major reason why vaccine-aided eradication succeeded. Epidemics in the preindustrial world were difficult to sustain because aggressive diseases inoculated populations or burned out altogether, failing to gain a permanent foothold. Some diseases, however, found the sweet spot and settled into endemicity. Whatever disease was behind the Antonine plague, the circumstances suggest it hit the eastern Empire before the west, perhaps years in advance. Not only was the east more populous than the west, but it was more urbanized as well. The links between cities and their hinterlands were stronger in the east.[86] It is conceivable that when Lucius's troops returned from the Parthian War, they marched through at least some areas which had already encountered the disease that spawned the Antonine plague, with local populations who may even have enjoyed some level of population immunity.

Galen himself, our best witness to the Antonine plague, seems to have strangely never fell victim to the disease. Or, if he caught the contagion, he failed to note it in his extensive corpus. Did the Pergamese doctor obtain immunity somehow? Galen was a showman—gaining notoriety by dissecting and vivisecting the corpses of livestock and other animals in public. It is plausible that he encountered some less lethal relative of the Antonine plague pathogen through the offal of some animal and even developed a form of cross immunity. Such luck would not be unheard of. The eighteenth-century English physician Edward Jenner observed that people who regularly worked around cowpox-infected cattle did not catch smallpox during the epidemic outbreaks of that era. Jenner would go on to purposefully inject willing volunteers with cowpox as a way to inoculate them against smallpox. His experiments not only produced smallpox immunity but sparked the eventual development of a smallpox vaccine, and vaccination more generally. Unfortunately, for the Romans, vaccination technology arrived about 1,500 years too late.

The Antonine plague pathogen seemingly lingered in the Roman Empire for years, maybe even more than a decade. Even if only a small percentage died in each wave, the numbers would have compounded in successive outbreaks. The dynamics of natural immunity in a pre-industrial empire made the pandemic seem capricious. It spurted and then subsided throughout the Empire in sporadic fashion. A city with a naive population might endure a spike while a nearby city with recent exposure simultaneously enjoyed a reprieve. Smallpox, for example, behaved this way in early modern populations—giving the disease the reputation for persistence it still enjoys, even decades after its eradication.[87] Early modern populations struggled to muster the levels of population density necessary to force smallpox into an endemic state; recurring waves hit preindustrial cities again and again.[88] Even in eighteenth-century Central America, for example, smallpox was at best "semi-endemic." Devastating outbreaks hit Mexico City at intervals in 1737, 1761, 1779, and 1797.[89] Smallpox-based simulations of the Antonine plague suggest a minimum of sixteen years before the Roman population would again become susceptible.[90] Disease endemicity is dynamic and complex, a function of the attributes of particular diseases as well as social and demographic processes of host populations (including non-humans!).[91] But sustained high densities in human populations often aid disease transmission, and therefore increase mortality.

To better understand the Antonine plague, therefore, we must consider population densities in the Roman Empire. But historians hardly agree on the Empire's total population, let alone density figures for individual cities, including Rome itself. Still, archaeologists such as Andrew Wilson have put forward probable ranges based upon house sizes and floor plans at sites across the Empire. In general, most Roman cities packed people in at around 100 to 400 persons per square hectare, with a handful of large cities reaching tens of thousands per square kilometer.[92] Such numbers were more than enough to spawn epidemic surges of even the most slowly spreading diseases. But reaching endemicity for some diseases required not only high densities but sustained high densities.[93] Based on figures for the Roman Empire, a novel density-sensitive disease would have announced its presence with a bang in a sudden and deadly epidemic outbreak. After the initial burst, however, infections would have dropped precipitously as the disease struggled to find susceptible hosts. Smallpox epidemics in the early modern period, for example, often died out quickly in low-density rural settings.[94] In the few cities with large and dense urban populations, however, smallpox sustained itself as a childhood infection. Surviving on a slow trickle of victims, endemic diseases could lurk in a high-density population for years while new births and immigrants gradually built up the non-immune population. At some point, a critical mass would be reached, and the disease would pounce again in another epidemic wave.[95] With smallpox in eighteenth-century Mexico City, for example, the deadly cycle occurred about every decade or two. During the Antonine plague, the interval in the Empire's densest cities may have been similar.

In the Roman Empire, only a fraction of the Empire's inhabitants lived in cities. Did demographic realities keep the pandemic's aggregate lethality at bay? To compete with history's deadliest pandemics, the disease needed sufficient transmissibility to churn through the majority rural population. But the evidence for rural spread during the Antonine plague is almost nonexistent. Survival bias may be at work here. The elites who wrote our surviving sources were hyperfocused on cities and the military; they cared little for the countryside. One source, however, implies universal spread, although only vaguely. Fourth-century historian Ammianus Marcellinus claims that the ravages of the Antonine plague reached "from the frontiers of Persia all the way to the Rhine and to Gaul."[96] Ammianus may have been looking for a creative way to say that the Roman world experienced a pandemic; the term, however, had not yet been invented.[97] Instead, he improvised by referencing the boundary zones of the Rhine and Persian frontier as representative thresholds of Roman civilization.

Still, we should consider the pandemic's rural impact, even if only speculatively, especially in the western provinces. Much of the population of the western Roman Empire inhabited small villages or self-sustaining family farms. The exceptions were the coastal cities along the Mediterranean and the permanent military forts and settlements near the boundaries of Roman influence, especially along the Rhine and Danube rivers. Gallic cities enjoyed the same high densities as their eastern counterparts but at lower overall populations and with large swathes of uninhabited land in between. Around 800,000 city-dwellers in total lived in the nearly 500,000 square kilometers of territory in the Gallic provinces.[98] Perhaps ten or fifteen times this number were scattered throughout the Gallic countryside—with heavier concentrations in the south and east and far fewer people in the north and west. Only about ten Gallic cities had populations near or slightly above 20,000 people. The region's most populous city, Lugdunum (modern Lyon, France), was home to a mere 35,000 at most.[99] Roman Gaul was like an archipelago of small cities and settlements dotted throughout a sea of forests and meadows. Even highly transmissible diseases were unlikely to become endemic in such areas. Epidemic bursts, however, would have flared up in the cities from time to time with slow and limited transmission occurring in the vast countryside.[100]

In parts of rural North Africa, it seems as though the pandemic never arrived at all. Some have even called the second century a "golden age" for the region.[101] Ceramic evidence from surveys of rural Tripolitanian sites suggests impressive stability and resilience among rural populations during and immediately after the Antonine plague, especially

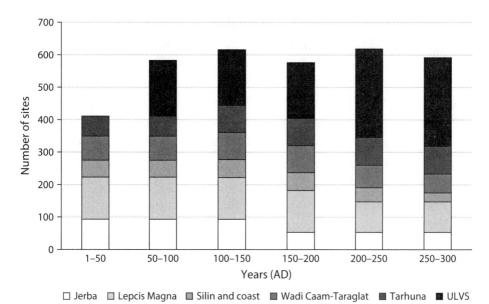

FIG. 4.3. Rural settlements in North Africa (Tripolitania), AD 1–300.
Data from Sheldrick 2021, 29, 194. ULVS is the UNESCO Libyan Valleys Survey.
Data are largely composed of scattered artefact finds difficult to date—hence
the 50-year periods. For sites dated to an entire century, Sheldrick presented
these data twice in two 50-year periods.

those inland from the coast. Only settlements on the Island of Jerba
show a major drop during the latter half of the second century—from
93 to 53 sites. The 514-square-kilometer island's capital was Meninx, a
well-linked port city famed for its purple dyes, fish sauce, and sweet
wine.[102] Jerba's island-bound inhabitants may very well have suffered a
plague outbreak due to these trade links as well as increased manufac-
turing in the cities. Settlements along the Tripolitanian mainland, however, seemed to have otherwise escaped the pandemic unharmed—
including settlements near the major port city of Lepcis Magna. The
Antonine plague apparently had little effect in rural North Africa. Perhaps the Empire's many other rural inhabitants also largely escaped the
tragic fate of the Empire's cities?

The most tantalizing evidence for the spread of plague in the western
Roman Empire is also some of the most puzzling. A set of near-identical
but undated inscriptions appear in Italy, Dalmatia, Sardinia, Numidia,

Mauretania, Hispania, and Britain, and one in Asia Minor (Pisidia). The inscriptions beseech "the gods and goddesses" in accordance with an oracle of Apollo—god of plague and healing. Curiously, no individual claims responsibility for setting up the inscriptions save one; the etched stone near Hadrian's Wall in Britain was posted by an auxiliary cohort—the *cohors* I *Tungrorum*.[103] Typically, only a decree from an emperor enjoyed such thorough reverberation in stone.[104] Did Marcus Aurelius himself consult Apollo during the pandemic? Possibly. As the next chapter shows, the unprecedented endurance of the Antonine plague triggered petitions to Apollo in numerous eastern cities. Why not in the west?

The inscriptions to "the gods and goddesses" seem to have been meant for placement in the walls of buildings. Walls marked physical boundaries; inscribing them with divine words secured not only the inscribed building or temple itself but the whole community. Did Marcus attempt to inoculate the whole of the Empire against pestilence with dedicatory inscriptions at strategic locations? Perhaps the contagion could be thus driven back across the boundaries of the Empire? Such a thing was not unheard of. The first-century BC poet Horace wrote that if Apollo was moved by the prayers of the emperor Augustus, the god would "drive away . . . wretched famine and plague from our people and Caesar, our leader, and direct them against the Persians and Britons."[105] Marcus's religiosity is well-documented.[106] Ancient sources record how Marcus "summoned priests from every quarter, carried out foreign rites, and cleansed Rome in every way" on the eve of his Germanic war and otherwise "most scrupulously restored the worship of the gods."[107] And, as we shall see in the next chapter, as the Pax Romana faltered, Marcus even sought the aid of a popular plague-curing charlatan who commanded the Empire's populations to inscribe dedications to Apollo. So while these undated inscriptions reference no disease, the cultural context is highly suggestive.

But inscriptions, like appearances, can be deceiving. A fragmentary inscription—just a few letters in fact—found in the Tuscan city of Cosa undermines the connection between the mysterious dedications and the Antonine plague.[108] The Cosa inscription in both form and content seems to be yet another petition to "the gods and goddesses," but its location is curious.[109] Cosa was an old Roman colony—founded before the Punic wars of the third century BC. But by the time of the Antonine plague, the city had fallen into decline and shows evidence of desertion.[110] Yes, Cosa's failing port may have received a few traders, as well as their goods and diseases, but mid-second-century AD Cosa was an unlikely site for an imperial inscription at the time of the Antonine plague. Several decades later, however, during the early third-century reign of the crazed emperor Caracalla, Cosa's fortunes changed dramatically. The city was rebuilt—receiving a new forum and several temples. Could it have been Caracalla who initiated *all* the inscriptions, and not Marcus Aurelius during the Antonine plague?

Caracalla was a haunted man. He not only murdered his own brother and co-emperor in cold blood at a banquet with their mother in AD 211 but damned his brother's memory to boot. Over the following years, Caracalla suffered persistent physical and mental sickness—including the belief that the spirits of his father and murdered brother hounded him. The exasperated emperor made frantic offerings and sacrifices, sent prayers to deities by courier, and visited scattered shrines of gods and goddesses in person, especially those of Apollo.[111] Caracalla even saturated his coinage with images of Apollo; the deity shows up on 29 percent of the troubled emperor's silver coins in 214, and 22 percent of those struck in 215.[112] No such iconographic burst, by the way, has been noted in the coinage at the time of the Antonine plague. It may be during the early 210s that Caracalla propagated the Cosa inscription—and potentially all the inscriptions to "the gods and goddesses," since they are so similar—throughout the Empire. But in the end, this alternative theory is just that. It does not disprove the possibility that the inscriptions represent Marcus's fear of epidemics during the Antonine plague—but it does complicate matters. Besides, other circumstantial evidence may speak to the pandemic's deadly reach into the rural provinces of the Roman Empire.[113]

The pandemic may have in fact made landfall on the island of Great Britain. Excavations near an old Roman road in the city of Gloucester—the *colonia* of Glevum (population ~10,000) in the Antonine Age—revealed a mass grave of ninety-one men, women, and children.[114] As with the catacombs of Saint Peter and Marcellinus, the skeletons at Glevum were tangled together, suggesting bodies tossed irreverently into the grave. Although hastily buried, none of the remains show evidence of trauma or violence. Artefacts found with the skeletons, as well as radio-carbon dating, place the time of burial firmly in the late second or early third century AD. In their report, the team of excavators notes the mass grave's chronological correlation with the Antonine plague, positing that the dead could have been plague victims. At the same time, the team notes that "other interpretations may be equally valid, particularly the possibility that the pit was used for the disposal of the corpses of individuals too poor to afford a proper burial."[115] How do historians even begin to solve this 1,800-year-old cold case?

Demography may hold some clues. If these were plague victims, their ages suggest an outbreak of a novel rather than an endemic disease. Most victims in the mass grave were adults. Those aged approximately between 18 and 35 account for 36.4 percent of the bodies while adults over the age of 45 make up a further 15.8 percent. Adult skeletons too fragmented to fit into an age or sex category make up a further 28.5 percent of identifiable skeletons. Only slightly less than 13 percent of the victims were under age 18.[116] While every pathogen is different, endemic diseases tend to kill children, not middle-aged adults. When smallpox, for example, became endemic in London sometime in the seventeenth century, most of its victims were children.[117] Burials in the west London parish of St. Martin's-in-the-Fields reflect this grim reality: victims under age four represent over two-thirds of the burials from 1752 to 1766 and 85 percent of burials from 1775 to 1799.[118] In the later series, only 3.5 percent of victims were adults aged 20 to 49. By contrast, most victims in the mass grave at Roman Glevum died in the prime of their lives. If a disease killed these people, it must have been a novel scourge.

Glevum was a confluence point in Roman Britain—as likely a city as any to endure an epidemic. The main land route between the nearby military and mining communities (in modern South Wales and England) crossed a north-south road near the city before reaching the population center of Corinium Dobunnorum (modern Cirencester).

Glevum was also well situated as a waypoint for river traffic to and from the Bristol Channel along the River Severn. Workers in such places were especially vulnerable to diseases imported by ship crews or with cargo, including insect and rodent reservoirs. The city was a staging point for transitory workers: crews of small ships, operators of land transport, hired guards, prostitutes, migrant workers from the hinterland, and others who lacked local connections to the permanent population. When such transient people died—whatever the cause—who buried them and where? Open pits were dug in many Roman cities for such tragic purposes.[119] Isotopic analyses of several skeletons from both the mass grave and "regular" burials in nearby cemeteries confirm that nearly one-third of those buried were from outside of Britain.[120] The mass grave found at Glevum—located in a marginal location in the Roman cemetery—indeed may be filled with Antonine plague victims, or maybe victims of some local epidemic surge. Yet the grave also serves as another sad reminder of the harsh realities of poverty and transience in the Roman world.[121]

Did the Antonine plague fan further afield? At the opposite end of the Eurasian landmass, in lands the Romans thought almost mythological, obscure hints in Chinese sources suggest that cities of the Han Empire too suffered under the dark shadow of a persistent pestilence during the middle and late second century AD. Signs of emergency pop out of the source material: the imperial court offered tax rebates, food relief, and distributed medicine.[122] Unfortunately, chronicles of the period, many of which were compiled centuries later, offer scant details of disease symptoms—certainly not enough to compare with the disease described by Galen. But the chronological confluence is certainly curious.

The few surviving details about the Chinese outbreaks suggest a winter/spring seasonality and scattered epidemic bursts in cities and armies—similar to the epidemics associated with the Antonine plague in the Roman Empire. The first regional flare-up in the cluster of Chinese epidemics occurred in the Han capital of Luoyang in the spring of AD 151. This was the same city which would receive the Roman "embassy" fifteen years later. From Luoyang, the pestilence reportedly struck the major cities of Jiujiang and Lujiang before burning out. Ten years later, Luoyang was again wracked by disease. Then, the following year, in the middle of intense border wars in China's westernmost region of Xinjiang, Chinese chroniclers record the February arrival of what they call the "great pestilence."[123] Whatever disease was responsible, it had made its way into the army, and around one-third of the soldiers reportedly died.[124]

Subsequent outbreaks followed. In AD 166—the year the Antonine plague raged in Rome—a report to the emperor Huan proclaimed: "Heaven is displaying strange signs, earth spits forth uncanny creations, and mankind has pestilence and disease."[125] For naming the troubles of the age, and insinuating Heaven's displeasure with the emperor, the author of that report barely escaped prison. But outbreaks continued to pummel China, many unrestricted to specific regions.[126] Another "great pestilence" struck in AD 171.[127] Regional reports note epidemics following in 173, 179, 182, and 185, and usually during the colder seasons.[128] In fact, Chinese physician Zhang Ji, who lived through the string of late second-century plagues, theorized in his *Treatise on Cold Damage and Miscellaneous Disorders* that cold and wind caused the outbreaks.[129] The last of these major epidemics coincided with the Yellow Turban Rebellion. For the rebels, the sheer number of epidemics, famines, and floods in the previous decades confirmed that the Han emperor had lost the "Mandate of Heaven." By contrast, the faith healer Zhang Jue—due to his miraculous ability to use incantations, holy water, and confessions of sin to ward off disease during the 170s—verified his credentials to lead the rebellion.[130]

The near synchronous chronology of epidemics in similar populations in both the Roman and Han empires seems too close to be a coincidence, but historians lack the details to make an indisputable connection. Just one tantalizing description of a Han-era pestilence is known, and it comes several decades too late to connect with the Antonine plague directly.[131] And yet, the account, authored by early fourth-century AD Chinese alchemist Ge Hong, echoes Galen remarkably in its description of a disease that had become endemic and seasonal in parts of Han China:

Recently there have been persons suffering from epidemic sores which attack the head, face and trunk. In a short time, these sores spread all over the body. They have the appearance of hot boils containing some white matter. While some of these pustules are drying up a fresh crop appears. If not treated early the patients usually die. Those who recover are disfigured by purplish scars which do not fade until after a year.[132]

Ge Hong adds a key detail in his description that never appears in any Roman account, including Galen's: pustule scars remained visible at least a year after infection. Was this pox a remnant of the epidemics that swept throughout China in the mid- to late second century? And was it also the same disease that flared up in the Roman Empire at the same time? As with so much about the Antonine plague, what is plausible is still never quite provable.

Dots litter the ancient map of epidemic outbreaks—from Persia to Rome, from Italy to Britain, and even to China—but does the Antonine plague connect them? If only a fraction of these fragmented sources originate with the Antonine plague, historians should consider the disease a true pandemic—even if its specific path cannot be traced, its pathogen cannot be pinpointed, and its death toll cannot be counted.

Mortality during the Antonine plague was probably different from location to location, and population to population. City-dwellers probably suffered far more than those in the countryside, not unlike populations during the pre-vaccination smallpox era. Surveys of cemeteries in eighteenth-century Britain, where smallpox was the most lethal disease on record, show this pattern clearly. In the cities of the industrializing north, smallpox accounted for 10–20 percent of burials. In rural southern populations, smallpox burials were under 5 percent. And smallpox victims in the north tended to be children—a strong sign of endemicity. Southern smallpox burials tended to be adults—victims who never obtained immunity as village children and subsequently caught the disease when they traveled to large cities like London.[133] The disease responsible for the Antonine plague too seems primarily an urban affliction—unprecedented at the time but certainly nowhere near as deadly and universal as subsequent pandemics such as the Black Death or early modern smallpox pandemics. The Antonine plague undoubtedly made appearances in the villages and hamlets of the Roman Empire, but perhaps without the same sustained deadly ferocity as occurred in Rome and other high-density cities. While absence of evidence is not evidence of absence, historians must balance ancient authors' most brazen claims—that the disease spread just about everywhere and killed just about everyone—against the curious fact that the Antonine plague also left behind so little obvious and direct evidence, even at a time when Roman sources in general survive in high numbers.

Amid such paucity, mortality estimates of 20 or 30 percent (or even higher) are unsustainable. Overall mortality in the Roman Empire had to be much lower. Even if all ninety-one skeletons found in the mass grave at Glevum were plague victims, for example, the loss would represent less than 1 percent of the city's estimated population of around 10,000. Of course, there would have been other victims buried elsewhere—perhaps most were cremated—and probably multiple epidemic waves. A disease that killed 30 percent of urban victims, for example—a mortality comparable to preindustrial smallpox—would have drowned Glevum with thousands of bodies. During the Justinianic plague in Constantinople, for example, the bodies were so numerous that the government paid people to trample the corpses cast in the pits, crushing the diseased flesh like the grapes of wrath in John's apocalyptic vision in Revelation.[134] Such descriptions exaggerate of course, but they rest on much more plausible foundations than much of the literary evidence for the Antonine plague.

Still, as the next chapter shows, the pandemic's body count was at least sufficiently high that, when combined with its pandemic novelty—that the disease could strike anywhere—panic ensued. The disease certainly put a serious scare into Galen when he finally faced it in Italy during the winter of AD 168. It was after this—his first recorded encounter with the disease—that he invented a novel name for an unprecedented sickness: "the everlasting pestilence."[135]

The Everlasting Pestilence

Despite his fame, Galen could not ignore the summons of his emperor. One and a half years had passed since the doctor's hasty departure from Rome mere months ahead of the contagion. The pandemic's first wave in the capital killed untold numbers. Now, the disease's deadly tendrils fanned out into the western Empire. All roads led to Rome, but those same roads also led *from* Rome.[136] Along those routes, Roman soldiers once again marched toward another massive war, this time along the Danube. With them, no doubt, the Antonine plague's microbes hitched rides to yet more unconquered frontier populations.

From the opposite direction, a cacophony of Celts and Germans overran the Empire's northern defenses. The hordes pillaged cities in the Balkans, defeated several Roman legions, killed a Roman governor, and, most symbolically devastating, the northern tribes crossed into the heartland province of Italy. It had been over two and a half centuries since a foreign army entered Italy—an unthinkable development to a generation that knew nothing but the Pax Romana. The Parthian War may have been vainglorious foreign adventurism mixed with a little contrived vengeance, but this new war seemed more immediate, more menacing. But if anything, most Romans probably underestimated the war's long-term significance. In fact, leading authorities on Rome's centuries-long struggle against northern invaders pin the beginning of Rome's end on the war in Germany under Marcus and Lucius.[137]

Just before the Antonine plague broke out, the emperors recruited two legions of Italian soldiers and stationed them along the Danube in the provinces of Noricum and Pannonia. While only Lucius went to Parthian territory (well, near it anyway), this new war was so urgent that both emperors attended to the German front. The emperors set up their command headquarters in the northern Italian city of Aquileia, which the invaders may have recently besieged.[138] Epitaphs of Roman soldiers suggest the city was a destination for veterans from across the Empire.[139] The city's location near the front and its veteran population made it an ideal staging point for the offensive. But these same factors, along with the flood of new soldiers in anticipation of the war, also made the city the Antonine plague's next ground zero.

The center of empire was where its emperors resided.[140] And there Galen was wanted. When he received his marching orders, however, the doctor was over a thousand kilometers east of Aquileia in his hometown of Pergamum "minding my own business," he says. The pompous physician begrudged the command to return west—no doubt he had heard about the epidemic in Italy—so Galen took a few detours. Instead of hitching a ride on a crowded ship—a journey of three weeks at most in high summer—Galen simply walked the less trafficked country roads, and maybe even that slowly. The Aegean, of course, he could not cross by foot, so he took a boat. Still, he somehow managed to get lost on the island of Lemnos (an accident, I'm sure). After making landfall in Europe, he plodded across much of Macedonia and Dalmatia, taking the over one-thousand-kilometer Via Egnatia by foot, despite the fact that ships were readily available, cheaper, and faster.

Galen's delay tactics kept him out of Italy as the disease presumably moved north, likely carried by imperial troops mustering at Aquileia. Soldiers marched to the northern frontier along a road that went straight through the wealthy northern Italian city of Iulia Concordia. Much like Glevum, the city was a crossroads for land traffic and military movements. Around the time of the mobilization effort, an inscription records unspecified "difficulties" in the city.[141] We know the problem was much more severe than the sanitized official source lets on because the emperors personally intervened, sending a judicial official of praetorian rank (*iuridicus*). Such high-level intervention was abnormal. Praetorian officials were only sent to address the most worrying crises, such as severe grain shortages that required imperial officials' personal threats to coerce local elites into selling or "donating" any reserve stores of grain.[142] Concurrent pestilence and grain shortage, as the attested "difficulties" may have been, had occurred in Italy before. Cassius Dio tells us that "a pestilence raged throughout all Italy so that no one tilled the land" back in 22 BC.[143] That outbreak had followed severe flooding, so it was probably some nasty concoction of fecal-oral pathogens. The deaths must have been high, but even those who survived would have struggled to produce at previous levels during the sowing season that followed. Had the pandemic worked its way into cities and settlements in northern Italy, disrupting grain production or distribution? What Galen tells us about the long dark winter that year leaves little doubt.

Aquileia was a mere forty kilometers east of Iulia Concordia by road. In the fall of 168, over half a year after he was first summoned, Galen finally wandered into Aquileia.[144] As the launching point for the northern campaign, the city was crammed with soldiers, not to mention the retinues of both emperors. The weather may have just turned cold. Amid the uncharacteristically dense and diverse population, the Antonine plague pathogen pounced upon the populace. Galen remarks that the outbreak in Aquileia "caused destruction on a scale previously unknown" and that "a majority" of the population died.[145]

The doctor was clearly terrified, and for good reason. Marcus and Lucius, too, having endured the Roman epidemic wave of 166/7, recognized the horrors that were upon them. This time, the emperors did not linger. Neither did they attempt to rally the city's spirits or inspire pro-social behavior. No, both men immediately fled the city. The long-planned-for war was suddenly abandoned. The emperors departed with such speed that only a precious few were allowed to accompany them. Galen was not among the fortunate. The ability to flee pandemic outbreak was a mark of privilege then as now. Abandoned in a city saturated with sickness, suffering soldiers, and Aquileia's poor urban masses, Galen reports that "survival became very difficult over a long period"—"the effects of the plague being compounded by the fact that all this was taking place in the middle of winter." After traveling for months across thousands of kilometers, Galen settled in for the hardest winter of his life.

But even those who escaped the city could not outrun death. Lucius Verus, age thirty-nine and in the prime of his life, never made it back to Rome. The emperor died on the journey home, but strangely no contemporary record reveals the cause of death.[146] Much later authors ascribe the emperor's demise to a "surge of blood."[147] But Galen connects the emperor's death to his narrative of the epidemic at Aquileia. Marcus was left alone to perform the rights of deification for his late adoptive brother. Only after the epidemic had burned out for the season did Galen rejoin Marcus in Rome. There the doctor settled back into writing, finishing a treatise on pulses. The work, which survives into the present, reflects the looming threat of plague. At one point, Galen exclaims that he hopes people will "never experience a pestilence like the one we endured, and which is still raging."[148] Unfortunately, his hopes were dashed. Not only would the Antonine plague continue to hound Galen into the AD 170s, but it terrorized the Roman Empire itself.

5

THE AGE OF
ANGST

Lucius Verus was dead. Even if the emperor had not succumbed to plague directly, the rumor mill among Rome's elite undoubtedly began to turn at the dawn of AD 169. It still turns to this day. Modern historians know about as much of Lucius's final days as his contemporaries did back in Rome 1,800 years ago. Gossip and conjecture must have swarmed in the streets, as it seems only a few facts were widely known. Plague had swept through Rome a couple of years earlier, and had then spread through Italy into Aquileia. As the outbreak overwhelmed the city, both emperors took sudden flight—leaving most of their entourage behind. Lucius then died shortly after leaving. Was the emperor struck down by "the great pestilence"? Or did he die of an apoplexy, as later sources suspect?[1] Could he even have been poisoned? Conspiracy theories wilder than these surely ran rampant in Rome. But rightly or wrongly, Lucius's death is forever linked with the Antonine plague. And if the disease could (purportedly) kill an emperor—as perhaps many Romans suspected occurred—then it could kill anyone.

Panic gripped the cities. Like the emperors, many fled urban outbreaks. Elites left for country villas. Non-elites had far fewer options. Some people may have wandered weeks or months hoping epidemic waves would die down. Others may have taken work on country estates. Those with additional problems—especially overdue tax bills— vanished entirely to eke out a meager existence in the countryside.

Across the Empire, plague remedies proliferated—many of which were ineffective and even toxic. Supernatural solutions were especially popular, as people petitioned the old gods for healing. But this pandemic was unlike any local plague that had come before. It endured. Temporary mitigation strategies became normalized—inducing lasting cultural changes.

But the rites and rituals that had seemingly suppressed the local plagues of the past failed to fend off a threat that could strike anyone anywhere. As a culture-shaping force, the Antonine plague's potential for death was perhaps even more powerful than the disease itself. And so, the desperate turned to opportunistic folk healers who proffered magical incantations, prophetic utterances, and talismans. Religious changes were especially pronounced—so much so that classicist Eric R. Dodds believed the Roman Empire entered "an age of anxiety" which lasted for centuries.[2] Historians have rightly objected to this term as an all-encompassing explanation for the religious innovations that swept across such a wide temporality and geography.[3] Others have used more pointed language and limited time scales, calling the mid-second century alone "an age of hypochondriacs," for example.[4] I prefer the language of religious historian Luther Martin, who labels the anxiety of the era not as mere worry or tenseness but as a fundamental existential condition of *angst*. And incurable diseases, including the one responsible for the Antonine plague, were crucial ingredients in an emerging zeitgeist. The era's angst became expressed in what Martin calls "obsessive-compulsive behaviors" meant to ward against unspecific threats or even "perceptions of an uncertain and unpredictable cosmological and political environment . . . [which] manifest as a wide range of behavioral and cognitive changes."[5] As the pandemic settled in for the long haul, it seems as though the preexisting obsession with health revved into overdrive.

The enduring disease and an ancillary string of disasters struck at the very foundations of traditional Roman religions. In broad terms, the relationship between ancient peoples and their gods—the Pax Deorum—was both contractual and logical. Appropriate human piety obliged divine favor. So when the plague-fearing set up statues of Apollo, wore magical amulets, inscribed verses over their doors, or stoned scapegoated citizens to death, they genuinely believed the gods would respond by ending the pestilence. The gods *had* to; it was a matter of obligation and honor. But what happened when the gods did not keep their end of the bargain? During the Athenian plague, Greeks met their absentee gods in kind: "those who saw all perishing alike thought that the worship or neglect of the gods made no difference," Thucydides wrote.[6] The Romans, however, could become outright nasty when their deities failed them. Following the inexplicable death of the much beloved Roman general Germanicus in the prime of his life in AD 19, for example, Romans pelted statues of the gods with stones.[7] Similarly, each day the Antonine plague persisted, the angst of Roman populations ratcheted up. The search for sacrifices to appease the gods widened into strange and dark places.

As religious anxiety frothed and boiled, a small but widespread enigmatic group of radical mystery cultists attracted attention. These zealous devotees of a crucified Jewish carpenter distributed money to their destitute and cared for those of their number who caught diseases. The young religion of Christianity grew as the pandemic era ascended, but Christians also earned hostility for their deviations from accepted plague mitigation measures. Many Christians already avoided mainstream religious feasts and festivals; they outright refused to sacrifice to the traditional gods. To the Romans, such rituals were surefire ways to expiate divine wrath. Traditional rites inoculated both the participants and the broader public from disaster. To question established rituals and remedies was to indulge in baseless and dangerous conspiracy theories. The religious logic of the Pax Deorum was settled science. Christian unwillingness to participate endangered not only the Christians and the cities in which they lived but the safety of the Empire itself. And so during the Antonine plague years, vague hostility against Christians transformed into deadly persecutions. The era kicked off a crisis of faith that would last more than a century, fundamentally altering the relationship between the inhabitants of the Roman world and their gods.

Migration as Mitigation

Just shy of a year following Lucius's death, Marcus relaunched the war against the Germanic tribes still pressing against the Empire's northern boundaries. This time, he wanted Galen to go with him. Galen, however, came up with a clever out. He claimed that one even greater than the emperor—the god Asclepius himself, patron deity of physicians—had supposedly appeared to the doctor in a dream and told him not to follow Marcus.[8] Whether the dream was real or not, the supernatural visitation provided Galen a religious exemption to cover what was otherwise naked insubordination. Instead of cowardice or selfishness, Galen could claim the opposite—piety—supposedly guided him as he fled his duty as both doctor and subject to his emperor. Flight became fidelity. A skeptic might say that Galen discovered double-speak nearly two millennia before the appearance of George Orwell's famous dystopian novel.

Galen's excuse carried weight with Marcus. The emperor, like most people of his era, took the gods seriously. Even an emperor would never dream of upsetting a god of medicine in the middle of a seemingly unending pandemic. Marcus especially respected the strange workings of Asclepius.[9] The emperor admitted in his *Meditations* "that remedies have been granted to me through dreams" by the god.[10] In the end, Galen avoided the military camps, and thus escaped the Antonine plague's main crucible.

Galen was not the only runner. Germ theory was unknown in antiquity, but the prevailing miasmatic theory of disease still provoked flight from pestilence.[11] Ancient peoples often associated sickness with the "bad air" that lingered in particular places or even in sick people themselves.[12] Avoiding such air was crucial, as Galen himself remarked: "it is dangerous to share the daily life of pestilential patients."[13] A decade later, when Marcus was on his deathbed, sick with an unnamed feverish disease, he sent his son Commodus away from him "in case the disease should be passed on to him."[14] Even as early as the fifth-century BC Athenian plague, Thucydides tells of people "afraid to visit one another."[15] Basic contagion was understood in the ancient world, even if it was badly explained.[16] For all these reasons then, those who could afford to leave the area of an outbreak usually took flight. Migration was the most common mitigation strategy for dealing with disease among all social classes.[17]

Elites were often the first to flee; their opulent country villas offered a comfortable quarantine while those forced to remain in the city suffered. Seneca, for example, recounts in a personal letter: "I have run off to my villa at Nomentum . . . to shake off a fever which was surely working its way into my system . . . the disease was not of the body but of the place."[18] Seneca was already symptomatic when he took flight. So too was one of Galen's elite Roman victims of the Antonine plague. That patient, despite a high fever, nevertheless boarded a ship down the Tiber and sailed out to sea—no doubt spreading the disease to his shipmates and perhaps many others.[19] Even emperors abandoned their people when outbreaks flared up, as Marcus and Lucius had done at Aquileia, and Marcus's son Commodus would do during an epidemic outbreak in Rome in AD 190.[20] Perhaps such flight transmitted as much disease as it prevented?

With the Antonine plague, however, elites could not always escape. In Athens, for example, the noble population had died in such numbers from what Marcus called "disasters . . . of chance" that the emperor himself gave the citizens permission to reduce the barriers for entry into the Areopagus—the city's governing council.[21] Such elevations were not uncommon, to be sure, and in fact may have even been enacted just prior to the Antonine plague.[22] But there was clearly something abnormal happening as well. Marcus's surviving decree to the Athenians is impressive in many ways, showing both humility and mercy; after all, Marcus himself had placed the restrictions on Areopagus membership in the first place. In his inscribed words, the emperor extends his sympathy to the city for their losses while also acknowledging that many other cities had also sought relief due to the unnamed "disasters." Why did Marcus not utter the word "plague" anywhere in his letter? Yes, it could be that the pandemic had no role in the deaths at Athens, but that seems unlikely. Rather, some historians believe that the emperor deployed a polite form of code, so as not to suggest that the Athenians were to blame for the pestilence that struck their city and decimated their noble class.[23] If impiety brought disease, then naming the source of Athens's suffering may very well have stigmatized a city Marcus the philosopher dearly loved. The superstitious fears at the time may have become so intense that even acknowledging the disease seemed accursed. Marcus was undoubtedly aware of the social panic in his empire, if not the outright scapegoating of undesirable groups to propitiate the divine wrath which many believed was behind the epidemic waves. It would not be the last time that victims of a pandemic suffered from both the disease and stigmatization.

Common people had even fewer options for flight. There were no public hospitals as such to go to—at least outside of the military camps—until the Christianization of the Empire in the fourth century AD.[24] Many soldiers on active duty, however, could access medical staff and basic therapeutics.[25] Camps were set up near fresh water, and rules and regulations governed waste disposal. Standards of medical care in military facilities may have been low compared to modern hospitals, but according to preindustrial standards of care, Roman legionary hospitals were not too shabby. Military units appointed an officer (*optio valetudinarii*) to supervise camp hospitals and ensure the provision of equipment and medicine. The similarity of medical tools found at camps all across the former empire suggests a network of military physicians who shared knowledge and practices. Soldiers who suffered from the Antonine plague's sickness would have received some meaningful aid in these facilities. And yet military hospitals and traveling military physicians could have been a source of transmission as well, especially among soldiers.

Denied access to military hospitals, civilians instead sought healing in temples and shrines. At sanctuaries of Asclepius in the eastern Empire, ill people gathered and slept overnight in temple *adyta* (sacred rooms for healing) or, if those were full, they crowded the courtyards.[26] During the famous plague in Athens, Lucretius claims that "all the sacred shrines of the gods had been filled . . . and all the temples of the celestials . . . were continually littered with corpses."[27] Sacred spaces abounded in cities, and the disease-ridden crowds during the Antonine plague's epidemics must have been terrifying to behold. But some who feared the pestilence likely flocked to rural sites as well. One such place was Soknopaiou Nesos, an Egyptian tourist village populated by priests and home to a popular old temple to a local crocodile deity. Late in the Antonine plague years, the town lost about one-third of its inhabitants—down from 244 men in September of AD 178 to a mere 169 men in August of the following year.[28] It is impossible to know whether the pandemic was responsible for the sudden depopulation, but the village never recovered. Indeed, as Lucretius said of an earlier disease: "neither the worship of the gods nor their divinity counted for much."[29]

Egypt, in fact, is the only Roman region which leaves behind quantifiable numbers of those who departed villages during the Antonine plague. Thanks to a rare census record from the Nile Delta, we know that what happened in Soknopaiou Nesos was not an isolated incident. Such papyrus documents rarely survive the Delta's marshes, which tend to devour organic material. This unique papyrus, however, was burned and carbonized, sealing it against the decay of the local environment. The figures in the census document are stunning. Villages in the Delta lost 33 to 93 percent of registered inhabitants in the mid- to late 160s—the years of the Antonine plague's opening wave.[30] Historians are tempted to count these losses as plague deaths, but the real tragedy was in fact far more complex. Even during normal times, the inhabitants of Delta villages lived desperate lives on the edge of crisis. They were routinely hounded by starvation, local diseases, violent bandits, and oppression by greedy officials. Indeed, the document clearly shows that the villages were already in decline decades prior to the Antonine plague; the local climatological variability discussed in this book's second chapter must have been a major factor.[31] When the disease finally arrived, however, the region tipped into chaos.

A novel disease would have run rampant in Egypt. The overall population density in the Delta, Nile Valley, and Fayyum Oasis averaged somewhere near 300 people per square kilometer.[32] The city of Alexandria was a crowded mess. Its population of between 300,000 and 750,000 was so crammed together that some neighborhoods contained upwards of 50,000 people per square kilometer—a staggering press of people rivaled only by Rome.[33] On the whole, as much as 30 percent of the Egyptian population lived in high-density settings—perhaps the highest urbanization rate in the entire Roman Empire.[34] Even Egypt's villages were crowded, and thus were far more susceptible to transmission of many of nature's most deadly pathogens.

In AD 166—the same year of Rome's first epidemic wave—the Egyptian economy tanked. Records from the local real estate market show the blazing speed of deterioration. Prior to that year, Egyptian landowners had little trouble finding lessees, and these for large parcels of land. Starting in the late 160s and lasting through the early 180s, however, the size of individual land parcels dropped by more than half.[35] What does this change mean? As villages depopulated—whether from crop failures, banditry, or plague deaths—fieldworkers became difficult to find.[36] Also, the duration of leases more than quadrupled in the same period. Before the Antonine plague, one-year leases were common. From 166, landlords rented parcels for four years or longer. Markets had been destabilized, and landowners realized that rents might not arrive in the short term. Long-term guarantees were required. The ensuing real estate crisis lasted decades.

Plague also contributed to—but again did not solely cause— insurgent unrest in Egypt. Around AD 169, for example, every single male inhabitant of the Nile Delta village of Kerkenouphis either died or migrated. First, raiders attacked and burned the village.[37] In the aftermath of the tragedy, plague struck, killing most of the survivors. Destitute and desperate, the handful of people that remained abandoned their homes. There were few options available to those ruined by the chaos in Egypt. Some swarmed into the cities to beg. Others wandered the marshy wilderness of the Delta, living off the land. But the hopelessness of the times also presented migrants a third option: form into gangs of bandits. That choice turned out to be the popular one.

As the "plague situation"—as it was named in the census document— deepened, a wave of brigandage flooded Egypt. Economic desperation had bred criminality. Within a few years, groups of migrants, bandits, nomads, marsh-dwellers, and others coalesced into a powerful force. The dissidents overwhelmed Roman soldiers in the area.[38] Then, they set their sights on the capital itself: Alexandria. In the end, Avidius Cassius—victorious lieutenant under Lucius Verus in the Parthian War—was called upon in AD 172 to rescue Egypt's capital. Following the death of Lucius Verus, Cassius became Marcus's second-in-command, having been given the extraordinary title of *Rector Orbis* ("Supreme Commander of the Orient"). As leader over much of the eastern Empire, the rebellion was Cassius's to deal with. The throng of rural Egyptian rebels, however, was too large to confront directly. Instead, Cassius employed the tried-and-true strategy of divide and conquer. The sources do not tell us how Cassius sowed division, but the rebels were a diverse group, and old animosities and prejudices must have been easy to stir up. As the infighting boiled over, the veteran general attacked the divided rebels, and the uprising soon melted away.

Imperial powers rarely muse upon the causes of contemporary insurrections. Doing so might expose oppression or corruption or, even worse, prompt decentralization of power and resources. As such, no Roman source connects the Antonine plague to what happened in Egypt. Reliable accounts are in fact nowhere to be found. The clearest commentary is from Cassius Dio, but even he unrealistically paints the rebels as crafty but dishonorable—turning to cannibalism and cross-dressing to survive and succeed in the siege.[39] Avidius Cassius himself may have played up the event as an "insurrection" for his own benefit. It had been years since the general had confronted a credible threat, and defeating a so-called "insurrection" allowed him to claim a meaningful military victory. Alexandria, if not the Empire, now owed him. And the ambitious general would cash in that debt three years later when Marcus was diseased and on his deathbed and the reigns of the Roman Empire seemed ready for a healthier hand to take hold.

It is worth investigating the pandemic's unclear role in the revolt: how did such a disturbance—one severe enough to require major military intervention—spring up in a province so peaceful that a single Roman legion policed it? Egypt was normally no hotbed of extremism. But context mattered, and it in fact had changed drastically from the AD 150s. Wounded by drought and then plague, Roman taxation policies further ratcheted up the populace's pain.[40] The Romans taxed all Egyptian males aged fourteen to sixty-two (or sixty-five in some cases), including slaves, at a flat regressive rate. Every fourteen years, officials counted the number of taxpayers in each village and then slapped a collective tax bill for the total amount on the community as a whole.[41] But what happened if a deadly pestilence reduced the number of taxpayers responsible to foot the bill? The survivors, still reeling from loss of loved ones, suddenly bore the tax burden of the deceased. Poor villagers could not come up with that kind of extra cash, especially in the midst of a crisis. There was no alternative but to run. Flight further compounded the problem for those who remained. Here too, inflexible Roman policies exasperated the effects of plague and directly undermined economic recovery.

Initially during the pandemic, authorities were lenient with taxpayers. But by the early 170s, the Roman prefect's patience wore thin. Instead of reflecting on the inherent flaws in the taxation system and the damage done to the social fabric, the prefect demanded repayment of all taxes, present and past. Authorities increased coercive measures— making it illegal for men to flee their registered areas. In some cases, as one witness corroborates, officials would kidnap, torture, and even murder the family members of those who fled tax obligations.[42] But even such brutality failed to stem the tide of migration; the calamity was too overwhelming. So tax flight, already common prior to the Antonine plague, blossomed into a crisis in Egypt as disease ravaged the province.

Should the revolt that followed really surprise us? Law-abiding people had been arbitrarily robbed of their ability to earn livelihoods in legitimate society. Even worse, they were branded as criminals by their professed protectors. It would have only been rational—a matter of survival even—for such "desperate" people (a word Cassius Dio himself uses to describe the dissidents) to ally with or even join groups of bandits and other outcasts.[43] Even some Christians—yet another marginalized group—may have joined with the rebels in the hopes of escaping growing persecution in the province.[44] But elites, and undoubtedly their hangers-on in lower-level officialdom, refused to reflect on the conditions that pushed people to such extremes. Instead, elites drew

upon stereotypes and crass characterizations—lumping all the disaffected together as "godless" *Boukoloi* ("herdsmen")—a term that con-
noted backward, rural, semi-nomadic hicks. It was widely held among
civilized urbanites that such rural deplorables should be feared, avoided,
and even shunned.[45] Yet without question, many of these men were
pushed into banditry by the very people who hated them. The villages
of Egypt, already decimated by hunger and plague, must have been easy
pickings. In response to the dour conditions of the age, migration and
movement in the Nile Delta took off. Did such movements keep disease
outbreaks alive and circulating in the area? However long the epidemic
itself lasted, Egypt remained a province in turmoil for years. Soon the
same signs of distress, both direct and indirect, spewed westward as the
pandemic dispensed devastation.

Pharmacology, Folk Healing, and Cult Leaders

Even before the Antonine plague broke out in the Roman Empire, elites
were preoccupied with health, sickness, mysticism, and even magical
healing. Galen remarks that shrines and temples to Apollo and Asclepius had popped up everywhere.[46] Aelius Aristides—the same orator
who praised Rome in the court of the emperor Antoninus Pius—
captured the zeitgeist of the Antonine plague era by writing a self-
absorbed account of his personal history with diseases. When he finished the book in the late AD 170s, he called it *Sacred Tales*, but its title
could just as easily have been *The Mystical Musings of an Upper-Class
Twit*.[47] In the book, Aristides not only mentions the Antonine plague
but claims the distinct honor of being among the pandemic's first victims.[48] Way back in the summer of 165, Aristides tells us, his neighbors
in Smyrna—a Greek city on the western coast of Asia Minor—caught
a mysterious disease. Soon his own household servants were bedridden
with fever; some even died. Aristides himself then became sick, and
feared that the end was finally upon him. But a miracle occurred. Aristides received visions from deities such as Athena and Asclepius. Aristides's life was to be spared but at a high and terrible cost. A boy in
Aristides's household died on the same day that the orator recovered.

Aristides felt that it was an exchange of life for life. The orator was a paragon of piety; the gods owed him protection. For Aristides, surviving plague was not a source of stigmatization but evidence of the gods' favor. The orator was so proud that around a year later, Aristides says he endured a second bout of "the great plague" (as he and many others called it). That time, as before, the gods charged a hefty price for healing their valued noble devotee; they stole the life of a young woman.

Aristides may have indeed witnessed the Antonine plague's early onset in the Roman Empire, although he distinctly notes a summer outbreak—a divergence from other accounts, especially Galen's reliable testimony. It may be that Smyrnans' lack of immunity encouraged the disease to spread even against typical seasonal constraints. Still, Aristides records the high infectiousness and mortality seen in other Antonine plague sources. He even notes that the livestock in Smyrna were sick—details consistent with accounts of an epidemic in Rome that some believe represents the Antonine plague's final wave in AD 190. An inscription to Apollo the "Warder-off-of-Evil" erected in 164 in nearby Hierapolis also suggests a regional outbreak of some kind—maybe the Antonine plague disease, but maybe not.[49] Unfortunately, apart from contagiousness and deadliness, as well as the fact that the disease infected livestock, Aristides gives us no other meaningful details (besides his own dramatic thoughts on his uncomfortable ordeal).

The rest of his story, however, is hogwash. Aristides was plagued by fear more than any disease. Despite the rabid pestilence around him, Aristides's symptoms were in fact quite benign: a mild sore throat, perceived stomach upset, a feeling of fever, anxiety, and fear of death. Medical historian and classicist Danielle Gourevitch offered an apt diagnosis of Aristides's true condition:

> Aristides desperately wanted to be sick when the plague reached his place. . . . To his regret, he did not contract the plague but, regardless of his excellent health, he described himself as if he had contracted it. He listed symptoms he knew quite well, because he had so often experienced them, but which were not those of smallpox: not one of the items in his list of ailments fits the bill.[50]

The fact that Aristides claims to have caught the sickness associated with the Antonine plague *again* the following year is suspicious. Even without knowing the pathogen (Gourevitch thought it smallpox), surviving the disease must have produced some degree of immunity. The preindustrial context of the Roman Empire seems unfavorable to rapid pathogen mutation. Aristides may have lied with conviction and flair, but he still lied.[51]

Those who *actually* contracted the disease circulating during the Antonine plague had few treatment options. The minutes of a Senate meeting posted more than a decade after the pandemic's beginning speak of a "pestilence so great" which "could not be cured by any medicine."[52] Indeed, Roman medical practice was backward and often even counterproductive in the face of normal diseases, let alone this persistent pestilence. Galen, however, claimed to have found plague cures that worked. While wandering vaguely toward Aquileia in 168, Galen's dalliances allowed him to collect the exotic *Terra Lemnia* ("Lemnian Earth")—small sealed tabs of dried earth from the Greek island of Lemnos which Galen believed could treat skin ulcers.[53] The doctor evidently suspected what he might encounter in pestilential Italy—perhaps even the telltale pustules of the pox responsible for the Antonine plague. As he gained more experience treating plague victims over the years, Galen transitioned to the use of red, iron-rich earth from Armenia ("Armenian bole"). "During the Great Pestilence," Galen reflects, "all those who drank this drug were swiftly cured." Although he then adds: "while those whom it did not help all died. Nor were they helped by anything else, from which it is clear that the only people it did not benefit were those in an incurable state."[54] So drinking mixtures of earth cured the Antonine plague sickness, except when it didn't. Makes sense.

The other common plague treatment was a concoction called theriac. Most theriac recipes contained exotic ingredients such as viper's flesh, saffron, cinnamon, myrrh, and—the most crucial ingredient of all—opium.[55] After being mixed into a paste, the concoction would be left to mature for at least half a year but often much longer. Obviously, this was a drug exclusively for the rich. A treatise swept up in the Galenic material, although not authored by Galen himself, notes that teachers in Rome prescribed theriac to plague victims.[56] Galen too was a believer in the drug, calling it "the only antidote during the plague which was able to help those who drink it."[57] Galen's theriac became so desired that the doctor was made the exclusive supplier for the emperor himself.

The rich also tried various kinds of smell therapies. In the Roman epidemic of AD 190, doctors claimed that strong scents could block the disease. The emperor, for example, took in the scent of his laurel groves in one of his country villas. Imitators followed. The less affluent owned no laurel-lined villas, and many could not even leave Rome, but according to the Greek historian Herodian, they "filled their nostrils and ears with fragrant oils and used perfume and incense constantly." Like most off-the-cuff medical advice dispensed by unqualified political leaders, such treatments failed, and "the plague, however, continued to rage unchecked for a long time, and many men died."[58]

Those who could not afford the designer drugs and rare perfumes proscribed by imperial physicians still had treatment options, but these were, frankly, disgusting. As the pandemic swept through Syria, many locals decided that drinking urine—especially that produced by young boys—was the proper cure.[59] Galen says that at least some local elites refused such treatments. Still, Galen was not opposed to using urine as medicine. Antiquity's greatest doctor boastfully tells us that he ordered some of his patients to urinate on their own skin sores.[60] It was best, however, he claimed, to have a young boy do the deed. No doubt, more than a few mischievous lads stifled snickers as they gleefully pissed upon their betters.

Such a pitiful list of treatments tells us that the Antonine plague baffled even the Empire's best medical experts. After all, medicine in the High Roman Empire was quackery, plain and simple. Galen himself, for all his bluster, offers contradictory and confused solutions. The cacophony of medical interventions seems to have both worked and at the same time not worked. When Galen returned to Rome after enduring the dark winter in pestilential Aquileia, the typically proud doctor made a rare and startling admission: the regular people who survived the disease, because of their experience and common sense, sometimes offered better advice than professional doctors.[61] This confession is shocking considering it comes from the same doctor who claimed to be the medical establishment's equivalent to the emperor Trajan. Galen's candor indicates that the Antonine plague was truly beyond the powers of ancient medicine. There would be no miracle cure.

Opportunistic charlatans took advantage as conventional medicine failed. The panic induced by the Antonine plague was a literal godsend for folk healers and would-be cult leaders. While Galen was treating the sickness with Hippocratic medicine in Rome and Italy, an equally famous Greek prophet named Alexander took up the ancient equivalent of selling snake oil. Alexander had been a traveling "doctor." In reality he was something between a magician and a messiah—gaining notoriety for his claims that Asclepius had taken the form of Alexander's own pet snake. This snake-god, Glycon, sported human hair and maybe even a fake head with a movable mouth. In exchange for coin, Alexander allowed his followers to ask Glycon any question they wished, and the snake would respond either from his own mouth or in writing. Alexander's tricks wowed many in the Hellenistic East during the years preceding the Antonine plague—even earning Glycon a place on a coin minted in Alexander's hometown of Abonoteichus (modern İnebolu on the north coast of Turkey).

Alexander cleverly mixed magical healing with the symbols of the established medical-religious order. He may have known, for example, that Asclepius was first welcomed in Rome following three years of widespread sickness in 293 BC. Back then, the god also took the form of a snake (but a real one, however)—eventually swimming to the island in the middle of the Tiber. The pestilence subsequently vanished.[62] Asclepius became the patron god of legitimate doctors. In fact, the deity himself was a trained physician—the only member of the pantheon with such practical skills.[63] Alexander took the ascendant Asclepius's brand—one built on the success of Hippocratic medicine—and repackaged it into a kind of faith healing that appealed to the ignorant mystical obsessions of the age.

As the pandemic moved from city to city, Alexander sent minions "all over the Roman Empire," we're told by the eyewitness Lucian of Samosata. These apostles repeated Alexander's instructions to copy a magical verse: "Unshorn Phoebus [Apollo] keeps away the cloud of pestilence!"[64] Many in the panicked Empire blindly followed Alexander's advice. Lucian tells us the verse "was to be seen everywhere written over doorways as a charm against the plague."[65] We know that Lucian spoke the truth because the inscriptions survive to this day. For example, the base of a statue at Antioch bears Alexander's verse nearly word-for-word. The lines are followed by the seven vowels of the Greek alphabet—a common magical device used to call upon divine protection from sickness.[66] In fact, many instances of the verse, such as the one discovered at Hierapolis in southwest Asia Minor, include additional wards against pestilence—a sign of people's desperate desire to control that which could not be contained. The Hierapolians posted a lengthy oracle received from Apollo: "you are not alone in being injured by the destructive miseries of a deadly plague; many are the cities and people which are grieved at the wrathful displeasures of the gods."[67] Apollo demanded a number of rites, including sacrifices of animals, food, and drink. Finally, the Hierapolians were to set up statues of Apollo with bow in hand "as though he was shooting at the unfertile plague from afar with his arrows."[68] Such measures go beyond a general concern for health. When whole cities enacted reactionary religious mitigation measures, it was due to widespread pestilence.[69]

Alexander's influence reached the furthest corners of the Empire. In 1989, a pewter amulet was discovered in London at the Roman foreshore of the Thames River.[70] On it was inscribed thirty lines of Greek which contained not only Alexander's famous verse but a variety of magical invocations (even some with Hebrew origins) designed to "send away the discordant clatter of raging plague, air-borne . . . infiltrating pain, heavy-spiriting, flesh-wasting, melting, from the hollows of the veins." The amulet also includes a warning against kissing. Evidently some Romans believed that disease spread in this way.[71]

Inhabitants of Roman London (Londinium) seem to have been utterly terrified of the disease. The densely populated port town was frequented by soldiers. While archaeological surveys show substantial increases in temple-building in general during the time of the Antonine plague, a new local iteration of Apollo (Apollo Cunomaglus) received a monumental temple on the eastern edge of the city.[72] The god was sought in Londinium and other parts of Britain for plague healing. His image in Londinium was accompanied by dogs, sacred to Asclepius, their saliva able to heal infected wounds—perhaps an acknowledgment of the disease's pustules.[73] In line with Asia Minor dedications, Apollo Cunomaglus's statues in Londinium were also set up outside the city on the south side of the Thames, a place whereby the god could defend the city from contamination.[74] And yet, even as Londinium enjoyed the most substantial religious building program in the whole of the Roman period in the mid- to late second century AD, its population nevertheless rapidly shrunk at exactly the same time. Within a single generation, many buildings were abandoned and whole neighborhoods became desolate.[75]

Alexander's quasi-magical mitigations gained credence with a panic-stricken population. Government officials, even the emperor himself, came under his seductive sway. One senator offered his daughter in marriage to the "prophet." The organs of the state peddled product and propaganda for Alexander. Images of Glycon proliferated on coinage—the mass media of the Roman world—alongside Lucius and Marcus.[76]

Marcus sought Glycon's help through Alexander for the (re)commencement of his war in Magna Germania. The pandemic had thwarted the war's initial launch in Aquileia in 168—sending Marcus back to Rome in a carriage, while Lucius returned in a coffin. Marcus took no chances the second time, asking Alexander for an oracle on behalf of his legions. Alexander foretold "victory" provided two lions were cast into the Danube.[77] Marcus followed the oracle's bizarre instructions, but the lions swam to the opposing shore where the German army clubbed them to death. Twenty thousand Roman soldiers died in the disastrous battle that followed. The Germans then rampaged through Roman territory. Alexander escaped accountability for the debacle by the age-old excuse of oracular ambiguity: he simply promised "victory"; he never specified to which side.

Alexander's other so-called remedies also failed spectacularly. In the central Asia Minor city of Aizanoi, a horse breeder named Menogenes died "of a cloud of pestilence."[78] Here, the reference to Alexander's

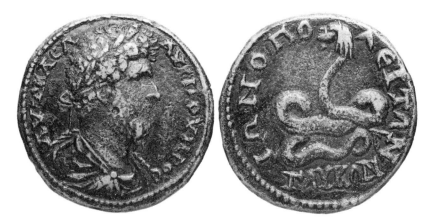

FIG. 5.1. Glycon appears on this provincial bronze coin of Lucius Verus dated from between AD 161 and 169 (RPC IV.1 5364). Bibliothèque nationale de France, https://gallica.bnf.fr/ark:/12148/btv1b85610787.

bogus charm is unmistakable. Were those who inscribed the tombstone noting the irony? According to Lucian—one of the few recorded skeptics of the superstitions that sprang up around the time of the Antonine plague—those who relied on Alexander's magic verse seemed to have worse results than those who did. Why? Lucian's answer is prescient:

> Do not suppose me to mean that they were stricken on account of the verse—by some chance or other it turned out that way, and perhaps, too, people neglected precautions because of their confidence in the line and lived too carelessly, giving the oracle no assistance against the disease because they were going to have the syllables to defend them and "unshorn Phoebus" to drive away the plague with his arrows![79]

Here is Lucian, almost 1,800 years before economist Sam Peltzman codified the concept of risk compensation (otherwise known as the "Peltzman effect"), describing the phenomenon perfectly. People are prone to take more risks when they perceive they are safe (even if their precautions do not make them any safer). Drivers who wear seatbelts, for example, drive faster and more recklessly than those who do not.[80] The Peltzman effect also works in reverse. In the mid-2010s, the town of

Poynton in the United Kingdom resolved congestion and dramatically increased safety at a busy downtown intersection by removing all traffic lights, signs, and road markings. Drivers perceived that risk was higher than before, so they drove far more cautiously and attentively. Accidents at the intersection plummeted, while traffic simultaneously eased.[81] By bravely pointing out that the charms, statues, and incantations that spread throughout the Roman world merely provided people with a false sense of safety, Lucian was a voice of reason in a society captivated by fear. He understood an uncomfortable truth: uncontained pandemics will run their course, and trendy mitigations—even those promoted by the experts and authorities of the age—may turn out to have been ineffective or even harmful.

Why then were such failed mitigation measures so widely adopted? One answer is that people did not distinguish between medicine and religion. The same doctors who empirically tested medicines and treatments also worshipped Asclepius with festivals and sacrifices. The wealthiest doctors spent vast sums of money on shrines and temples to the god.[82] But there were limits to superstition in Rome's medical community. Galen, for example, routinely criticized those who overrelied on the dreams given by Asclepius or the advice of his priests, especially in instances where sound, tested medical treatments were available.[83] The irony, of course, is that Galen used just such a dream to get out of returning to Aquileia after its epidemic outbreak. When authorities hypocritically fail to follow their own medical advice, it does incalculable damage to public trust. Besides, doctors' approaches seemed bizarre and their medical reasoning was difficult for laymen to grasp. The contradictions in plague mitigations must have also been obvious and troublesome. By contrast, simplistic talismans, charms, and oracles like those provided by Alexander and his ilk were more comprehensible in a culture captured by anxiety.

The age of angst was in full blossom. And anxious people tend to make irrational decisions. As sociologist Frank Furedi observes:

When fear assumes a morally unrestrained form, communities responding to threats often seek refuge in simplistic black-and-white answers to their predicament. Unease with uncertainty can encourage the attitude of "certainty at any cost," and intolerance toward those who question dogma is often one of the regrettable outcomes of this cause.[84]

Societies might press even harder into the same mitigation measures that have already failed, refusing to accept uncomfortable realities in the face of nature's uncontrollable power. And when the talismans of a superstitious society inevitably falter, the search for scapegoats intensifies. In the same way that individuals purged diseases, whole cities in the ancient world attempted to purify the body civic. Scapegoating (*pharmakos*) rituals were already standard practice in cities across the ancient world by the time of the Antonine plague.[85] The Massilians (modern Marseille, France), for example, rounded up a member of the underclass and fed him at state expense for a year. At the end of his period of feasting, however, the man was led around the city to receive the abuse of onlookers.[86] At the end of this trial, the citizens summarily kicked the man out of the city and barred him from ever returning. The citizens of Abdera in Thrace were far more violent. When pestilence broke out in that city, instead of feasting a man for a year, they pelted him with stones until he either died or fled the city.[87] The philosopher Apollonius of Tyana (in south-central Asia Minor) convinced a crowd in Ephesus to murder a beggar with stones to ward off a local plague.[88] Some cities performed such rituals annually; after all, an ounce of prevention is worth a pound of cure.

The Antonine plague coincided with eccentric and strange turns in conventional purification rituals in Asia Minor. The gods ordered all the citizens of Caesarea to wash the city buildings—not for sanitation but to purify them so that "the not yet diseased men that are left over in the fields" could obtain food for both future sacrifices and the suffering city.[89] Inscriptions from the cities of Hierapolis and Kallipolis call for black-haired animals to be burned whole and then buried in the ground.[90] Such rites imply that demonic underworld forces were responsible for the pestilence, perhaps including Hades himself. Life must be destroyed to purify the city. A small town in Lydia was instructed not only to set up a statue of Artemis to "free them from the man-slaying poisons of plague" but to also seek out and burn wax puppets to counteract acts of sorcery and evil magic.[91]

Ephesus went all-in to fight the pandemic. There the citizens called upon Artemis "the ancestral leader of the town from its origin"— crafting her a statue of gold rather than stone or bronze. The inscription then demanded dark rites, numerous sacrifices, and complex ritual chants. But most serious of all, the oracle threatened divine vengeance in the form of fiery fevers upon those citizens who did not fulfill the demanded practices.[92] Unlike many other oracles, this one directed blame to members of the community who did not participate in collective purification. Pandemic had clearly bred panic, and panic could easily inflame persecution. No one seemed to know what the gods wanted, only that they were furious. And fear of divine wrath was a powerful motivator.

Scapegoats and Saints

During the Antonine plague, some Christians stuck out from the panicked populations of the Roman world. When charlatans like Alexander arrived in town, enthralling the gullible masses by appealing to their fears of plague, many Christians balked. Indeed, even the satirical Lucian was impressed. In his invective against Alexander, Lucian singled out Christians as one of only two groups immune to Alexander's charms.[93] Even Galen, who thought Christians simple-minded because they overrelied on "undemonstrated laws," admired Christians for being "free from the fear of death."[94]

By the middle of the second century, followers of Christ had dispersed to all corners of the Roman Empire. Reasonable estimates put the Christian population at around forty or fifty thousand on the eve of the Antonine plague.[95] Despite such relatively small numbers, however, reports suggest a stunningly diverse membership. Pliny wrote to the emperor Trajan in the early second century, saying that he had found Christians of "every age, every rank, and also of both sexes."[96] Later Christian authors quote second-century contemporaries who claim that even the imperial court at the time included Christians.[97] The church grappled with a stunning array of theologies, and some Christian leaders became established public intellectuals.[98] By the age of angst, the church was both sufficiently pugnacious and sizable to become a public nuisance.

As the stresses of the mid-second century accumulated, some wondered if Christians bore some of the blame. Improper worship, no matter how slight, wrecked the Pax Deorum.[99] The free-floating anxieties of the age no doubt encouraged hypersensitivity to unconventional religion. Christians worshiped no god but their own, and they worshipped him in strange new ways rather than through traditional animal sacrifice.[100] To the Romans, the Christians seemed like atheists and blasphemers. Christian practices like baptism and the Eucharist were perceived as "superstitions" (*superstitio*) that corrupted the mind and led people away from proper worship.[101] And as both Christians and calamities both proliferated, Romans readily drew a connection.

A pivotal moment in attitudes toward Christians predates the Antonine plague by just a few years. Around AD 160 or 161, "an astonishing succession of earthquakes and terrors" struck cities in Asia Minor, according to one ancient source.[102] Local citizens blamed the Christians in their communities—among the earliest instances of Romans affixing responsibility for a natural disaster to Christians. Even then, however, Marcus intervened on behalf of the Christian minority, imploring the mob to avoid vigilante justice.[103] Desire for law and order may have motivated Marcus more than any sympathy for the Christians. The emperor enacted harsh penalties against anyone who "does anything whereby men's light minds are frightened by superstition"—a law which may well have been partially aimed at Christians.[104]

The pandemic seemingly stoked popular prejudices, and a burst of outright persecution followed.[105] Care, however, is warranted here, as no source directly connects the Antonine plague to Christian persecutions or deaths. And although governors and other officials oversaw trials and executions of Christians during the Antonine plague and immediately following, "popular hostility" was still the driving force; official and systematic "top-down" imperial persecution did not arrive until the mid-third century.[106] Still, the surge in apologetics and increasing mob violence against Christians suggest growing tension in the Empire's religious milieu during the mid- to late second century. By the end of the Antonine plague, the Christian author Tertullian frames a church beset by many dangers, toils, and snares:

> They think the Christians the cause of every public disaster, of every affliction with which the people are visited. If the Tiber rises as high as the city walls, if the Nile does not send its waters up over the fields, if the heavens give no rain, if there is an earthquake, if there is famine or pestilence, straightway the cry is, "Away with the Christians to the lions!"[107]

Tertullian's list of calamities was not random. Each of these items afflicted the Empire during the first decade of Marcus's reign, from the flood of the Tiber in 162 to the Antonine plague's initial epidemic surge. All were serious threats, and according to Tertullian, Christians had become somehow implicated.

How might developments during the Antonine plague have influenced the trajectory of the early church and its Roman context? As with so many of the pandemic's social, economic, and cultural effects, it seems less that the pandemic alone stimulated a sudden change of direction but rather that the general troubles of the era intensified and accelerated existing movements and trends. Even as the cities in Asia Minor erected statues to Apollo to ward off plague, for example, some also granted legal immunity to those who persecuted Christians. A fragment of an address to Marcus by Melito, bishop of Sardis, asks the emperor to intervene to stop "new decrees" against Christians in the cities of the region. These laws empowered "shameless informers and coveters of the property of others" to "openly carry on robbery night and day, despoiling those who are guilty of no wrong."[108] We do not know what these "new decrees" were, and it seems that local Christians were also unsure whether or not the emperor had officially sanctioned them. Nevertheless, the laws provided cover to "lawless plundering by the populace" not necessarily because of the disease but certainly during the panic the contagion's pandemic potential helped induce.

Around the time of the pandemic's arrival in Rome, the high-profile apologist Justin Martyr was murdered. The emperors likely knew of Justin; he had delivered a defense of Christianity to Marcus and Lucius's adopted father, the emperor Antoninus Pius. But Marcus did not intervene when Justin and several companions—male and female, slave and free—were brought before the urban prefect Quintus Junius Rusticus. Although a record of the Christians' trial survives, the specific charges against them remain unknown.[109] The record simply notes that the prefect examined the Christians on their doctrine and their meetings before demanding they "sacrifice to the gods." After refusing, Justin and his companions were summarily beaten and beheaded. This injustice was but a foretaste of the persecutions to come.

After a decade of plague, the mass murders began. In AD 177, some fifty Christians in Lugdunum in Gaul were tortured and killed for unknown reasons. The account of their demise—a firsthand letter preserved in Eusebius's fourth-century *Ecclesiastical History*—does not mention disease or sickness.[110] And gladiators had become expensive by that time—putting pressure on officials to find alternative "entertainments."[111] And yet, the circumstances of the mass public killing of men, women, and children hint at fear of contagion and even expiation of divine wrath not unlike strange purification and warding rituals in Asia Minor at the time. The first abnormality in the Lugdunum persecution is that even those who recanted their Christian beliefs were killed. Victims' bodies were burned and thrown into the Rhone River—an indignity to be sure, but also a form that aligns with both ritual sacrifice to underworld deities and purging contamination. Such desecration also prevented Christians from collecting and venerating the martyrs' bodies. Just prior to the mass execution, local authorities banned Christians from bathhouses and markets. Many of Lugdunum's Christians were recent arrivals from Asia Minor, and one was even a doctor. At some point, Lugdunum—Gaul's most populous city—probably suffered an epidemic that a frightened population could attach to the pestilence shaking the Roman world.[112] Did the citizens of Lugdunum conclude that the Christians had brought some evil with them? Such speculation aligns with the context provided by other source material. False and baseless conspiracy theories about Christians ran rife in elite circles. Marcus and Lucius's teacher Fronto, for example, was convinced that Christians devoured infants and engaged in incestuous orgies.[113] Similar charges are named in Athenagoras's *Embassy for the Christians*, published contemporary with the massacre in Lugdunum. Such rumors had become sufficiently widespread by the end of the Antonine plague that Tertullian was forced to address them in his *Apology*.[114]

Christians had grown accustomed to ad hoc degradations and persecutions over the first century and a half of the church's existence. Religious historian James Rives argues that second-century Christians came to expect that popular violence against them "might occur at any time, especially during periods of stress."[115] Persecution was for the Christians what the pandemic was to the rest of the Empire's inhabitants: a potential killer that might strike at any time and any place. Persecution in some ways had prepared the Christians for the pandemic. Some Christians, therefore, responded to contemporary crises with acceptance rather than angst, at least according to Christian accounts.

Perceptions of Christian resilience, however, were mixed. Some Roman officials believed Christians' tolerance for pain and death seemed smug, deranged, and even dangerous. Pliny the Younger, when he was governor of Bithynia in the early second century, was certainly put off. Pliny impatiently executed a small number of Christians on account of their "stubbornness and inflexible obstinacy" even before he received the emperor's confirmation on the exact legal status of his Christian prisoners.[116] Similarly, Marcus Aurelius described Christians' embrace of death as "sheer obstinacy"—the opposite of a philosophy informed "by reason and dignity."[117] Some Christians actively courted persecution as the surest means to follow Christ and obtain eternal life, reinforcing the idea that Christian views on the resurrection derived from a sure and steady hope.

As the fear of disease and death infected the cities of the Roman Empire during the Antonine plague, Christianity offered both the hope of bodily healing and compelling frameworks to accommodate suffering and a comparably concrete perspective on the afterlife. While he was alive, Jesus healed the blind, the deaf, and the leprous and even resurrected the dead. After his crucifixion, Jesus himself came back to life and gave his followers instructions and mighty promises. "You will receive power when the Holy Spirit comes on you," he assured them, "and you will be my witnesses in Jerusalem, and in all Judea and Samaria, and to the ends of the earth."[118] This delegated power included the ability to heal sickness, as the accounts in Luke's *Acts of the Apostles* demonstrate. As with all ancient religions, Christianity featured many local varieties of beliefs and practices, some of which modified existing pagan ideas. Some in the church, for example, believed that disease was the result of demonic forces, not necessarily personal impiety—unburdening the sick and their family members from guilt.[119] Some Christians thought rites such as baptism and the Eucharist were magical wards against demons and the diseases they caused. But perhaps more meaningful than rituals were the glorious promises given to those Christians who perished: "[God] will wipe away every tear from their eyes, and death shall be no more, neither shall there be mourning, nor crying, nor pain anymore, for the former things have passed away."[120] If death—even painful and excruciating death from plague—led to such glory, was it not worth the cost of suffering?

Christians broadly—despite many different theologies and ritual practices—enjoyed confidence concerning the final destination of their departed friends and family. Those who endured sickness could draw upon the notion that their anguish was sanctifying. The visionary words of Paul the Apostle, for example, must have been frequently on the lips of Christians as they endured the ravages of plague:

> I count everything as loss because of the surpassing worth of knowing Christ Jesus my Lord. For his sake I have suffered the loss of all things and count them as rubbish, in order that I may gain Christ and be found in him . . . that I may know him and the power of his resurrection, and may share his sufferings, becoming like him in his death, that by any means possible I may attain the resurrection from the dead.[121]

For many Christians, suffering prior to death was akin to the agony of a final sprint before winning a race. Yes, it was exhausting; but such misery translated to victory. The Carthaginian bishop Cyprian, in the middle of the third-century pandemic which bears his name, called suffering through disease an "exercise." "We are learning not to fear death," he said. "These are trying exercises for us, not deaths; they give to the mind the glory of fortitude; by contempt of death they prepare for the crown."[122] It is unlikely that contemporary philosophers could compete with such logic. Marcus himself said that suffering was found "in your capacity to see it. Stop doing that and everything will be fine."[123] Would such trite advice have provided much comfort to those in pain? Would the statues of Apollo set up at the gates of pestilence-stricken cities have inspired confidence, especially once those elites and priests who erected them fled or even perished themselves despite the gods' empty promises? The Antonine plague must have provided Christianity with its most demanding test up to that point; its subsequent growth, and perhaps the brief peace the church enjoyed in the 180s, suggests it passed with flying colors.[124]

But Christianity provided more than mere perspective on plague. The church's sacrificial care for the sick and dying would have spoken volumes to non-Christian communities. Christianity, from its inception, was constructed on communal principles which emphasized material and spiritual care for the helpless and hopeless. In a famous passage in the book of John, Jesus commands his disciples to "love one another as I have loved you"—a command repeated many places in New Testament writings.[125] Jesus denotes a "love" (agapē) without condition or the expectation of return—a radical concept in a world defined by patronage and reciprocity. Christians were to love in this self-sacrificing way because "[God] first loved us" by sending Christ.[126] Here was an entirely different logic than the Pax Deorum. Human love was to reflect divine love, which was self-sacrificial rather than contractual.[127] Even non-Christian sources, such as the letters of the hostile emperor Julian, tell that "the impious Galilaeans support not only their own poor but ours as well, all men see that our people lack aid from us."[128] Sociologist and scholar of early Christianity Rodney Stark summarizes the situation in the second century best: "these were revolutionary ideas."[129]

What would such radical compassion have looked like during the Antonine plague? We have no direct sources to tell us. But a letter written by the Alexandrian bishop Dionysius describing an outbreak of the Cyprianic plague in the early 250s may not be far from the truth:

> Many of our brothers, because of their exceeding love and brotherly affection, taking no thought for themselves and caring for one another, unhesitatingly oversaw the sick, readily waiting on them and serving them in Christ. When they contracted the disease from others and drew the sickness upon themselves for their neighbors and readily accepted the pain they departed along with them most gladly. And many who cared for the sick and strengthened others died themselves, transferring their death to themselves . . . the best of our brothers departed life in this manner, and some presbyters, deacons, and even some of the laity were greatly lauded, with the result that this form of death, on account of its requiring great piety and strong faith, seemed to lack nothing in relation to martyrdom.[130]

Formal Christian charitable institutions did not arise until the fourth century, but a combination of rituals, redistributions, and social networking gave the early church an impressive ability to care for their sick.[131] Thus, when the Antonine plague pandemic swept through a city, the Christians there did not need to suddenly invent programs for helping the sick, the suffering, and even the dead. It was as though the church had been prepared for just such a purpose.

Even the earliest Christian sources confirm the radical charity practiced by Christians before the Antonine plague, and then during its early years. A defense of Christianity composed by a converted Athenian philosopher during the mid-second century, for example, lists several forms of benevolence:

> When they see a stranger, they take him in to their homes and rejoice over him as a very brother; for they do not call them brethren after the flesh, but brethren after the spirit and in God. And whenever one of their poor passes from the world, each one of them according to his ability gives heed to him and carefully sees to his burial. . . . And

if there is among them any that is poor and needy, and if they have no spare food, they fast two or three days in order to supply to the needy their lack of food.[132]

Justin, who was martyred in Rome just prior to or even during the Antonine plague, noted that Christians regularly collected and redistributed to the needy, including those who were sick.[133] We have confirmation of ongoing Christian charity contemporary with the Antoine plague in Rome from a letter from the Corinthian bishop Dionysius. In AD 171, just a few years after the first epidemic wave in Rome, Dionysius commends the Christians in the capital for their generosity to thousands of poor and needy both within and outside the community of the church.[134] Undoubtedly, Christian accounts cast the church in the best light. And some Christian leaders, like Clement of Alexandria, advocated limiting Christian philanthropy to "all who are enrolled as God's disciples"—not necessarily the wider non-Christian community.[135] But even if Christian charity was largely inward focused, such acts still delivered a powerful witness compared to the flight and folk healing seen outside the church.

The Antonine plague pathogen must have killed many Christians as they ministered to the sick and dying. It seems, however, that such sacrifices only strengthened Christian faith and practice. Writing less than a decade after a major epidemic in Rome, Tertullian notes that Christians took up regular monthly contributions for the poor, the orphans, the elderly, mine workers, prisoners, and the dead and dying.[136] In AD 215, Hippolytus of Rome reminded Christian deacons to keep tabs on who was sick so that the bishop could visit them at their homes.[137] And when plague victims died, Christians treated their bodies with reverence and care. They performed this service, moreover, knowing the danger of the act. When pandemic disease returned in the mid-third century, such acts of compassion cost Christians their lives:

And they took up the bodies of the saints with welcoming hands and bosoms, cleaned them and closed their eyes and mouths, placed them on their shoulders and laid them down. They clung to them, wrapped themselves around them, and adorned them with washings and funeral wrappings, and a short time later they received the same, for those left behind always followed those who died before them.[138]

Elite Romans had long professed honor and respect for the deceased, and corpses were to be treated with dignity.[139] But during the Antonine plague, sources describe widespread neglect of the bodies of those who lacked the social or economic resources to secure proper funerary rites. Christians, however, motivated by a belief in the bodily resurrection of all God's elect—no matter their status or resources on earth—would have respected the bodies of Christian plague victims.[140] Such reverence for the dead was something even non-Christian Romans could understand and admire.

While Christian willingness to visit the sick exposed them to enormous danger, it also made the survivors more likely to gain immunity. In Thucydides's description of the Athenian plague of 429 BC, for example, we learn that "more often the sick and the dying were tended by the pitying care of those who had recovered, because they knew the course of the disease and were themselves free from apprehension. For no one was ever attacked a second time, or not with a fatal result."[141] Whatever the disease behind the Antonine plague, survivors would have been immune for at least some time afterward. If immunity was long-lasting, as it is with many orthopoxviruses, Christians would have survived subsequent pandemic waves in higher proportions. Christian survival over time might have seemed miraculous to onlookers. As for Christians themselves, even if they did not understand the causes of their immunity, they no doubt credited survival to divine affirmation of their charitable efforts.

Indeed, distinctions between Christians and their contemporaries were not lost on Christian writers. Several made much of how plague outbreaks revealed a qualitative difference between those inside and outside of the church. Cyprian, for example, notes that "plague and pestilence, which seems horrible and deadly, searches out the justice of each and everyone and examines the minds of the human race."[142] Non-Christians failed such tests, he claims: the healthy forsook the sick, relatives abandoned their kin, masters failed to care for diseased slaves, and even doctors deserted those who begged for their help. Similarly, Dionysius of Alexandria did not mince words in his letter describing behavior seen in Egypt:

> Those who began to fall ill [the non-Christians] set apart, and they fled from those dearest to them. They even threw them in the roads half-dead and treated the unburied dead like garbage as they tried to avoid the spread of death and its fellowship, which was not an easy thing to avoid.[143]

Undoubtedly, Christian authors exaggerated the selfishness of non-Christians as well as their own altruism, but not wholesale. After all, even the emperors had turned tail and run from pestilence. But the Christian framework for death, let alone plague, transcended the preservation of mere biological life. Whether they lived or died, many Christians—despite their differences with one another—assigned high spiritual value to risk-taking acts of compassion during epidemics. The Antonine plague must have been no exception. In a world which increasingly reviled and persecuted them, Christians could point to their faithfulness in the midst of epidemics as evidence of their *agapē* love and, therefore, of the effectiveness of Christ's own selfless sacrifice to liberate their once sin-stained souls.

A Pestilential World

As the age of angst dragged on, one thing became abundantly clear: there was no stopping this new disease. Nor could people run from it. No mitigation strategy worked. Drugs failed. Folk healing failed. And scapegoating Christians and others certainly failed. If the evidence thus far gives us a keyhole view into the effects of the Antonine plague pandemic broadly, then pestilence and especially panic settled into cities across the Empire by the mid-170s. The stresses introduced during the pre-plague years proliferated, catching the Roman Empire off guard. The toxic mixture of preexisting conditions and an active pandemic altered the social and cultural fabric of the Empire. The pandemic became the symbolic vanguard of a full-blown crisis.

It was an age marinated in pestilence and panic. In addition to Aristides's dream journal and inscriptions to Apollo, references to plague seasoned Marcus's own *Meditations* on life and philosophy—suggesting intimate knowledge of the symptoms. "In the mind of one who has been chastened and thoroughly purified you will find no infected tissue, no contamination, no festering sore beneath the skin," the emperor wrote in the late 170s.[144] Galen too would allude to the Antonine plague in his *On Avoiding Distress*, a treatise on how to maintain composure in the midst of a world where death and loss seemed to be lurking around every corner.[145] A senatorial speech delivered in the late 170s contains perhaps the most telling plague reference: "our Princes, whose only desire is to revive and restore public health, now overwhelmed and worn out by such a great disease, have first turned their attention to finding out what gives the disease its strength."[146] The unnamed senator, however, was not speaking about the pandemic but high gladiator prices. The realities of ever-present pestilence had so soaked daily life that its rhetoric seasoned discussion of even seemingly unrelated matters.

Art imitated life, however. The trauma of the age derived from real tragedies—and these continued to accumulate. Violence—a kind of plague in its own right—metastasized as the Pax Romana crumbled, weathered by ecological and systemic stresses, pummeled by plague, and then torn down in part by the terrified descendants of those who constructed it. Around AD 170, war once again broke out. After retreating from plague-infested Aquileia, Marcus relaunched his northern campaign. Again, the soldiers gathered. Again, the destructive power of the pandemic sowed sickness among the armies. But very real troubles of the age also contaminated the Roman economy. Mines, quarries, and agricultural estates show signs of stoppage as the pandemic wore on. These enterprises were key engines of imperial power, and they all faltered before the end of Marcus's reign. Rome's golden age was rapidly rusting. The long-term consequences of the age of angst loomed on the darkening horizon.

6

AN EMPIRE
EXHAUSTED

No one could have known that the economic challenges and social strife that multiplied under Marcus would cascade into crises that would permanently restructure Roman society. An era was ending. Mighty as Rome was, it lacked any man-made mechanism to arrest the evolution and transmission of pathogens. No emperor, pronouncement, or institution was powerful enough to alter the Empire's changing ecological context. The Antonine plague was not behind all the Pax Romana's problems, but the pandemic gashed Rome's ideological veneer, exposing the underlying fragility of the Roman system. In the end, the real scandal was not the collapse of the Pax Romana but the fact that it survived so long.[1]

Roman soldiers pooled near the Danube in the autumn of AD 170. After enduring the loss of his co-emperor and brother the previous winter, Marcus, alone, relaunched his war against the Germanic tribes harassing Rome's northern provinces. Historian Peter Heather's account of Rome's centuries-long battle with European invaders commences with this moment for good reason. Indeed, unbeknownst to Roman military leaders, northern tribes had been migrating toward Roman borders in untold numbers. Rome's allies in the region—the Marcomanni and Victuali, among others—were under severe pressures and demanded admission into the Roman Empire for protection.[2] Marcus answered their request with a declaration of war . . . against them.

The war morphed into a series of conflicts historians refer to as the "Marcomannic Wars." This name underplays the full scope of the conflict, as more than a dozen different German tribes became involved. One Roman source named the struggle "The War of Many Nations" as "all the peoples from beyond the Rhine and Danube conspired against Rome."[3] But at least some Romans initially thought the campaign would be something of a cakewalk.[4] Galen, for example, expected Marcus to return to Rome victorious after just one campaign season.[5] The ferocity and desperation of the Germanic tribes, however—their own territory beset by invaders from still further north and east—pressed them up against Roman boundaries for the remainder of Marcus's life. The ensuing military quagmire so consumed the emperor's attention that Marcus would not see Rome for a full seven years.

In the thick of this sea of soldiers—Roman and German alike—plague foamed and frothed. Several sources confirm the devastation among the Roman troops. The least reliable of these characterizes the years of the Marcomannic Wars as "a time when a grievous pestilence carried away thousands of civilians and soldiers."[6] The more trustworthy imperial secretary Eutropius, writing in the middle of the fourth century AD, interrupts his summary of Marcus's Germanic war with these chilling words: "there occurred so destructive a pestilence that at Rome, and throughout Italy and the provinces, most of the Empire's inhabitants, and almost all the soldiers, sunk under the disease."[7] Similarly flamboyant, the Christian author Jerome says that an outbreak in AD 172 "slaughtered the Roman army almost to extinction."[8] These later authors relied on earlier accounts which have since been lost. And while their interjections are exaggerated, and therefore suspect, there should be little doubt that the Roman army—beleaguered by barbarians—suffered concurrent terrors of war and pestilence during the early 170s.

A wider crisis spread into social and economic systems across the Empire. Supplies of metal, stone, and other goods were disrupted. Food shortages in several regions continued unabated. Violence became endemic in parts of Egypt and Asia Minor. In this chaotic moment, one of Marcus's most capable generals turned renegade and openly proclaimed himself ruler of the Empire. But he was not the only one to go rogue. Many rank-and-file soldiers also betrayed their allegiances and turned to pillaging and terrorizing their own countrymen. Rampant disease, unending war, the lack of money, the supply shortages—all these things destroyed morale and loyalty in soldier and citizen alike. Gangs of ex-soldiers and runaway slaves proliferated in the countryside like parasites, devouring the waning resources of an exhausted Empire. Eventually, the worst occurred: Marcus himself became sick. After generations of apparent glory, the Pax Romana crashed in one horrific decade.

Shortage and Scarcity

In the summer of 1812, Napoleon's Grande Armée marched into Russia with over half a million soldiers—a portable metropolis of men from all over France's newly acquired empire.[9] But in the winter of that same year, less than a hundred thousand returned. Lost battles, starvation, and the cold decimated Napoleon's army, but the most prevalent killer was infectious disease. A large-scale genetic study of French soldier burials confirmed widespread louse-transmitted diseases among the troops, including scourges like trench fever and epidemic typhus.[10] The scale of death seems shocking—80 percent of Napoleon's soldiers died in just six monstrous months—but in historical terms, the fate of the Grande Armée is in fact typical rather than exceptional. Prior to World War II, more American soldiers died of diseases than from bullets or bayonets.[11] Military conflicts have been among the most prolific transmitters of pathogens in all of human history.[12]

The AD 160s was a decade of rapid, massive movements of soldiers to and from numerous hot spots along Roman borders. Vexillations from as many as ten legions fought in both the Parthian and Marcomannic campaigns—providing the cross-fertilization necessary to root and grow the surging Antonine plague in the otherwise sparsely populated provinces of Germania, Raetia, Noricum, Pannonia, and Moesia.[13] With the Marcomannic Wars, Rome unwittingly flung fresh meat to the pandemic. With regular units deployed in Parthia, the emperors formed two new legions of Italian soldiers—Legio II and III Italica—and sent them to fortify the northern borders. And in the north, just as in Parthian territory, conditions were perfect for pathogen transmission. Large populations of soldiers moved into an area with a similarly large migrant population. Whichever group first contracted the Antonine plague pathogen probably doesn't matter much. Few on the frontiers likely had immunity to the disease. Very quickly, the Empire's now crowded northern border became a chaotic mixer for various forms of death and misery, but especially disease.

Marcus's army rivaled Napoleon's as a cultural and ethnic melting pot. A study of the names of Roman auxiliaries in Britain reveals how the British-born soldiers that dominated local military units in the first century AD were gradually replaced by a more diverse set of soldiers from various Italian and Balkan regions in the second century.[14] These soldiers from all over the known world shared close contact with their comrades. Most too would have engaged the wider community around them. Members of the military were routinely deployed to aid in resource extraction and management. They policed local settlements. They worked on infrastructure projects.[15] There is plenty of evidence that Roman troops bought from local merchants and drank in nearby establishments, and they certainly slept with local women.[16] Rape was likely commonplace, and camp followers were in high demand, as Roman citizen-soldiers were legally forbidden to marry. In spite of the prohibition, perhaps around one-third of legionaries took "unofficial" wives.[17] Many fathered children, although their sons were illegitimate by default and therefore ineligible to follow their fathers directly into the legions. In and near the camps or in nearby towns, therefore, were large communities of women, children, and servants. These, along with the soldiers themselves, could have sustained and transferred the Antonine plague disease as it circulated in military settings, especially in the camps along the northern frontier during the wars of the 170s.

Plague deaths in those early years of the Marcomannic Wars must have been significant.[18] Even rough mortality figures, however, are impossible to deduce. Multiple sources suggest a recruitment crisis in the late 160s and early 170s—signaling massive losses in the military beyond the normal casualties of war, and thus a desperate need to fill gaps in the legions. Fourth-century AD priest and historian Paulus Orosius makes the strongest claim:

> A plague now spread over many provinces, and a great pestilence devastated all Italy. Everywhere country houses, fields, and towns were left without a tiller of the land or an inhabitant, and nothing remained but ruins and forests. It is said that the Roman troops and all the legions stationed far and near in winter quarters were so depleted that the war against the Marcomanni, which broke out immediately, could not be carried on without a new levy of soldiers. At Carnuntum, Marcus Aurelius held the levy continuously for three years.[19]

Orosius's claims sound outlandish, but hints of mass death in Marcus's northern army can be found, if one knows where to look. A rare list of recruits for one Danubian legion (Legio VII Claudia) shows the legion took in nearly double its annual intake in the year 169.[20] These men may have replaced soldiers who died suddenly during the epidemic the previous year. At the same time, the Empire had been waging near constant war in the 160s, and perhaps the high number of recruits reflects the pressing needs of the moment. Also, the Romans often doubled the manpower of their legions' first cohort, from 400 to 800 men. But the list of Legio VII Claudia soldiers shows other cohorts with similarly high numbers of recruits—so it would seem that some atypical recruitment needs prompted the influx.

There are other indicators of trouble in the Roman military in the pandemic's opening years. It seems that far fewer soldiers obtained official discharge from the army during and after the Antonine plague. Upon discharge, emperors themselves awarded rights and privileges to veterans of several classes of soldiers (auxiliaries, praetorian guardsmen, urban cohorts, naval soldiers, etc.)—the decrees preserved for all to see on a wall atop the Palatine hill in Rome.[21] These valuable privileges might include citizenship itself, the right to openly marry, the ability to pass on inheritances to children, citizenship for children, and other benefits. Soldiers also received individual copies of the imperial decree on a bronze tablet, whether by gift or purchase.[22] Many of these diplomas

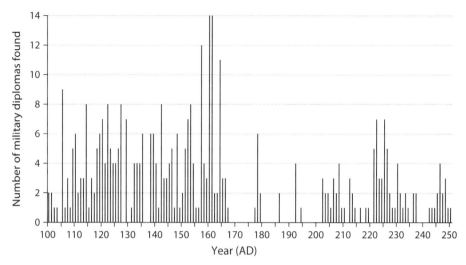

FIG. 6.1. Recovered military diplomas, AD 100–250.
Based on data from Holder 2006, 681–98. Diplomas that cannot be dated to
specific years are not included. A small number of additional diplomas have been
found or published since, but it is impossible to collect all of them in the scope of
this study. Moreover, their inclusion would not alter the impression from the
2006 data. For comparable counts, see Eck 2012a; Duncan-Jones 2018, 53.

have been found, the majority of which date to between the mid-first
and mid-third century AD. But there is a noteworthy gap in this bounty
of bronze certificates.

If these diplomas are a proxy for soldier survival, then the sudden
drop after AD 165 seems an unmistakable indicator of mass death in the
army.[23] But as is often the case with this persnickety pandemic, the evidence is more complicated than it might appear. Discharge occurred
after around twenty-five years of service, so it is worth asking: was there
a significant change in recruitment terms around the year AD 140 when
these missing soldiers first enlisted? In fact, there was: the privileges
offered to some veteran classes were sharply reduced, creating far less
demand for many veterans to acquire diplomas upon retirement from
around 165.[24] And diplomas would have been of less use for veterans
who settled near the camp where they had served, as people in the community would have known them and their status.[25] Finally, as will be
discussed below, even the raw materials to make the bronze diplomas

may have been in short supply from the time of plague onward.[26] Still, diploma survival returns to more consistent levels from the beginning of the third century among non-auxiliary soldiers, suggesting that the dearth of diplomas during the Antonine plague and the decades following may be due at least in part to unprecedented deaths, or perhaps desertions (see "Plague's Fugitives" below) in the army.

As it was, Marcus struggled to obtain sufficient soldiers to prosecute his war. Such recruitment crises were not unprecedented in Roman history, but they were nevertheless rare. Major losses to Hannibal in the Second Punic War (218–201 BC), for example, required emergency levies. But there is no evidence that battle losses in Parthia were out of the ordinary. The Marcomannic Wars likely elevated soldier casualties, but then plague deaths could have tipped Marcus to trawl the dregs of Roman society for recruits.[27] The normal standards for military service were summarily dropped. Slaves filled the spaces in the ranks. Gladiators were taken from the arena and formed into combat units. Supposedly, even highway robbers and brigands were given some degree of legal immunity and allowed to join the war effort, their crimes momentarily forgotten in the emergency. An Egyptian inscription shows that recruiters for Legio II Traiana in Alexandria obtained over half of their recruits in AD 168 from "the camps"—that is, from the illegitimate children of soldiers, defying existing prohibitions on such men serving.[28] Prior to the pandemic, recruits arrived into the military from named cities only.[29] This deviation from normal recruitment suggests not only the pressing needs of the military as it waged two major wars but also serious limits in available manpower—perhaps due to plague casualties.[30] Officials also incentivized military service by passing out honorifics and prestige like candy. Commoners from the Greek city of Thespiae who joined the war effort, for example, and their parents too, were granted elite status and allowed to serve on the city council.[31] Finally, Marcus's recruiters even hired men from the very tribes Rome intended to subdue. The desperation was palpable. Only a few years earlier in 165 Italy had easily supplied thousands of fresh recruits to form Legio II and III Italica. But after only a few years into the Antonine plague, the mighty Roman army had withered to a shell of its former power.

Adding to the shortage of military men was a fiscal crisis. The treasury became exhausted. It was easy for emperors to promise money; it was another thing to deliver when payment came due. The wages of Roman soldiers were good, but they had recently hit a plateau. Legionary salaries had been fixed at 300 silver denarii per year since the reign of Domitian (AD 81–96) nearly a century prior.[32] But each soldier could expect bonuses (*donativa*) of gold and silver coins every few years. It had not always been this way. In the early decades of the Empire, such donatives were reserved for special occasions. Yet in their first years in office, Marcus and Lucius spent lavishly on soldier bonuses—passing out 5,000 denarii to each member of the Praetorian Guard, with smaller amounts to hundreds of thousands of regular soldiers stationed throughout the Empire.[33] The grandiose spending spree continued throughout the 160s, especially as the victories against Parthia began to stack up. In summary, Marcus and Lucius paid out military donatives at an average of about one per year—a pace without precedent.[34] Then, inexplicably, the prodigality stopped dead in 170. After nearly a decade of distributions, Marcus refused to pay even one single bonus until 175. That donative and only one other are the only known bonuses that Marcus gave his soldiers for the remainder of his nearly twenty-year reign.[35] The spending stoppage is astonishing.

Just a few years into the Antonine plague, the imperial finances entered fiscal freefall. The dire situation forced creative solutions so that a population decimated by plague, panicked by their superstitions, and embroiled in war might not face additional tax burdens. Perhaps inspired by his own stoic disregard for luxuries and frills, Marcus pulled a stunt which was both practical and politically savvy. He had various knickknacks from his imperial palace trucked out to Trajan's Forum—Rome's economic hub. There everything from eating utensils to fine art and statuary was auctioned off to the highest bidder.[36] So much property was on offer that bits and bobs were still selling a full two months later. In reality, Marcus may have dragged out the auction on purpose, thus projecting a constant image of imperial sacrifice. But in any fiscal crisis, redistributing the coffers of the wealthy is a short-term solution at best. Even Marcus's vast personal wealth could not rescue the Empire from the root causes of its economic malaise.

Marcus could barely afford to pay his soldiers. That did not stop them from demanding handouts anyway. The emperor raged against the nagging troops, informing his men that "whatever they obtained above their regular pay would be wrung from the blood of their parents and kinsmen."[37] And so legionaries were forced to make do with their standard pay, and that alone. Besides, even if Marcus wished to maintain his prodigal military spending of earlier years, he now lacked the necessary silver and gold to mint the coins. As a result, Roman officials must have crammed as many workers as they could find into the mines. Large numbers of people in enclosed spaces, working together on a daily basis; within mining communities, antiquity's communicable diseases must have hit paydirt. And mine workers came from a surprisingly diverse range of places, according to sources.[38] Roman soldiers, furthermore—undoubtedly a vector of transmission—were often garrisoned in resource-rich regions, if not near or even around extraction facilities themselves. Soldiers routinely administered and even labored in mines throughout the Roman Empire.[39] At the large gold mines at Alburnus Maior in Dacia (western Transylvania), for instance, not only was Legio V Macedonica in the vicinity according to literary sources and inscriptions, but bricks found near the site bear the mark of a second legion: Legio XIII Gemina.[40] Soldiers in both units fought in the Parthian and Marcomannic Wars. So even without knowing the Antonine plague pathogen, the case for transmission at mines seems rock solid.

Numerous sources indicate mass abandonment of mining operations at the time of the pandemic. No source, however, gives sufficient details to clarify the extent to which disease deaths contributed to the pause. Sometime around the start of the 170s, for example, the massive mining operations at Rio Tinto in southern Hispania slowed down—or at least the amount of pottery on the site declines sharply around that time, suggesting a general hiatus in operations.[41] At Alburnus Maior, a college of miners which paid members' funeral costs mysteriously dissolved in the winter of early AD 167. The depopulation is eye-opening: a stunning two-thirds of the college's members were no longer at the mine.[42] A wax tablet recounts the group's misfortunes but gives not a single detail as to what exactly happened to the men; it merely laments their absence. Then, just a few months later, *all* source material from the mine dries up. Some galleries were never mined again. Several historians believe that the pandemic made it to Dacia, and the missing miners were in fact disease victims.[43] This is a plausible theory. Recall that Legio V Macedonica—freshly returned from disease-ridden Parthian cities—was sent to the fort at Potaissa in Dacia, a mere sixty kilometers or so from Alburnus Maior. Soldiers and officers from the legion certainly visited the mines and some would have worked there. But local violence also must have been a factor. In the summer of 167, the Iazyges invaded the area, disrupting mining operations. Members of Legio V Macedonica eventually fought off the invaders, potentially transmitting plague to any Germanic tribesmen who survived.

New evidence now tells us even more about the state of Roman mines during the Antonine plague. For thousands of years, this evidence lay locked in ancient arctic ice. When Roman mines and mints smelted silver, lead particles wafted into the atmosphere. Each year, the snow that accumulated over Greenland deposited some of these particles on the frozen ground. Layers of pollutant-packed ice gradually formed, creating meter-by-meter an unimpeachable record of metallurgical activity (especially mining and coin production) in the territories of the northern and western Roman Empire. Recently a team of scientists, archaeologists, and historians reanalyzed cores from the Greenland ice showing thousands of years of lead emissions. Consistent with archaeological and numismatic evidence, the ice-core data reveal a clear decline in lead emissions during the second century AD, with an accelerated drop in the worst years of the Antonine plague.

These data are not perfect. Some Chinese emissions, for example, may also be present. But researchers were able to remove "background" emissions from natural causes and isolate emissions generated by human activity. The data seem sound because surges and sudden reversals in lead levels prior to the Antonine plague line up with significant numismatic events. Reflected in the data, for example, is Nero's massive spending splurge following Rome's Great Fire in the mid-60s. Another

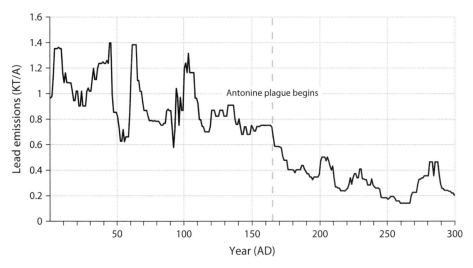

FIG. 6.2. Lead emissions in Greenland ice, AD 1–300.
McConnell et al. 2018. Line is 11-year median filtered estimated lead emissions
(kt/a).

peak in emissions occurs at the time when Trajan conquered Dacia and
ramped up mining and minting, whether to fund his wars or following
the windfall. Then, after fifty stable years during the retrenchment of the
mid-second century, the freefall began in AD 166. This time, however,
there would be no recovery until the time of Charlemagne. Lead emissions remained a fraction of what they were during the Pax Romana.
Whatever crisis struck mines and mints around the time of the Antonine plague, the damage outlasted the Roman Empire itself.

Statistical analyses of these data confirm two key turning points in
the second century AD which fit neatly with other data presented in this
book. A team of researchers at Stanford University performed a regres-
sion analysis which allowed the slope of the lead emission trendline to
change in the year AD 166—presumably the Antonine plague's most
severe year.[44] Indeed, the line turned down dramatically—from an average annual decrease of .25 percent to 1.4 percent—a nearly sixfold decrease, which suggests that AD 166 was a pivotal year in the data. But a
second statistical technique—change-point detection—is even more
sophisticated, and revealing. This approach applies a mathematical

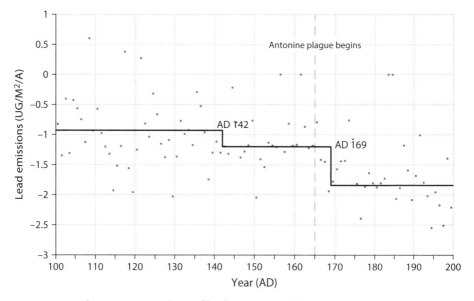

FIG. 6.3. Change-point analysis of lead emissions, AD 100–200.
The change-point detection was performed by Daniel Gaines of Indiana
University Department of Statistics on the logarithm of the non-background
lead flux data spanning AD 1–300. The R package change point was used to
create the model using the cpt.meanvar function with a BIC penalty on the
number of periods.

function to a data series in order to identify points in time where the
mean value of the data changes significantly. The Stanford team's analysis, as well as a second one performed by my Indiana University colleague Daniel Gaines (fig. 6.3), reveals not only a change point during
the Antonine plague period (Stanford: AD 174; Gaines: AD 169) but
also a mid-second-century change point (Stanford: AD 145; Gaines: AD
142). If these emissions figures are a proxy for mining and smelting activity, they seemingly confirm not only the impact of the Antonine
plague but also the stressful period that preceded it. The pandemic did
not attack a Pax Romana at its peak; rather, it accelerated a downturn
that was already gaining speed.

And both the pre-plague stresses and plague itself were not isolated to
mines. Quarries too—which like mines employed many laborers, from
numerous places, and in high-density working conditions—show similar

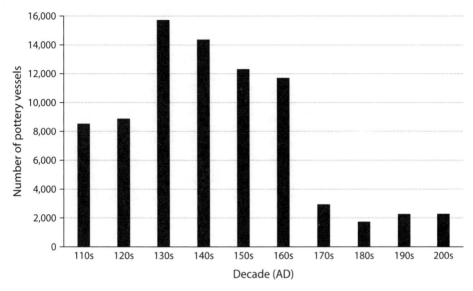

FIG. 6.4. Roman pottery vessels found in the City of London in the second century AD by decade.

These data, which were never published in full, are reproduced with the kind permission of Robin Symonds, who spent more than fourteen years working on Roman ceramics in London. Between 2001 and 2004, Symonds used these data to produce several graphs under the aegis of the Museum of London Archaeology Service. The wider data set includes 463,330 sherds and runs from AD 40 to 400. The reduction in discovered vessels (as well as sherds) following the decade AD 151–160 is sustained through the chronological end of the database (i.e., through AD 400). An explanation of the database can be found in Symonds 2008. See also Symonds 2006; Perring 2022, 283.

patterns of exhaustion and abandonment. The marble quarries at Docimium (in western Asia Minor), for example, seem to have shut down—or at least they produce no dated blocks after 165 through the year 173.[45] Another quarry in the same region—the *africano* marble quarry at Teos (on the western coast of Asia Minor) which provided beautiful black and red rock exclusively for the city of Rome—was similarly abandoned in or around 166.[46] Plenty of valuable stone was left in the ground at these sites, but there was seemingly no one to recover it.

In Londinium, many industries dramatically halted operations. Several mills were abandoned. Local kilns stopped producing tiles and bricks. Glass-making workshops near the city's amphitheater failed abruptly. Soil studies show that the once bustling industrial area became open land. The quarry on the east side of the city was filled in. Timber imports slowed. And perhaps most dramatically, an impressive database of some 463,330 Roman pottery sherds recovered from the City of London shows a sudden and permanent drop in the AD 160s (fig. 6.4). Lingering signs of depopulation include two coin hoards buried in AD 166 and 174 that went unrecovered. All told, between one- and two-thirds of urban plots in Londinium that were still occupied in the mid-second century were abandoned within two generations—a contraction which suggests that as many as 10,000–20,000 of the city's 30,000 inhabitants simply vanished. Where did the missing go? Excavations of Roman settlements in the surrounding countryside show similar signs of contraction; the missing Londoners, therefore, did not migrate to rural sites. The pandemic may very well have killed thousands in London. The permanent drop in pottery sherds, however, hints at a concurrent long-term evacuation of the entire region. Until the 160s, Londinium enjoyed a strong military presence—likely several thousand soldiers. In frontier provinces like Britain, the Roman military drove economic activity. Around the time of the Marcomannic Wars, however, many of London's soldiers were redeployed elsewhere, drying up demand for production in the city. Food shortages and reforms of the city's grain distribution scheme—modeled after Rome's—may too have aided in the city's late second-century demise.[47] Either way, Londinium never fully recovered.

Did the pandemic kill workers in mines, quarries, and other industries across the Empire? Certainly. But as with so much else in the era of the Antonine plague, the Empire's social and economic preconditions and comorbidities played a major role in the pandemic's broader effects. Imperial policy as well as climate change were likely involved. Readers may recall that Egyptian grain production became less stable from the 150s. We also know from Roman legal records that Marcus (and Lucius in one case) enacted laws privileging the Empire's largest maritime transportation operations toward servicing the Roman grain supply.[48] As the *annona* system fell under strain from poor Egyptian floods, the emperors did not suddenly build fleets of new ships; rather, they used state power to repurpose existing transportation resources and infrastructure. Ships that had moved stone from quarries and wood (for smelting metal), for instance, now moved fewer of those goods, and instead transported grain to soldiers and select cities. As a consequence, operations designed to extract and transport those same resources may have declined, or even paused. The reallocation of infrastructure may have been intended to be temporary, but if, as it seems, grain shortages endured for years or even decades, an increasingly permanent economic reorientation would usher in a more meager new normal. Mine and quarry workers may have indeed died en masse from plague, but a large-scale restructuring of the Roman economy to serve the military and Rome's insatiable food needs would have exacerbated economic woes.

Local factors, too—some of them directly caused by the Antonine plague, but some unrelated—may have been responsible for work stoppages. Flooding was a common problem in mines as well as quarries. The unexpected discovery of an aquifer could bring a quick and sustained halt to work. Any modern archaeologist will confirm that the fight against the water table at many excavations—even with modern pumping equipment—is a persistent threat. Flooding may have been behind the stoppage at the marble quarry at Teos, for example.[49] An engineer, if one was available, could employ screw systems for lifting water out of flooded areas, but such machines needed constant human labor for power. And even if the state somehow found and brought in emergency workers—forced laborers, prisoners of war, convicts, requisitioned slaves—there was still only so much that could be done once serious flooding began.[50] And stone production in Asia Minor was already falling decades before the Antonine plague's inaugural years.[51] The same is true of the Egyptian quarry at Mons Claudianus (in the eastern desert), which shows signs of a slowdown from the mid-150s (as do so many other proxies from Roman Egypt).[52] When the pandemic finally arrived and swept through communities of quarry workers, it was probably the deciding factor following years of pre-pandemic problems.

The warfare that sprang up under Marcus too cannot be ignored. The Marcomannic Wars alone would have been sufficient to halt mining operations in contested areas during the 170s, regardless of plague's impact. Alburnus Maior's shutdown was clearly connected to the war, although plague deaths almost certainly preceded the pause, and then stymied the resumption of operations. But what of mine stoppages in Hispania or Britain?[53] Germanic peoples did not invade those areas. And emissions from those mines factor most strongly in the Greenland ice cores according to regional wind patterns. Roman interests in Hispania, however, were faced with an incursion of raiders from Mauritania along the North African coast from AD 171. With only one legion left to defend the entire province—and a hot war in Magna Germania demanding the full attention of the Roman military—southern Hispania became overrun. Mines were abandoned, but so were the fields. Shipments of olive oil from Baetica in southern Iberia to Rome's port at Ostia decline by orders of magnitude contemporary with the mining disruption.[54] Mauri raiders remained an ongoing threat in the region through the 180s. Plague would have augmented and even prolonged the local crisis, of course, but clearly warfare was a decisive factor.

As deaths from disease and ever-growing military conflicts mounted, the value of labor would have increased through the AD 170s. Information on Roman wages from most parts of the Empire is either unavailable or simply too scarce to be statistically useful. Yet again, Egypt is the exception. Several hundred wage rates survive in papyri, showing what we would expect during and after a sudden surge in mortality. The few wages datable to the first years of the Antonine plague (AD 166–170) are 1.5 times the average from the previous decades of the second century (AD 104–165). Typically, the agricultural cycle must have driven wages of unskilled workers in Egypt: plentiful harvests placed higher demands on fieldworker labor, and years of poor flooding meant lower demand. In four out of the five years between 166 and 170, however, the floods were terrible. Demand would have been low, and hence so too should have been the wages offered to fieldworkers. So the high wages in that period truly are an anomaly and must be explained by factors exogenous to the agricultural cycle. A deadly outbreak of disease, therefore, seems a likely contributor to Egypt's problems during those years. But violence, climate change, and tax flight also afflicted the region.[55] The local silver coinage was also faltering.[56] Economic realities permanently changed. Nominal wages in third-century Egypt are more than double their equivalent counterparts in the second century.[57] If only we had more wage data from the rest of the Empire for comparison!

Did plague also drive labor costs to new heights elsewhere? Mine and quarry shutdowns in numerous regions suggest a general labor shortage.[58] In addition to requiring large numbers of unskilled workers, both slave and free, skilled workers were essential for restarting operations. After months or even years of abandonment, some mine galleries and quarries would have flooded or collapsed beyond repair. Resuming normal operations—if "normality" as such was even possible—required educated and experienced specialists. Indeed, according to an inscription found at the mines at Vipasca in southern Hispania, a "Restorer of Mines" (*restitutor metallorum*) was sent to the area sometime during Marcus's reign, likely in the late 170s.[59] Such specialists were hard to find under normal conditions, but if some were killed or displaced by the pandemic, the effects on economic production would have endured for years. The economic impact of the Antonine plague, therefore—even if direct mortality was not particularly high—may have reverberated for decades following its initial entrance into Roman territory.

But what about slave labor? Slaves required no wages, and could have filled gaps in the labor force. And yet, even slaves, gladiators, and other unpaid laborers seem to have become more difficult to find, and expensive too.[60] Economic theory offers one explanation: when one good or service becomes suddenly expensive, demand shifts to alternatives, driving prices up in those goods too. But Rome's wars typically drove slave prices downward, not upward. Romans used wars to capture new markets in human property, increasing supply. Julius Caesar's war in Gaul (58–50 BC) netted as many as one million slaves according to the Roman writer Appian—an obviously fictitious figure, but Caesar's captives must have numbered in the tens of thousands at least.[61] Images from Marcus's victory column suggest the Marcomannic Wars generated a windfall of enslaved men, women, and children. Still, the number of captured slaves was apparently dwarfed by slaves lost to emergency recruitment and killed by disease.

State intervention, as ever, burdened labor markets further. Sales taxes on gladiators, many of whom were slaves, were as high as 25 and 33 percent.[62] The high costs of gladiators created serious problems for priests of the imperial cult, governors, senators, and other public officials obligated by tradition and their station to fund lavish public entertainments (*munera*). One priest in the AD 170s complained that he "despaired of his fortune when he had been made priest" because his estate was "crushed" by the expenses associated with "provision of a public spectacle."[63] Government relief in the midst of soaring prices was slow to arrive, but finally in AD 177 Marcus enacted a series of reforms. First, the tax on gladiator sales was abolished. Second, the government set a mandatory price ceiling on the cost of booking gladiatorial combat. Finally, and most significant for its long-term effects, Marcus streamlined financial and legal barriers to performing public executions in the arena. Under the new laws, condemned men and women could now be sold for "not more than six gold pieces" to those who put on public spectacles.[64] Elites throughout the Empire celebrated the new laws, as senatorial proclamations of thanksgiving posted in Asia Minor and Hispania attest.[65] In reality, the consequences of these seemingly technical provisions were far-reaching indeed— perhaps escalating religious persecution.

All laws have unintended and often perverse effects; Marcus's new rules were no different. His tax cuts on gladiator sales lost the treasury between 5 and 7.5 million denarii per year—the equivalent of the annual pay of three to four legions.[66] At a time of poor military recruitment and soldiers agitating for higher wages, the revenue loss must have cut deep. As for the slave market, if anything, Marcus's tinkering made the situation even worse. The fixed prices of gladiators, like all price ceilings, would have backfired—exacerbating rather than alleviating the shortage. Why would a gladiator school or owner lease out his valuable performers at prices which failed to cover costs or generate a profit? But if gladiators became even scarcer due to the price ceilings, a ready-made alternative "entertainment" was provided by the provision allowing condemned criminals to be bought on the cheap for public execution. No gladiators available? Buy a few criminals at no more than six gold coins each; then design elaborate, torturous, and gruesome modes of death for mass enjoyment: a bloody spectacle for the whole family! All that was needed was an abundant supply of the condemned. And it just so happened that a growing movement of dangerous religious extremists was practically volunteering for execution at the time of the Antonine plague: Christians.[67] Convicting Christians of a capital crime was scandalously simple: drag them before the governor and accuse them of being Christians; demand they recant their faith and offer sacrifices; when they refuse, condemn them to death and sell them for peanuts to spectacle organizers for humiliation before crowds of anxiety-ridden onlookers eager to punish *someone* for the calamities of the age. It was all too easy. The Christians massacred in Gaul in AD 177 may have represented the law's pilot program.[68] Eusebius says as much: "And so, once their souls had endured the great contest for a long while, they reached the end, having become on that day a spectacle for the cosmos in place of all the various forms of single combat."[69] The Antonine plague, therefore, may have been the crucial link in the chain of events that led Roman officials to spill countless gallons of Christian blood upon the crimson sands of Roman arenas for decades to come.

A Faltering Food Supply

Even absent epidemics, economic life in the Roman Empire was precarious. And during the Antonine plague years too, some people simply fell on bad luck—and plague had little to do with their misfortunes. But pandemic is by definition all-encompassing, and historians too might be prone to give plagues, poxes, and other scourges undue credit for more complex economic and social ills. Some scholars associate the Antonine plague with an inscription from the Italian port of Puteoli, for example, in which a group of traders from the eastern Mediterranean city of Tyre note: "we are few in number" but "in the past [we] . . . were numerous and wealthy."[70] The lengthy inscription, dated to AD 174 or 175, goes on to record how the down-on-their-luck traders requested their home city subsidize the rent on the trading station in Puteoli. The inscription mentions neither plague nor death—a surprising omission if the whole point of the traders' request was to generate sympathy among their countrymen back in Tyre. Is this inscription really evidence that mass numbers of Tyrian traders in Puteoli died in the Antonine plague? Plague was no doubt woven into the Puteolians' plight but so too were drought, climate, and infrastructure problems. The inscription may thus be a prime example of the complex ecological, epidemiological, and economic crisis in full bloom in the 170s.

Despite being roughly 200 kilometers southeast of Rome, Puteoli had been the main port for receiving Egyptian tax grain in the first century AD. But under Claudius and then Trajan, the much nearer harbors of Portus and Ostia were vastly improved. Over time, deliveries of Egyptian grain shifted to those sites. But Puteoli still had grain warehouses in abundance, and so the port continued to receive Alexandrian grain— potentially after Portus and Ostia were full—even through the middle and late second century.[71] The Tyrians in Puteoli, however, did not trade in grain. We know this because their building rented for a mere 250 denarii a year.[72] Large grain warehouses would have rented for tens of thousands of denarii annually. So the Tyrians' building was a small clubhouse or storage building, likely holding small but expensive goods. We know that luxury goods tended to travel to Italian ports via the Alexandrian grain ships; such high-value cargoes were, in fact, crucial for making grain deliveries financially viable. But if the Egyptian grain harvest was in crisis in the 170s, then the transport of luxury goods to Puteoli would have also been disrupted. This was, in fact, exactly what was going on.

Droughts in Egypt were already a problem prior to the Antonine plague, as we saw earlier. Things seemingly got much worse in the AD 170s. Worker deaths from epidemics, and concomitant shortages and high wages, must have been a factor. But the cumulative effect of year after year of weak floods eventually exacerbated Egypt's ability to serve as Rome's chief breadbasket. We already saw the evidence for a serious drought. For the entire duration of the pandemic, a bountiful Nile flood occurred only once. But another surprising proxy also confirms the seriousness of the grain shortage in the 170s: Egyptian coinage.

Egypt had operated a successful independent coinage system for centuries—upheld by strong grain production. After the Roman gov-

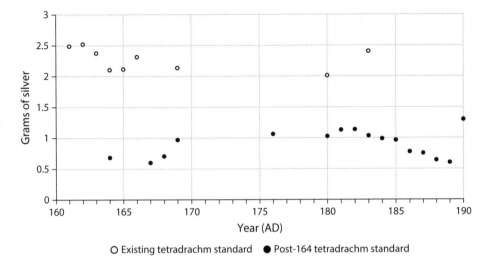

FIG. 6.5. Coin (tetradrachm) quality in Roman Egypt, AD 160–190.
Elliott 2020a; Howgego, Butcher, and Ponting, forthcoming.

ernment took its tax quota in grain from Egypt, any remaining grain was made available for sale at the discretion of the Egyptian prefect. But there was a catch. Anyone who wished to purchase leftover Egyptian grain had to first trade in their non-Egyptian coins for local Alexandria-produced tetradrachms. The mandatory currency exchange was a racket, and a lucrative one at that. Alexandrian tetradrachms were pinned as equal in value to Roman denarii, but in fact the tetradrachm contained only 75 percent of the silver compared to its supposed equivalent in the Roman denarius. This disparity in the two currencies generated a substantial profit in silver to the Alexandrian mint. The mint, in turn, diluted this silver into even more debased tetradrachms. But whenever the grain supply dropped, and outsiders took their money to buy grain elsewhere, Egypt's silver supply correspondingly diminished, and the quantity and sometimes quality of tetradrachms suffered. Foreign silver could still enter the province from other sources—especially trade in luxury goods—but the droughts that began before the Antonine plague seem to have affected the Alexandrian coinage.

With their silver stocks low by AD 164, the Alexandrian mint was forced to experiment with a sharply lower tetradrachm standard—cutting out

around two-thirds of the silver from some coins. The move was drastic
and desperate, and hardly fixed the real problem. So around 170, the
mint had no choice but to pause the production of coins altogether. The
hiatus lasted for the better part of the decade. Only one year, that which
followed the abundant flood in 174/5—the first excellent harvest in
years according to flood reports—saw *any* coins produced. Then the
bad years apparently returned, and regular coin production did not re-
sume until the 180s. By then, silver stocks were so low that the old tetradrachm standard disappeared forever.

Poor floods and then plague pummeled Egypt. The uptick in deaths
of fieldworkers and estate owners combined with monetary insecurity,
tax flight, banditry, and violence. Some landowners abandoned their
holdings or liquidated parcels at rock-bottom prices out of desperation.
We see this situation most clearly in real prices of Egyptian land
(measured against wheat rather than coinage due to the varying silver
standards and money supply).

Despite gaps in these data (see fig. 6.6.), a few trends are visible. First,
land prices prior to AD 165 average just shy of 60 hectoliters of wheat
per hectare of land (58.34 hL/hectare). From 165 to the 260s, the average
land price is half that figure (27.94 hL/hectare). To take another
measure: four of the five highest prices in the collection date between
AD 128 and 159, while three of the five lowest date during AD 170–184.[73]
The bubble in real estate values in the second quarter of the second
century correlates with the best floods of the entire century (see fig. 2.2).
With so many floods reaching the ideal of 14–16 cubits between AD 125
and 150, plots of land—especially those which only flooded under ideal
conditions—must have been flush with crop. The troubles of the 160s
and 170s had not yet arrived, and labor was plentiful. As a result, foreign
silver poured into Egypt as outsiders purchased the abundant grain. In
the years just ahead of the Antonine plague, however, the abundant
floods diminished, demand dried up, and land values began to drop. The
pandemic then shocked the labor market. Plague deaths brought on a
worker shortage; without workers, land was left fallow, sold, or abandoned, depressing land values even more. When occasional good floods
returned in the last decades of the second century, the worker shortage

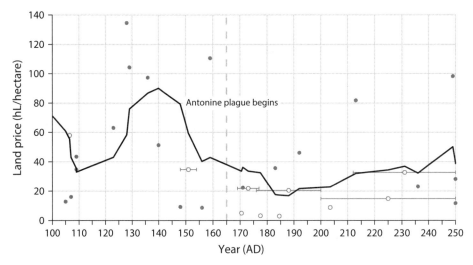

FIG. 6.6. Real land prices in Roman Egypt (hectoliters of wheat per hectare), AD 100–250.

The black line represents a 5-point moving average. Raw data: Harper 2016b. I have removed two prices which could not be dated to within half a century and added error bars in other prices to account for uncertain dates (hollow circles). For the rationale for such an approach, see Elliott 2020b. Harper's original graph and analysis, however, provide a good picture of changing land prices; see Harper 2016c, 820–22.

and high costs of labor likely kept overall crop yields in the province low. In the long run, therefore, Egyptian land values never recovered.

Real land rental prices in Egypt show a similar trend, only less pronounced, and with a noticeable lag (fig. 6.7). Again, prior to AD 165, rents average higher (8.23 hL/hectare) than the period following (5.96 hL/hectare), but the gap is less than that associated with land sales. And like land sales, the highest prices tend to cluster in the second quarter of the second century, with six of the top ten occurring between AD 125 and 163. But a cluster of the lowest prices (five of the bottom ten) appears not during or immediately after the Antonine plague but later in the first quarter of the third century. Despite plummeting land values, landowners were able to hold the line on rents. The rental market could be flexible; part of landlords' coping strategy involved lengthening lease terms and reducing parcel sizes.[74] But also, some dispossessed

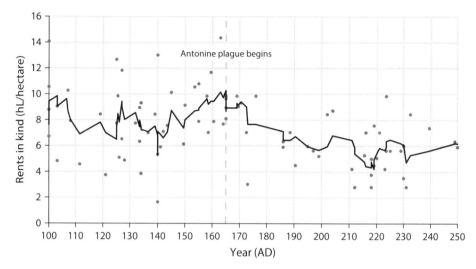

FIG. 6.7. Real rents in Roman Egypt (hectoliters of wheat per hectare), AD 100–250.
The dark line represents a 5-point moving average. Raw data: Harper 2016b. This chart includes some uncertain data that could not be removed.

smallholders undoubtedly had to turn around and rent land, perhaps even plots they used to own, to survive and pay taxes—keeping rents high against sale prices.

Egyptian data show in stark terms the exhaustion of both the local workforce and the land both before and then during the Antonine plague. But Egypt's problems gradually became the Empire's problems. Our Tyrian traders in Rome felt the pain, but so too did Marcus. In the spring of AD 175, the troubles in Egypt—plague, famine, worker shortages, tax flight, banditry—boiled over into outright revolution. Avidius Cassius—loyal general, hero of the Parthian War, defender of Alexandria, and "Supreme Commander of the Orient"—unexpectedly betrayed Marcus and proclaimed himself emperor.[75] The usurpation seemingly came out of nowhere, but Cassius had clearly prepared his coup because many of the eastern governors and their legions extended immediate allegiance to the usurper.

Cassius's motivations are mysterious, but the theory advanced at the time sees sickness as the catalyst. While on the presumably pestilential

German front, Marcus contracted a disease that no source names. It was the first of two times the emperor would be gravely ill. We cannot know if either instance was the disease associated with the Antonine plague, but a connection seems possible, if not probable. During this first sickness, at least some close to the emperor, including his wife Faustina, assumed Marcus would die. Indeed, in the sections of Marcus's *Meditations* composed around this time, the emperor spoke of being "on the verge of death."[76] In a panic, Faustina supposedly wrote Cassius—promising him both her hand and the Empire once Marcus inevitably succumbed to the disease.[77] Shortly after Cassius received Faustina's letter, a rumor followed claiming Marcus had died. Failing to fact-check the gossip, Cassius seized the moment, declaring himself emperor. There is at least one benign explanation for the move. Marcus's son and heir, Commodus, was a mere thirteen years old and ineligible to take over for his father. If Marcus had suddenly succumbed to sickness, Cassius's move would have spared the Empire a succession crisis and civil war.

Marcus, however, defied the odds and recovered. But the disease forever scarred him. His body, according to several sources, remained wracked and weak until his death five years later. Galen mixed theriac daily for the emperor—and the opium would have helped Marcus endure the lingering pain in his chest and stomach.[78] Eventually, the bedraggled emperor became well enough to address his soldiers on the coming civil war with Cassius, but even then he was vulnerable, revealing to his troops that he was "unable to take food without pain, and sleep without anxiety."[79]

Cassius's rebellion clearly sent waves of unrest through a panicked and exhausted Empire, and perhaps even threw martial fidelity into question. Retribution was nasty for anyone—even lowly legionaries— who chose the wrong side in a Roman civil war. The insecurity of the moment is captured in the coinage of that year. For the first and only time in his entire reign, Marcus issued coins proclaiming the "harmony of the soldiers" (CONCORD EXERC). Upholding the slogan was an image of clasped hands holding a legionary standard. As with most propaganda issued during a crisis, the official line is typically opposite the truth. In Roman numismatic history, legends proclaiming the "harmony

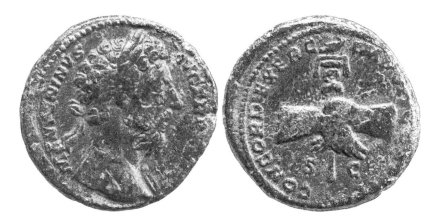

FIG. 6.8. Copper as of Marcus Aurelius minted in Rome in AD 174/5 (likely summer of 175). Clasped hands hold a legionary standard surrounded by a legend which proclaims, in part, the "harmony of the soldiers" (CONCORD EXERC). The British Museum Images. Coin, Marcus Aurelius, Roman Empire. IDs: 01613844684 and 01613844685.

of the soldiers" often appeared at times of rebellion or outright civil war. A similar inscription, for example, marked the coins of the short-lived emperor Vitellius (AD 69) after the eastern governor Vespasian was made emperor by his own troops in AD 69. The emperor Nerva (AD 96–98) dusted off the slogan and images around the time his own soldiers besieged him in the imperial palace in AD 97, not long after the assassination of his predecessor Domitian. Marcus's rare use of such propaganda suggests that he indeed feared his soldiers might abandon him. Cassius had been wildly successful as a commander—making swift work of the Parthians. Meanwhile, Marcus's soldiers, many of whom had formed battle-tested bonds with Cassius in Parthia, were languishing in a seemingly unwinnable war in the disease-ridden marshes and forests of Magna Germania.

A stroke of luck, however, enabled Marcus to keep both his soldiers and his empire for at least a little while longer. One of Cassius's own centurions murdered the usurper in the summer of 175. Before a single battle was even fought, Marcus received Cassius's head by courier. The new Syrian governor, Martius Verus, summarily burned all of Cassius's documents—protecting all who had been involved in the rebellion from accountability.

We do not know the extent to which the rebellion further disrupted Egyptian grain supplies to Rome. But with Egypt in turmoil, the overall health of the city's population—already precarious due to terrible sanitation, and weakened by apparent shortages in the 160s—could not have improved in the 170s. Other cities, towns, and settlements in the western Empire too, even if they escaped the direct effects of the pandemic, began to suffer as its indirect effects—shortages, unpayable rent, banditry—reached their communities. No doubt many of those impacted took to flight, swarming the major cities in a renewed surge of migrations. Eventually, even Rome's soldiers wavered—their loyalty to Marcus, his German war, and even the Empire itself became debased much like the coinage that bore the emperor's philosophic countenance and increasingly hollow honorifics and promises.

Plague's Fugitives

With Avidius Cassius's death in the summer of 175, Marcus may have realized that his myopic focus on a single frontier was unwise. The political fragmentation that had just occurred was a sign of a more foundational crisis. Egypt, at the very least, demanded his immediate personal attention. The emperor, therefore, made a hasty peace with the Germanic tribes and began an eastward march to shore up his crumbling Empire.[80]

It is from this time that direct evidence for a continuing pandemic becomes difficult to dig up. The final references to the Antonine plague come from Galen. In his book on pulses—composed during his second stay in Rome in the early to mid-170s—the doctor speaks of the pestilence "still raging" (presumably in Rome, but maybe elsewhere).[81] Then, sometime between 172 and 175, Galen published a therapeutic treatise in which he discusses a telltale symptom of the disease: ulcerations in the throat. In mid prose, Galen exclaims: "the great pestilence, may it cease someday!"[82] It may be no coincidence that the Antonine

plague's disappearance in the sources—even in Galen's writings—
follows directly after Avidius Cassius's failed coup d'état. Marcus nearly
died of disease, and remained weak. Commodus was too young to take
over. Speaking of sickness may have become taboo, at least for those in
the emperor's inner circle (or who aspired to remain there). Here is
another eerie parallel between ancient Rome and Han China. But
whereas talk of widespread pestilence threatened the Han emperor's
Mandate of Heaven, concerns among the court of Marcus Aurelius may
have been far more practical. Marcus's sickness reminded everyone that
the reigning dynasty was on life support until Commodus came of age
in AD 179. The suddenness of Avidius Cassius's usurpation evidenced
that even the faintest whiff of sickness or weakness in the reigning emperor or his heir could bring challengers, even open civil war.

Commodus, however, became sick around the same time as his father.
We should expect the emperor's sole heir's sickness to have been widely
reported, but only Galen's *On Prognosis*—published in the late 170s—
preserves a little of what happened.[83] Galen downplays Commodus's
ailment as not too dangerous—just a fever and an inflamed throat. In
other words: nothing to see here, folks. But Galen's recollection is odd,
to say the least. Galen describes two of Commodus's symptoms: "quite
a hot fever" and sores in the boy's throat. The doctor, ever aware of his
competition, is quick to blame the sores on another physician's efforts to
treat Commodus's condition with a mixture of honey and sumac. But
these ingredients were not known to cause such sores. Even more odd:
if Commodus had only just then become sick, why had he been taking
medicine for a throat condition? It would seem that Commodus then
had both a fever and sores in the throat—two known symptoms Galen
elsewhere associates with the Antonine plague. Did Commodus catch
the infamous disease but escape with a mild case?

Stranger still, while Galen dismisses Commodus's illness as unex-
ceptional, it is clear from Galen's own account that some believed the
boy's life was in jeopardy. Several days after Commodus first became
ill, his cousin Annia Faustina burst into the young prince's chamber
with a small army of physicians in an attempt to save the teenager's life.
Annia believed Commodus had caught something deadly, and ques-

tioned Galen for bathing him after only two days in his care. Galen treated fevers by proscribing baths, but this was also his treatment for skin conditions and "buboes."[84] In the early 1900s, archaeologists recovered a small jewel—a cameo of a youthful Commodus once embedded in a sacrificial bowl—from a monastery in northern Spain. A still-legible inscription in Greek suggests that the item not only had belonged to the imperial family but seems to commemorate the young prince's survival following a grave illness. The inscription, commissioned by a "Faustina" (His worried cousin? Perhaps his mother or sister?), reads: "with Commodus safe, Faustina is fortunate."[85] We cannot know how or even if the jewel is connected to Galen's strange story, but the doctor records no other childhood illness for Commodus. In fact, neither Cassius Dio nor the early third-century Greek historian Herodian says anything about Commodus being sick, ever. A later biography, however, written long after the reigns of both Marcus and Commodus, does. It claims that Commodus was "weak and diseased" and had a "conspicuous growth on his groin."[86] The biographer's source for this information is supposedly the biography of one Marius Maximus—who indeed lived during the reign of Commodus—but his work has vanished from the historical record.

Finally, *On Prognosis*—Galen's treatise in which the story appears—was written when Commodus had just been given full imperial power alongside his sickly father in the late 170s. Perhaps the aging and increasingly feeble Marcus did not wish it widely known that his only surviving son and heir—and now co-emperor—also had a history of serious illness, even plague? When Marcus himself had been weakened by disease in AD 175, he faced the first usurpation of a living emperor in generations. It would have been disastrous for his sole surviving son and heir to have had the same life-threatening sickness as well—the Antonine plague disease or otherwise—even if recovered. In fact, all mention of pestilence is curiously scrubbed from Galen's *On Prognosis*, including in places where it definitely should appear: in his account of Lucius's return from Parthian territory, his story of events in the city of Rome in 166, and especially his memories of the dark winter in Aquileia.[87] It is as though the Antonine plague itself never happened.

Maybe the worst of the pandemic was indeed behind the Romans. But the longer-term repercussions of cumulative plague mortality, even if the death count was finally slowing, translated into broader and long-lasting social disorder. At least one ongoing problem, however, temporarily diminished. Marcus formally "ended" the Marcomannic Wars by treaty. In reality, tens of thousands of Roman soldiers remained on the German front, and hostilities would flare up again in just a couple years. The temporary lull in the conflict, however, undoubtedly prompted new troop movements. Veterans of the Marcomannic Wars—both Romans and many Germanic tribesmen pushed into service for Rome as part of the conditions of the treaty—were redeployed elsewhere in the Empire. As after the Parthian War, it is worth asking: did some of these soldiers carry plague? Probably, but unlike accounts of the late 160s and early 170s, there is no mention of sickness in these soldiers.

A large number of soldiers traveled east with Marcus. No account gives the size of the force, but we know it was composed of detachments of recently mollified Marcomanni, Quadi, and Naristi as well as Roman legionaries from Pannonia.[88] The full group must have numbered in the thousands because two Roman legates were required to supervise the entourage. The emperor's family and the imperial court also tagged along. Here too, we can merely speculate about disease transmission. This group, however, due to its sheer size and also the seasons during which it traveled—autumn, winter, and spring—seems the most likely plague vector of all known troop dispersals following this pause amid the Marcomannic Wars. And, because of the group's high-profile members, ancient writers give details of the voyage. Modern historians have wondered if some of these details are at least suggestive of an ongoing plague. Faustina mysteriously died in the winter of late 175 in a Cappadocian village. Unfortunately, contemporary authors offer no cause of death. They speculate, of course. Cassius Dio, for example, wondered if she was murdered or committed suicide to cover her alleged involvement in the rebellion of Avidius Cassius.[89] Plague is not mentioned in any source. Marcus, however, mourned Faustina as a loyal wife and subject. He renamed the village of Halala, where she died, Faustinopolis. The Senate voted the late empress divine honors and the mint produced coins with her image and titles.[90] Faustina's death alone, however, is no clear indication that plague was active in the traveling party, or even in the eastern Empire for that matter.

Only one other tenuous link between Marcus's eastern travels and plague exists. Marcus arrived in Egypt sometime near the end of winter in early AD 176. He toured Alexandria's temples and public buildings, while members of his party explored other parts of the province.[91] Two winters later, after so many veteran soldiers visited and stayed in Egypt, the tourist village of Soknopaiou Nesos would see its male population drop by one-third.[92] As with so many other pieces of evidence, however, there is no direct mention of plague or even death in the account of the village's sudden change in population. The citizens simply are no longer *there*. And the two-year gap seems to prohibit a case for direct transmission from Marcus's party. Another dead end.

But the Antonine plague's ominous echoes continued to reverberate. The ongoing effects of mortality, combined with the comorbidities of the era, festered in broader Roman society. Other soldiers, for example, dispersed from the northern front, but these left secretly and in disgrace. Yes, deserters—but also fugitive slaves and bandits—began migrating through and subsequently terrorizing various parts of the Empire in large numbers in the 170s. As Marcus traversed his empire, it became impossible to ignore alarming reports of brigandage in previously pacified regions. The Pax Romana was breaking down.[93]

Even before returning to Rome, Marcus appointed one of his traveling legates—Marcus Valerius Maximianus—to ferret out the bandits rampaging in the Balkans south of Dacia.[94] Neighboring Dalmatia to the west was similarly beset by hostile groups on its borders, demanding the attention of its governor Didius Julianus.[95] In Sparta, inscriptions testify to "revolutions" in the area—almost certainly civil unrest—and the local coinage was debased.[96] Evidentially, the *Boukoloi* rebellion in Egypt—a product of plague, famine, taxes, and predatory officials— was no isolated incident. Rather, it was a canary in the mineshaft.

The Pax Romana had been poisoned by a pandemic, lengthy wars along the Empire's periphery, and the decade of stresses that preceded these tumultuous events. The desperation of the era soaked deeper into the Empire's basic social fabric, as organic uprisings of deserters and brigands spread like a virus. Not unlike the Egyptian *Boukoloi*, some brigands were tax evaders driven to flight—their normal burdens made suddenly onerous by depopulation from plague and wars. A contemporary inscription from Xanthos in Lycia (southwestern Asia Minor) commemorates a local elite who established a fund to supplement the population's inability to pay their standard taxes.[97] But few enjoyed the fortune of such benefactors; instead, they fled the predation of officials and landlords. Unlike the *Boukoloi*, however, who were largely pastoralists, the bands of brigands in Asia Minor and the Balkans were joined by former soldiers with military training and equipment. These groups were capable of acting tactically to ambush, plunder, and murder civilians as well as any soldiers sent against them.

Why might once loyal veterans have deserted their units in such large numbers? The penalties for desertion, after all, were severe. Breaking one's military oath brought a permanent and official curse. Deserters were hunted down and punished like runaway slaves.[98] But the consequences of the pandemic's initial sweep through the Roman military in the latter half of the 160s, and officials' short-sighted efforts to cope with the problem, were now bearing fruit. As readers may recall, Marcus's army had been seemingly decimated by plague even before the Marcomannic Wars formally began, forcing the emperor to take in slaves, gladiators, and even outlaws to fill the gaps in the military. With reduced numbers of soldiers, and many raw and unconventional recruits, the war warped into a quagmire. Casualties from crushing defeats—and the Romans clearly lost several battles—but ongoing deaths from epidemics too no doubt, depleted and demoralized military units. The new recruits—already of questionable fidelity to their commanders—as well as perhaps some regular soldiers with little to left to lose, performed the calculus and determined it was worthwhile to seek their fortunes elsewhere. Once they left, there was no going back.

Marcus's salary freeze at 300 denarii per year had not helped matters. Soldiers' equipment costs meanwhile, which were deducted from those stagnant salaries, must have been on the rise during the war.[99] Even under normal conditions, where soldiers spent much of their time garrisoned in camps, around half of soldiers' pay was lost to mandatory equipment, food, and supply deductions.[100] Even the Roman soldiers garrisoned in Judea in the early first century AD, for example, were tempted to break the law to alleviate their monetary troubles. Thus Jesus advised them: "do not extort money from anyone by threats of false accusation, and be content with your wages."[101] But Marcus's northern soldiers fought a hot war, where footwear, armor, and weapons were more easily lost or damaged. A set of armor, for example, was not cheap—likely priced at more than a year's salary. Faced with the choice of going into debt to replace such high-cost items or simply vanishing from the legions, some poor soldiers must have chosen the latter. During the chaotic third century AD, with its constant civil and foreign wars, emperors desperately tried to preserve military fidelity by paying out frequent and exorbitant bonuses—albeit in heavily debased coins (a woefully short-sighted solution). But as mentioned before, Marcus handed out not one single bonus in the worst years of the war between 170 and 175.[102] As a result, the once generous emperor gained a reputation as stingy and "economical," according to Cassius Dio.[103] But the lingering fumes of the Pax Romana ensured that Marcus avoided the nonstop civil war, rebellions, and invasions that sprang up in the third century AD. In fact, only a few decades after Marcus, the emperor Septimius Severus (AD 193–211)—who served as Marcus's legate—adopted a philosophy of rule that befitted the embryonic post-Pax era: "enrich the soldiers, and scorn all other men."[104]

Any of the factors concomitant with the troubles of the Antonine plague era—epidemic outbreaks, war fatigue, stagnant pay—would have been enough to generate low-level desertion even among regular troops, let alone hastily recruited former slaves, gladiators, and bandits. In the 170s, all these factors hit the legions simultaneously, and hard. The exodus must have been copious and constant. Mass desertion may explain the sudden downturn in finds of bronze military diplomas noted earlier in the chapter. The crime wave was so serious to elicit open elite complaints concerning the rise of criminality in Marcus's final years, even in the Empire's core territories. This was a serious development. Roman writers often evaded frank discussions of social disorder—slave revolts, rebellions, and brigandage—especially under "good" emperors like Marcus. Some emperors even interpreted such talk as treason, and punished it accordingly. Elites also remembered the chaos of the Late Republic, and thus imbibed a healthy fear of uprisings of any sort. One tactic contemporary Roman writers used to keep unrest under control was to ignore it and hope it went away. Writing about ongoing rebellion, even in a negative light, may inspire copycats. But brigandage went viral, and other disaffected groups joined the ranks of deserters and bandits.

Slaves appear to have run away in high numbers during the Antonine plague. Fear of plague mortality alone may have driven some slave flight, but even catching a non-lethal case posed a problem for slaves. Unwell slaves might be quietly killed by their masters, despite formal laws against such barbarity.[105] Some slaves may have also escaped when their masters succumbed to sickness. And if food was indeed as scarce as the evidence assembled in this book suggests, then the lowest-status members of Roman society, especially slaves, would have been the first to starve and the last to receive relief (if it even came). Like deserters, upon fleeing, fugitive slaves had little hope of rejoining civil society. But fugitive communities formed in times of crisis. The famous Spartacus—the former Thracian gladiator who terrorized Italy in the late 70s BC—gathered a following of tens of thousands even as the Republic crumbled around him. Likewise during the Antonine plague, the epidemics, famines, and the demoralizing war prompted a crisis sufficient to bring together a variety of disaffected and destitute peoples—deserters, slaves, bandits, and others—into communities which survived on low-level criminal activity.

Marcus seemed preoccupied with runaway slaves in a section of his *Meditations* composed at the time: "One who flees from his master is a runaway slave; now the law is our master, and one who departs from it is therefore a runaway slave."[106] Likely in response to increasing instances of slave flight, the emperor enacted strong and expansive fugitive slave laws in the late AD 170s. One edict, for example, required governors and magistrates "to assist any owner in seeking out runaway slaves and . . . they must give them up if they find them."[107] The problem was evidently so severe that it demanded the attention of even the highest officials. Marcus told the Senate that any slave catcher must be given full rights to "examine the sleeping-places or any traces of those who conceal them to enter on land of the Emperor or of Senators or private persons."[108] Elite property rights were typically paramount in the Roman legal tradition—but these extraordinary times called for extraordinary changes to once immutable norms.

Marcus's laws merely addressed the symptoms of the age's sickness, however, and not the causes. Pandemics have little respect for the decrees of political leaders. By the 180s, fugitive communities were seemingly even more prevalent. How much more prevalent? It is difficult to tell, because once the hated Commodus became sole emperor upon the death of Marcus in AD 180, elite writers went from timidly acknowledging social disorder to exaggerating and embellishing it. Roman elites loathed Commodus, and they drummed up calamities to affix blame to the new regime. Cassius Dio, for example, claims that some who died in an epidemic wave under Commodus were in fact poisoned "at the hands of criminals who smeared some deadly drugs on tiny needles, and for pay infected people with the poison by means of these instruments."[109] Here the senator engages in the age-old tradition of insulting an emperor by comparing him to a previously despised ruler. In this case, Dio adds: "the same thing had happened before in the reign of Domitian." The entire story of murderous assassins terrorizing the cities of the Empire under Commodus seems like a contrived excuse for Dio to vent his undisguised hatred for Marcus's unworthy son. How can we, 1,800 years later, sort fact from fiction?

The emperor's own words survive as testimony. Commodus acknowledged the brigandage under his reign in a surviving inscription from the town of Bubo in southwestern Asia Minor. Posted for all to see, the emperor praised the town for its "zeal and bravery" to "arrest the brigands, overcoming them, killing some and taking some alive."[110] Commodus went on to laud the town's actions for "encouraging [other towns and cities] to such brave deeds." Reading between the lines, the brigandage problem was clearly not limited to one settlement; it affected the entire region. Elites may have drummed up fake news to attack despised political leaders, but it really seems like banditry and brigandage were out of control in key regions: Egypt, Asia Minor, Gaul, and Spain at the very least.

Crime and desertion also proliferated in Italy itself. There, Roman authorities dealt with what one ancient biographer called the "Deserters' War" (Bellum Desertorum). As with the revolt of Spartacus during the waning decades of the Roman Republic, a charismatic leader—in this case, a former soldier named Maternus—amassed a significant following of fellow deserters, slaves, and other deplorables around AD 185. The historian Herodian—who likely embellished his story after reading an earlier source—claims that Maternus initially persuaded some of his fellow soldiers to flee with him and "attack and plunder villages and farms."[111] Trained men would have been more than capable of setting up ambushes and sieges to sack and loot whole settlements, even those guarded by militias and small detachments of Roman soldiers.[112] The easy profits in a time of economic uncertainty attracted followers, and soon the swelling mob "attacked the largest cities and released all the prisoners. . . . promising these men their freedom." In gratitude, the ex-cons (and presumably many slaves) joined the deserters. The growing force moved on to terrorize communities in Gaul and Spain before turning their sights on Italy, and even the emperor himself. Disguised as praetorian guardsmen, Maternus's band of former soldiers, prisoners, and slaves infiltrated Rome itself and attempted to kill Commodus. But, irony of ironies, the deserters were deserted. One of their own turned the criminals in to the authorities. Maternus was summarily beheaded—his captured followers executed shortly after.

Such blatant insurrection defies credulity. Had order really broken down to such an extent? Did Maternus and his band really try to assassinate the emperor, as Herodian claims? Most historians have doubts, although the numismatic evidence is curious. Coins proclaiming *fidei cohortium*—the loyalty of the urban garrison at Rome—were minted in AD 186/7. As with earlier issues, it is reasonable to wonder if the propaganda suggests that an uprising or rebellion occurred in Rome. Unsurprisingly, the exact same design was used in the coinage following another supposed "insurrection" in Rome under Commodus during the

AD 190 epidemic. Both coins of this type show a personification of Fides ("Loyalty") holding ears of grain, implying that the provision of grain ended the tumult. Certainly, the core elements in Herodian's tale of the Deserters' War—widespread desertion, unrest, and brigandage— are factual. An inscription records that a group of "new" enemies be-sieged the military camp at Argentoratum (modern Strasbourg). Many historians believe the besiegers were Maternus's deserters.[113] If so, then brigand forces were numerous enough to attack an entire legion (Legio VIII Augusta), and in its own camp no less! The inscription also tells us that the band of deserters roved through Upper Germania along the Rhine—information which provides a circumstantial link to the Anto-nine plague's effects on the northern frontier. Additional inscriptions from the region contemporary with the Deserters' War memorialize soldiers killed by "brigands" (*latrones*).[114] Perhaps most revealing: Commodus saw fit to dust off and deploy "loyalty of the soldiers" coin-age between AD 184 and 186—the coinage last used when his father faced troop desertion and brigandage following the revolt of Avidius Cassius. It was as much a bald-faced lie now as it was then.

History was repeating itself. And as with the desertion under Marcus, financial factors must have been at work. But this time it was far worse. First, the fundamental problems of the 170s remained unremedied. Le-gionary pay was still capped at 300 denarii per year. We can presume that pay for auxiliary units—the likely destination of many emergency recruits—was similarly frozen, and at slightly lower rates than the sala-ries of legionaries.[115] Commodus paid out token bonuses in the first two years of his reign, but literary sources and coin hoards suggest no additional military donatives until 186.[116] It may be no coincidence that Maternus's revolt began and flourished between those years. And over-all coin output under Commodus was chronically low, suggesting that the metal shortages which began under Marcus continued or even wors-ened under his son.[117]

But Commodus cut corners that his father did not. As happened with the Egyptian coinage in the 160s and 170s, the broader imperial coinage was debased in the 180s. Again, events in Egypt were prophetic, had anyone been keen enough to notice. The silver in Commodus's denarii

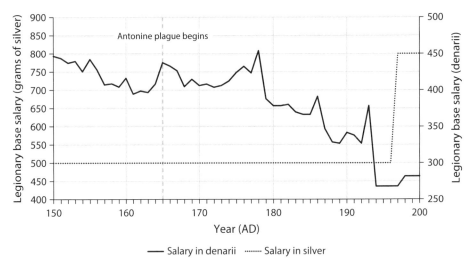

FIG. 6.9. Annual military pay in grams of silver and nominal denarii, AD 150–200.
After Elliott 2020b, 317.

dropped only a little, but coin weights were substantially reduced.[118] Money changers could easily spot the difference, so soon everyone was probably wise to the devaluation. From AD 178 to 190, wages in terms of silver would have dropped around 25 percent. Unlike the Egyptian debasement, however, the reduction in imperial coin quality would have been felt throughout the Empire—eroding the real value of military wages, and indeed all wages paid in imperial silver.

Unable to make ends meet, some soldiers, like Maternus and his comrades, left the military in search of plunder. Those that stayed, however, clamored for raises.[119] Eventually, the crisis in the military reached an absurd conclusion. After Commodus was assassinated in late AD 192, two candidates for emperor sought the endorsement of the Praetorian Guard by promising larger and larger bonuses. And "just as if it had been in some market or auction-room," Cassius Dio tells us, the highest bidder became emperor.[120] Finally, in 197, the soldiers received their due: a permanent raise of 50 percent. The bump had been a long time coming. But even then, this increase followed a severe currency debasement, and so its real value was negligible.[121]

Maternus's execution in AD 186 did not end the desertions. Again, the causes were systemic and deeply rooted in the short-sighted actions (or lack thereof) taken at the pandemic's opening act. Mass desertion, banditry, and brigandage carried on. Once it became clear that large gangs of thugs could essentially run rampant in the internal provinces of the Empire without consequence, imitators sprang up like weeds.[122] In what became a perverse and destructive cycle—a cycle which afflicts even modern imperial states—the Romans themselves ended up training, equipping, and radicalizing the very bandits, rebels, and insurrectionists that threatened peace and order in the cities of the Roman Empire.

It is worth considering one final consequence—one which feeds into the story of the last epidemic connected to the Antonine plague. As even rural settlements became increasingly unsafe, peasants would have flocked to the larger cities. A new inundation of migrants to Rome, for example, may have accompanied Maternus's march through Italy. We cannot know the numbers; and even if we had them, the transient nature of preindustrial life embedded instability in urban populations by default.[123] Instead, we can only identify and extrapolate from observations of events, circumstances, stresses, and crises that tended to displace the vulnerable. Grain shortages surely drove refugees in the 150s and 160s; crime and violence in the 170s and 180s likely had a similar effect, at least according to limited evidence. Numerous villa sites in central Italy show clear signs of decline and abandonment in the latter half of the second century.[124] The changes were severe and structural. Archaeological surveys of northern Italian urban centers turn up the same patterns: violently destroyed homes, with those still standing allowed to go derelict.[125] People left once prosperous settlements, and did not return. In the Sabina region of Italy, half of known rural settlements were abandoned by the mid-third century.[126] And genetic sampling from late second- and early third-century remains at a Roman necropolis (Isola Sacra at Portus) suggests a high rate of northern Italian migration to Rome, and these in family units.[127] If researchers are correct about the Italian origin of many of these migrants, it seems likely they were freeborn, and not captured slaves.[128] Further north and west, in Gallia Narbonensis, water mills, wineries, and vineyards all show signs of abandonment.[129] People seemingly left villas and rural settlements voluntarily, and in droves. This was not the work of a few raiders and bandits. The core of the Roman world was undergoing a painful transition.

Refugees displaced by the Pax Romana's metamorphosis would have joined the typical annual influx of migrants spawned by local famines, financial hardships, taxes, or myriad other routine challenges that accompanied daily life in the preindustrial world. There is no direct evidence that refugees carried plague into Rome, at least immediately. No source even hints of pestilence in Italy in the 180s. In fact, it may be reasonable to suspect that the rural migrants entering Rome at the time— especially any children—had not encountered the Antonine plague pathogen at all. Oxygen isotope analysis of those buried in the rural, working-class cemetery at Vagnari (southern Italy) suggests over 90 percent of those buried originate from the immediate region.[130] Immigrants, and their diseases, largely stayed out of rural settlements. The apparent population shifts in Italy in the 180s may have swelled Rome's streets with large numbers of people, many of whom were vulnerable to not only endemic urban diseases but also any traces of the Antonine plague still lurking in the city. Like Commodus's debased coinage, any population immunity won following the devastating epidemic of 166 would have been dangerously diluted. The pandemic was almost certainly well on its way to ending, but did it have one final trick to play?

PART III

CASUALTIES

The world has grown old, it does not enjoy that strength which it had formerly enjoyed, and does not flourish with the same vigor and strength with which it formerly prevailed. The world itself is now saying this, even as we are silent and offer no citations from Holy Scriptures and divine prophecies, and it testifies to its decline by the proof of its failing estate. . . . This sentence has been passed upon the world; this is the law of God; that all things which have come into existence die; and that those which have increased grow old; and that the strong be weakened; and that the large be diminished; and that when they have been weakened and diminished they come to an end.

—CYPRIAN'S *LETTER TO DEMETRIANUS,*
MID-THIRD CENTURY AD

7

REDUX?

Traditional histories of the Roman Empire tend to treat the transition from Marcus to Commodus as a major break. But if the pandemic was still kicking around the Empire, the change in regime did little to alter its course. Some, in fact, wonder if Marcus was himself among the disease's final victims.[1] In March of AD 180, as his empire withered before his very eyes, Marcus's fifty-eight-year-old body too began to fade. Five years prior, Marcus nearly died from an unnamed sickness. The disease that finally killed him is also a mystery. One fourth-century biography records that fear of the contagion was such that Commodus was sent away to preserve the health of Rome's next emperor. When Marcus's soldiers were told of the emperor's condition, they "lamented loudly, for they loved him singularly." They knew he was a goner. The ancient biography even claims Marcus spoke directly of his malady, and perhaps the Antonine plague: "Why do you weep for me, instead of thinking about the pestilence?" Marcus then starved himself as a way of accelerating his illness's deadly work.[2]

But in Cassius Dio's version of events, we get a much different and darker story. Eyewitnesses told Dio that Marcus died "not as a result of the disease from which he still suffered, but by the act of his physicians . . . who wished to do Commodus a favor."[3] In support of such a serious charge—murder—Dio provides no other evidence. In the end we cannot know what happened. But we have Marcus's own words on death, and these muse occasionally themes of plague:

> It would have been the mark of a better and a wiser man to depart from the human race without having had any taste of falsehood, pretense, luxury, and pride; but the next best course is to breathe your last when you have at least become sated with such things. Or do you prefer to settle down with vice, and has experience not yet persuaded you to flee from this pestilence? For corruption of the mind is a far graver pestilence than any comparable disturbance and alteration in the air that surrounds us; for the one is a plague to living creatures as mere animals, and the other to human beings in their nature as human beings. Do not despise death, but welcome it gladly, for this too is among the things that nature wishes.[4]

Whether or not it killed him, the Antonine plague had been a companion to Marcus during the final fifteen years of his life—so much so that his framework for death references pestilence. Sickness had taken his soldiers, his friends, perhaps members of his family, and maybe even his co-emperor Lucius. The relentlessness of "the everlasting pestilence" provoked extensive and meaningful reflection on what death was and was not, and how a courageous person should face this one sure thing about life: it must end.

Pandemics also must end. But did the Antonine plague die around the same time Marcus expired, or did it linger into the 180s? Just a few years before Marcus's death, the emperor held court in Sirmium (in modern Serbia). A delegation of Athenians, agitated over quarrels in their city, demanded Marcus intervene. As the discussion wore on, the impatient Athenians exclaimed: "Happy they who perished in the plague!"—a reference to the Antonine plague, not the pestilence under Pericles memorialized by Thucydides.[5] The sarcastic quip is revealing. To begin with, the plague was so severe and widespread as to imbue its memory with idiomatic currency. But an even more telling fact is implied in the Athenians' hyperbole: the plague was in fact *a memory*. The Athenians spoke in the past tense. In other words, the Antonine plague's epidemic phase was believed to be over. And yet, a major epidemic roared in Rome in the spring of AD 190. Many if not most historians describe that outbreak as the pandemic's final encore before it winked out of existence. But a close study of the decade prior to the 190 epidemic reveals very little sound evidence that the Antonine plague continued much past the mid-170s. The near silence in the sources need not mean that the pestilence was extinguished; it may very well be that the disease simply stopped grabbing the headlines. Commodus's reign was chock-full of scandal and intrigue. Some of those scandals, in fact, shaped the way our sources frame the Antonine plague's supposed curtain call in 190. It makes sense, therefore, to both examine the supposed plague evidence from the 180s and flesh out the strange politics that contextualized the final epidemic of the second century—the plots, insurrections, and ultimately Commodus's own transformation into Rome's infamous gladiator-emperor.

An End or a Respite?

Commodus's formative years were shaped by the age of angst—an age in which disease was a constant threat, both real and perceived. Even the nobility were not safe. An active and seemingly everlasting pestilence struck down family and friends around the boy in the mid-160s and 170s. As discussed in the previous chapter, Commodus himself became sick with a fever and throat condition in his teens. As Commodus's father knew, however, fear of disease is a kind of sickness in and of itself. Modern studies have since confirmed that anxiety-ridden parents and family members have a powerful influence on children's perceptions of the world around them.[6] Marcus and Fronto's letters were preoccupied with health and wellness—for both them and their family members.[7] Commodus's female relatives also worried for his health. We see similar anxieties when Commodus was whisked away from his father's deathbed, so that the young heir would not be contaminated by Marcus's deadly sickness. Such persistent fear is easily imbibed by impressionable children, and Commodus may have been no exception. Cassius Dio—a few years older than Commodus, and first appointed senator in the late 180s—unapologetically characterized Commodus as a coward.[8]

Cowardice was just one of many concerns about the new emperor. Although Commodus had reached the legal age of manhood, and had already accumulated all the honorifics and magistracies commensurate with his status as Marcus's sole heir, Roman elites held serious misgivings about entrusting absolute power to not only this teenager but teenagers in general. Even Rome's twenty-something emperors had thus far all been failures. The names of the three men that had taken the purple at or before the age of thirty prior to Commodus were among the most odious, and their reigns the most damnable, of all the emperors to have ruled Rome: Caligula, Nero, and Domitian.[9] Marcus doubtless thought that Commodus would need both dedicated mentors and wise, sober counsel to break the historical pattern. On his deathbed, Marcus charged his most trusted companions and advisors to "take my place as father" to the young Commodus. And Marcus cautioned his son directly: avoid the fatal mixture of idleness and power hunger that brought down Rome's infamous young emperors of the past.[10]

Almost immediately after Marcus died, however, Commodus broke from his father's plans. The new emperor reversed the course of the northern war—negotiating treaties with the leading Germanic tribes. Hawkish senators criticized the peace deals. But despite the hand-wringing of Rome's warmongering nobles, Commodus outperformed his father in the foreign policy arena. His deals with the Germanic peoples secured a lasting peace along the Romans' northern frontier. The diplomatic feat is all the more impressive considering that around half a century later, when Commodus's peace finally eroded, the Romans would never again control that border. In fact, even as contemporary writers claim that Commodus sued for peace out of laziness, cowardice, and a desire to indulge in the pleasures of life in the capital, they nevertheless begrudgingly admit that Commodus secured what seems to have been a beneficial settlement: the tribes gave the Romans at least twenty thousand soldiers and an annual grain tribute. And the treaties put in place meaningful safeguards against future insurrections. The agreements forbade tribal assemblies not supervised by a Roman centurion, for example. What probably most stabilized the region as a whole, however, were Commodus's non-aggression agreements between tribes; these prevented the kinds of proxy wars that tend to trap larger powers like Rome. Thus, far from "giving them everything they demanded"—as the historian Herodian alleges—Commodus in fact secured through prudent diplomacy what his father failed to obtain by a lengthy, costly war in the midst of a raging pandemic.[11]

But by the time Commodus took over the Empire, the Antonine plague was seemingly in remission. The contagion may have continued to circulate, but at muted levels beneath the radar of the elite writers who preserved the historical details of the era. In fact, by all appearances, Commodus's reign initially seemed poised to launch Rome into a new golden age. Commodus's treaty in AD 180 would have brought additional mass movements of soldiers and settlers, but presumably these would have diminished after the initial flurry of activity. And, unlike after the Parthian War, we know almost nothing of where Commodus sent his soldiers. More than twenty thousand Germans joined the Roman army.[12] Tens of thousands of Roman captives were also returned to Roman territory. And more tribes settled in Dacia.[13] Otherwise, it is a mystery as to where most soldiers—legionary, auxiliary, or foreign—went after Commodus's peace treaty.

Instead of Roman armies reinforcing the Empire's borders, gangs of deserters, slaves, and bandits roved about internal provinces of the Empire in the 180s. But did these groups of mobile marauders have the density to sustain plague transmission among themselves? And did they travel from settlement to settlement with enough frequency to keep contagion moving to naive populations, thus preserving the pandemic's lingering presence in the Empire? I think not. Ongoing brigandage may have been more a consequence rather than a direct cause of plague—but we just do not have the evidence to say much more. Only a few sources hint of a pestilence lying in wait in the provinces of the Empire in the 180s. All, however, have their flaws and irregularities.

An inscription from the province of Noricum (modern Austria, and parts of Slovenia) lists the names of four family members, one of whom was a thirty-year-old soldier in Legio II Italica. That legion was in the thick of the Marcomannic Wars, and therefore was likely exposed to the Antonine plague pathogen. Remarkably, the inscription says that the family members "died through the plague" in AD 182.[14] This is the only inscription in existence that explicitly references the Antonine plague. Several historians have used it to make the case for the pandemic's severity and endurance into the 180s.[15] But even this most valuable piece of evidence—which was unfortunately destroyed in 1944—has a major catch. Surviving images of the inscription show a curious feature: the reference to the plague and the year seem to have been written in a different hand, in smaller text, in the space which occupied a single line of the original inscription.[16] Could the epitaph's most valuable information have been added or even forged in more recent times? The motivations for such an addition are readily discernible: with no direct epigraphic evidence for the Antonine plague, this inscription, were it genuine, would be both financially valuable and historically without precedent. Instead of proof the pandemic lingered into the 180s, the inscription merely confirms that members of this family met some tragic end in a time of increasing turmoil, but perhaps not from the pandemic.

In the same part of the world—Noricum's capital city Virunum—a bronze plaque dated to June 26, AD 184 speaks of a "mortality" (*mortalitatis causa*) that killed five members of a mystery cult.[17] The "mortality" was severe enough that the cultists memorialized the deaths of their members during a meeting on the day after the summer solstice. Some historians believe the generic language of "mortality" served as code for an epidemic connected to the Antonine plague. After all, the mystery cult—Mithraism—is known for using esoteric language. But the cult also associated exit and entrance into mortality with the solstices on June 25 and December 25. A leading expert on Mithraism, Roger Beck, argues that complex and even paradoxical religious values prompted the Mithraists to commemorate their recent dead in a single meeting the day after the summer solstice.[18] In other words, the inscription merely tells us that five men—most or potentially all of them soldiers—died sometime during the year prior to the inscription. They *might* have died of the Antonine plague disease, but this inscription offers historians no concrete evidence of such a thing.

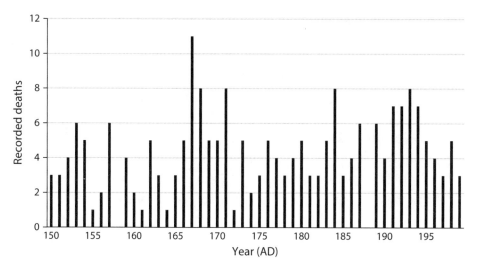

FIG. 7.1. Deaths recorded on funerary stelae in the Hermos valley in Lydia, AD 150–200.

Data from the Trismegistos database (https://www.trismegistos.org /tmcorpusdata/21/) as first published and discussed in Broux and Clarysee 2009. Subsequently discussed in Duncan-Jones 2018, 48–50. The new years on stelae begin on either Sulla's conquest of the province (September 24) or the battle of Actium (September 2). Converting from Sulla/Actium years to calendar years, therefore, results in split years (i.e., Sulla Year 250 = 165/6), which are difficult to graph. Because more of the Sulla/Actium year falls in the second calendar year, I have graphed split years based on the second calendar year (i.e., Sulla Year 250 = 166). Readers, however, should keep in mind that deaths dated to 166, for example, may have in fact occurred as early as September of 165. I do not know if Duncan-Jones took the opposite approach (shifting split years to the former year). His chart shows a far more prominent spike in 183, whereas in my graph, the spike occurs in 184 and is less prominent. My graph also omits a small number of undated or ambiguously dated inscriptions (which typically did not specify whether the year was of Actium or Sulla).

The most robust evidence for plague's lingering presence in the Roman Empire in the 180s may come from Lydia in western Asia Minor. A series of more than six hundred surviving tombstones dated by year offers historians an impression of years of low and high death counts in the region.

The two major epidemic waves associated with the Antonine plague in literary sources—one in the mid- to late 160s and another in the

190s—seem reflected in the tombstones. The year 166/7 shows a high single-year spike, which may be consistent with an epidemic outbreak. In the 190s, there is no single year that stands out (depending on how the inscriptions are dated) but rather a cluster of years with slightly elevated levels of death. Perhaps these latter inscriptions indicate a slower-moving wave of pestilence? The anomaly is in 183/4, which sees an uptick in deaths followed by the crescendo in the early 190s. The sample size, however, is small, and therefore prone to distortions. The inscriptions themselves also say nothing of pestilence or plague. One would think that if some ninety or so victims of the pandemic died and left tombstones, at least *one* of them might have listed plague as a cause of death. Did a wave of pestilence—whether local or associated with the latent pandemic—sweep through Asia Minor in the winter of late 183 and early 184? An extra few grave markers in one year is not much evidence upon which to build such a claim.

It could be that some apparent excess deaths in the 180s were caused by famine. Grain shortages seemed to have continued in the 180s. A scrap of papyrus dated to AD 185 shows that only about one-third of the required annual grain taxes in one of Egypt's most fertile regions had been collected.[19] The annual quota of 900,000 *artabas* (~27,000,000 kg) was consistent with taxation levels prior to the pandemic. Rome's greed for grain was apparently unmoderated by reality. Flood records are incomplete, but it is conceivable that the province may have gone more than a decade without a 15–16 cubit flood by the mid-180s. The pandemic's ongoing role during the food shortage is less well known, but Egypt's agricultural economy floundered well into the 180s.

Despite the relative silence in the 180s, many historians believe the Antonine plague disease remerged in AD 190. Yet it is difficult to bridge the fifteen-year gap between that epidemic (which seems to have only hit the city of Rome) and Galen's final datable comments on the pestilence from the early to mid-170s. Why would a major pandemic seemingly vanish from the sources, only to suddenly roar back to life over a decade later? Maybe the Antonine plague truly was over, and the outbreak of 190 represents the rise of yet another novel disease? Or maybe the migrants and refugees of the 180s crowded Rome in sufficient numbers to prompt an epidemic surge in one of Rome's many endemic maladies? Historians must accept such possibilities.

Whether the pandemic ended by the reign of Commodus or merely escaped notice of elite writers we cannot know. Political events captivate our sources for the period; ancient writers may have lost interest in the apparently diminishing pestilence. Driven by personalities and politics, developments in Rome under Commodus might at first seem to have had little to do with epidemic disease. And yet, with full awareness of the significant factors that drove the emergence of the Antonine plague pandemic in its initial waves, it is possible to read between the lines in political accounts and find similar elements. Distracted by political scandals, corruption, and conspiracies, the Roman population was unknowingly being primed for one final and unexpected onslaught of pestilence.

The Final Epidemic

Having concluded the Marcomannic Wars in autumn of AD 180, Commodus returned to Rome in triumph. The capital received the new emperor as though he had won the war his father fought. Showers of laurel leaves and garlands of flowers met the emperor. Commodus paraded through the streets of Rome in a chariot as though he were a god. In fact, he probably would have been clothed as Jupiter himself—his face even painted red to mimic the Capitoline statue of Rome's supreme deity. But Commodus was no god, and a slave likely stood over his shoulder whispering the reminder offered to all Roman triumphators: "Look behind you. Remember that you are a man."[20] Subsequent events would show the warning fell upon deaf ears.

But for the moment, the laurel-crowned Commodus was indeed the first man in Rome. A popular spirit of optimism followed the young emperor in the honeymoon of his reign. Not only was he the son of Marcus Aurelius, groomed for rule by Rome's philosopher-emperor, but Commodus was the grandson (through his mother) of Antoninus

Pius—an emperor remembered for his fidelity to family, Senate, and people. The new emperor even looked the part, as Herodian writes:

> He was in the prime of youth, striking in appearance, with a well-developed body and a face that was handsome without being pretty. His commanding eyes flashed like lightning; his hair, naturally blond and curly, gleamed in the sunlight as if it were on fire; some thought that he sprinkled his hair with gold dust before appearing in public, while others saw in it something divine, saying that a heavenly light shone round his head. To add to his beauty, the first down was just beginning to appear on his cheeks.[21]

Commodus's physical presence in Rome prompted celebration, but it also secured and legitimized his rule. He made personal appearances before the crowds—culminating in the triumphal parade in October. In the Senate House, he gave a formal address to the Roman nobility, where he shared touching stories about his beloved and now divine father. Marcus, like many emperors before him, officially became a god upon his death. Commodus would have sacrificed to his now divine father, and dutifully met with Rome's traditional deities—Jupiter in his palatial temple on the Capitoline Hill, but Commodus also visited other religious sites and shrines in the city. These acts not only demonstrated the new emperor's piety but confirmed his status as Rome's chief protector and savior—a man who deservedly commanded the military and civil organs of the Roman state. As subsequent events would show, Commodus needed to draw heavily upon these broader bases of imperial authority—as almost before he settled into the imperial palace, he faced serious threats from disgruntled senators, ambitious advisors, and even members of his own family.

Cassius Dio, only a few years older than Commodus, witnessed first-hand many of the events in Rome during Commodus's reign, including a conspiracy against the young emperor's life in the early 180s. Unsuccessful coup d'états had driven previous emperors to reclusion, even paranoia—especially when family members and close confidants were behind the plots. Commodus was no exception. In 182, his older sister Lucilla hatched a conspiracy to assassinate her lord and brother. As

Commodus entered an arena one day—his bodyguards either inatten-
tive or at a slight distance—a relative named Quintianus quietly drew
near, unnoticed. When the moment to strike arrived, Quintianus burst
from hiding. But instead of stabbing the surprised young emperor, the
would-be assassin dramatically but foolishly announced his intentions—
shouting that the Senate sent the blade that was about to strike Commodus down.[22] The short speech gave the emperor and, more impor-
tantly, his guards time to recover. The plot failed in spectacular fashion.
And the fallout brought a purge in the imperial court. Quintianus as
well as several co-conspirators were summarily executed.[23] Lucilla,
however—former empress and daughter of Marcus Aurelius—was
dealt with quietly. After exiling Lucilla to the island of Capri, Commodus sent a centurion to murder his sister several months later.

Although Commodus survived this first attempt on his life, he seems
to have been permanently scarred by Quintianus's claim that the Senate
wanted the emperor dead. Commodus, bereft of father, mother, and
now elder sister, reasonably came to see the Senate as hostile. Fear took
over, and Commodus went into hiding. Accounts of the first ten years
of Commodus's reign suggest a withdrawn and even frightened husk of
a man who, at the first sign of danger, fled to his villas and sent out assassins to defeat monstrous plots both real and imagined. Dio describes
Commodus as being "guileless as any man that ever lived" and called
him a "coward" outright.[24] But even as Commodus lived an adult life
consistent with a traumatized childhood in the age of angst, he nevertheless dreamed of being a hero. Commodus secretly play-acted as both
a gladiator and chariot racer. Before 190, Commodus never raced horses
in public. Instead, he would sneak out and race by himself "on moonless
nights . . . ashamed to be seen doing so." His gladiator moves too he
practiced behind closed doors, albeit with live playmates—and occasionally the emperor would slip and slice off a nose, ear, or other "sundry
features" as Dio claims.[25] Yet Commodus's full descent into madness
and megalomania—and the excessive antics which led to his reputation
as "the gladiator"—did not manifest until an epidemic in AD 190. Ancient and modern historians focus on the roles played by personalities
and politics during the 180s, as must be the case here as well. But the

contextual forces highlighted in this book—plague, famine, migration, and others—also set the stage for the drama that unfolded in Commodus's final years.

While out of the public eye, the young emperor established a reputation not as a sober stoic, like his father, but a derelict debaucher. To be sure, Commodus continued to fulfill the basic duties required of an emperor, or was at least sufficiently able to take credit for the accomplishments of his underlings. He also continued to hold the approval of the Roman people—perhaps won not by character or acumen but by his profligate handouts to citizens.[26] Even the hostile Cassius Dio admits that Commodus performed acts of beneficence and beautification in the capital.[27] And although Dio peppers his account with invectives against Commodus for racing chariots and living licentiously, the senator also acknowledges that the emperor at least kept in office a few of the competent men raised by his father, including the man who would succeed Commodus as emperor: Publius Helvius Pertinax.

But not all holdovers from the previous regime were well-thought-of by Rome's elite. By the mid-180s, Cleander, a former slave freed by Marcus Aurelius, had murdered his way to the top—becoming Commodus's *cubicularius* (a household manager or chamberlain) and *pugione* ("dagger man").[28] As a former slave, Cleander was barred from any higher station, such as leading the Praetorian Guard, joining the Senate, or holding high office in Rome. And yet Commodus's dagger man was, in effect, second in power only to the emperor himself. Like a few emperors before him and many after, Commodus banked on Rome's strict social hierarchy even as he pushed against its limits. Low-born dependents who owed their positions exclusively to imperial patronage were unlikely to make a play for ultimate power.[29] Cleander's position as "dagger man" was outside typical cultural or constitutional arrangements, but the appointment offered security to a frightened emperor who had already faced assassination attempts from Rome's traditional nobility.

Cleander was a veteran of two imperial households. The shrewd manipulator and social climber killed the previous *cubicularius*. He then used the rampant banditry of the age to bring soldiers from Britain into

Rome; these conveniently denounced the current praetorian prefect, one of Cleander's rivals. The next prefect, Cleander murdered. Cleander lacked the pedigree to qualify for prefect himself, but the former slave's influence was such that both the Praetorian Guard and even its supervising officers now reported to him. He could not himself become a high magistrate, but he used his power to dole out appointments to military commands, governorships, and even membership the Senate itself, for the right price. Most audaciously, Cleander sold the Roman consulship—the pinnacle magistracy reserved for the most elite of senators—to two dozen different men in a single year, although some historians doubt the ancient sources on this point.[30] Still, something strange was afoot. Normally, two consuls were elected each year, and emperors would then appoint two additional consuls midyear. In AD 190, however, the consulship reportedly rotated among a whopping twenty-five men: two for each month of the year, plus the emperor himself. Was Cleander debasing Rome's highest office? Or, alternatively, had the plague's resurgence led to a dearth of ex-consuls to fill governorships and other essential posts, and the unprecedented number of consular appointments was in fact an emergency measure to fast-track men qualified to meet the shortfall?[31] The wild story is yet another tall tale that further muddies the waters of the Antonine plague mystery.

Cleander himself became an indirect casualty of the epidemic many historians believe to have been the Antonine plague's final act. Violence and food shortages in the countryside had driven high numbers of refugees into Rome throughout the 180s. These of course added to the normal influx of bodies. Each spring, Rome's population swelled with artisans, seasonal workers, and migrants.[32] Few of these transient inhabitants dwelt in permanent housing. Most would have crammed into already occupied private spaces in apartment blocks or, in some cases, they lived on the streets. Indeed, Herodian tells us that Rome, "which received people from all over the world, was overcrowded" on the eve of that final outbreak.[33] How many of these people had preexisting immunity to the Antonine plague pathogen? Many of the Romans who survived the epidemic of 166 would have died by 190. And many in the rural parts of Italy and other western provinces likely never caught

the disease in its earlier waves. By the spring of 190, the city must have
been bursting at the seams with vulnerable hosts. Population immunity
had effectively been reset.[34]

What sparked the epidemic in Rome? We do not know. But two familiar authors, Dio and Herodian, provide us with tantalizing clues, but
also problematic exaggerations. Herodian dedicates a large section in
his opening book to the epidemic of 190:

> About this time, plague struck all Italy. The suffering was especially
> severe in Rome, since the city, which received people from all over
> the world, was overcrowded. The city suffered great loss of both men
> and animals. Then, on the advice of his physicians, Commodus left
> Rome for Laurentum. This region enjoyed the shade from extensive
> laurel groves (whence the area derives its name); it was cooler there
> and seemed to be a safe haven. The emperor is said to have counter-
> acted the pollution in the air by the fragrant scent of the laurels and
> the refreshing shade of the trees. At the direction of their doctors,
> those who remained in Rome filled their nostrils and ears with fra-
> grant oils and used perfume and incense constantly, for some said
> that the sweet odor, entering first, filled up the sensory passages and
> kept out the poison in the air; or, if any poison should enter, it would
> be neutralized by the stronger odors. The plague, however, contin-
> ued to rage unchecked for a long time, and many men died, as well
> as domestic animals of all kinds. Famine gripped the city at the
> same time.[35]

If we take Herodian at face value, then the pestilence affected the whole
of Italy and especially the city of Rome because of overcrowding. We
should also note a key bit of information corroborated in two accounts
associated with the Antonine plague, and many sources that concern
ancient diseases generally: the epidemic spread to both animals and
people—a fact Herodian mentions twice in this passage. Also, the conditions of disease endured for "a long time," although Herodian does
not quantify what he means. It is unclear whether Herodian refers here
to the outbreak in Rome only or in "all Italy." We also are not given any
sense of the numbers of dead, including people or animals. Finally, a

famine was concurrent with plague. All of these details are worth investigating, but we must look at our other source first to get the full picture.

The second, and likely earlier, account comes from Cassius Dio. The Roman senator, who may have witnessed all or part of the outbreak in Rome, is unfortunately brief in his prose, although he hints at high plague mortality: "a pestilence occurred, the greatest of any of which I have knowledge; for two thousand persons often died in Rome in a single day."[36] Taken at face value, Dio tells us that this plague was worse than any he knew about—which presumably includes the epidemic of 166 and following. Dio also gives a daily death count, although the senator had no disease mortality statistics to consult that we know of.[37] But Dio's guess at daily mortality stresses that many people died in the epidemic—and we can probably trust him on this point.

What Dio does not say is even more revealing. Conditions outside Rome are not discussed. Whereas Herodian, who was seemingly not in Rome or even Italy at the time of the outbreak, and was no older than a teenager anyway, adds that Italy was also affected. Dio's silence on this matter need not be taken as evidence of plague absence elsewhere. After all, Dio's account survives largely in a medieval summary; he may have said more about the outbreak and its context. But it is nevertheless curious that such a massive surge of infectious disease in Rome did not leave behind the kinds of circumstantial evidence in the epigraphic or papyrological record that accompanied the outbreaks in the 160s and early 170s. This outbreak—whatever was behind it—seemingly remained regional, or was at least perceived to do so.

Dio also says nothing about livestock, but Herodian implies twice that animals died in the epidemic. The purported earliest source for the pandemic in the Roman Empire—the overly dramatic and self-focused memoir of Aelius Aristides—says something quite similar: "the livestock too became sick."[38] This connection provides at least a circumstantial link between the first round of pestilence in the 160s and this later epidemic. More speculatively, aVARV—the ancient orthopoxvirus discovered in Viking Age human remains—shows genetic markers consistent with a wider range of animal reservoirs than modern smallpox.[39]

We do not know if aVARV was behind the Antonine plague; most likely, it emerged a century or two after. But orthopoxviruses and variants can and have emerged regularly and repeatedly in recent millennia. At the same time, livestock deaths in reports of ancient plagues are so common as to be a trope. Two iconic and oft-imitated texts—Homer's *Iliad* and Thucydides's *Peloponnesian War*—feature plagues which afflicted both livestock and humans.[40] Roman historical accounts, too, are replete with such instances.[41] So Herodian may have embellished for dramatic effect, as if to say: this was a disease on par with the worst diseases in the history books.[42]

Sources, however, confirm an even more familiar pattern. Rome suffered from two calamities simultaneously: disease and food shortage. The coincidence of famine with disease has been a refrain throughout this book. Herodian and Dio blame different causes, but both authors describe a starving and unruly populace in the midst of deadly pestilence. The 180s offered Rome neither respite nor recovery from the shortages of previous decades. Ostraca found at the quarry of Mons Claudianus in Egypt show that grain was unavailable there in March of AD 189.[43] That site was fed with local grain, signaling shortages that may have hit Rome the following spring in 190—the exact moment of the outbreak.[44]

It was a perfect storm: a sea of migrants, a wave of pestilence, and now famine pummeled the population. Rome's one million plus inhabitants somehow had to endure sickness and starvation for several months. As the hardships became unbearable and bodies began to pile up, the Romans presumably looked to their emperor for hope. But Commodus vanished. In the torrent of crises, Rome's captain abandoned ship—leaving the city to the concurrent horrors of famine and plague. This would not end well.

A Riot at the Capital

Commodus retreated from Rome—leaving the capital to suffer the pestilence without its head of state. Doctors told Commodus to isolate in the nearby coastal city of Laurentum some twenty-five kilometers from Rome. The city was named for its abundant groves of laurel, and the emperor's physicians believed that Commodus would do well to walk among the shady trees and smell the laurels' sweet aroma. The leaves of the laurel tree are both pleasant and pungent—its scent supposedly strong enough to create a wall of smell—a fragrant barrier that blocked any noxious and disease-laden fumes from entering the body.[45] In fact, dried laurel leaves—along with incenses and essential oils—were placed around infected persons in the hopes that the healthy smells would enter the body and push out diseases trapped there.

Commodus took few people with him into isolation. His main companion was his mistress Marcia—a powerful political figure in her own right. Marcia interposed herself between Commodus and the world outside the tranquil estate—isolating Commodus, but also, perhaps not coincidentally, isolating Commodus's "dagger man" Cleander as well. With Commodus away, Cleander was left in Rome all by himself to manage a hostile Senate, praetorians led by prefects who despised the freedman's authority, a severe grain shortage, and a deadly plague. But Commodus's right-hand man had a nemesis in the city as well: Papirius Dionysius, Rome's *Praefectus Annonae*. As grain commissioner, Papirius was supposed to ensure that stores of grain were rationed out carefully to the population to prevent riots. Papirius was a well-pedigreed elite. He had been an equestrian advisor to Marcus Aurelius—on track for a stellar career in the Empire. But Cleander had blocked Papirius from taking up the lucrative and prestigious governorship of Egypt.[46] Embittered from the setback, and free to meddle while Commodus quarantined, Papirius claimed the city's grain shortage was not his fault but that Cleander had bought up the grain and was hoarding it. We know Papirius's lie was successful, in part, because Herodian's secondhand account reflects the grain commissioner's spin—potentially the exact narrative concocted to bring down Cleander:

[Cleander] bought up most of the grain supply and put it in storage; he hoped in this way to get control of the people and the army by making a generous distribution of grain at the first sign of a food shortage, anticipating that he would win the support of the people when they were suffering from a scarcity of food.[47]

Even now, modern historians might believe Papirius's side of the story but for an ironic source for the truth: Cassius Dio—the senator who hated both Commodus and his freedman dagger man. It must have pained the senator to admit that the freedman he so despised was nevertheless innocent of the lies that had become accepted as history. And so Dio corrected the official record decades later:

> A famine occurred, sufficiently grievous in itself; but its severity was vastly increased by Papirius Dionysius, the grain commissioner, in order that Cleander, whose thefts would seem chiefly responsible for it, might incur the hatred of the Romans and be destroyed by them.[48]

The best misinformation often contains kernels of truth. Stories of Cleander's lust for wealth and power had apparently been circulating for some time among both elites and the wider population. Anyone could see, for example, the unprecedented speed at which new consuls were being appointed each month by the Senate (if that story is to be believed).[49] Surely these men were paying Cleander for the privilege? And what was he doing with this wealth? Again, our sources give us the spin: Cleander had bilked Rome's aristocrats to fund lavish parties for the emperor and his groupies. Cleander also used the money to increase his economic and social capital—buying up properties and handing out benefactions, the latter of which came with reciprocal obligations should their freedman patron come calling. It is easy to imagine Roman elites taking the rostrum and proffering such claims to a hungry, agitated crowd. Whether or not there was any hard evidence of Cleander's guilt, it did not much matter; mobs typically apply dangerously low standards of justice to their scapegoats.

With Papirius's lies embedded in their minds, nothing in their bellies, and plague surrounding them in the city, the seething crowds were ready to erupt. All they needed was a little push toward open violence. Cleander's enemies orchestrated the climax in mid-April when the city of Rome celebrated the Cerealia—a major festival of Ceres, goddess of grain, agriculture, and the harvest. Many of the festival's events took place in the Circus Maximus, Rome's largest entertainment venue with a capacity of around 150,000 spectators. Such events were both highly political and personal.[50] Emperors and elites shared the same physical space with commoners and criminals. The crowds used the opportunity to shout requests at emperors, and sometimes to heckle them. These spring races should have been a hopeful, forward-looking celebration of the grain set to arrive in the city in a few months. Instead, the crowds were hungry, disease-ridden, and desperate. The setting for a large-scale riot could not have been better.[51] The tinder had been carefully prepared and collected by Cleander's enemies, but the strike that set Rome's masses ablaze employed the oldest political trick in the book: using children to manipulate public opinion. And so into the Circus marched a group of boys and girls led by a motherly matron—chanting praises for Commodus and insults toward Cleander. The agitated crowd took up the chants and soon a riot broke out.[52] The urban prefect Pertinax—the official responsible for deploying the urban cohorts to control riots in Rome—strangely ordered his troops to stand down.[53] Sources even hint that members of the Praetorian Guard crept into the crowds, encouraging violence.[54] In the absence of law enforcement, and potentially with their explicit encouragement, the crowd poured forth from the Circus Maximus and terrorized the city, committing arson, assault, murder, and other acts of violence. The few soldiers Cleander sent against the mob had no effect. Herodian framed the episode as an outright "civil war."[55] Modern biographer Olivier Hekster more accurately called it an "engineered riot."[56]

Commodus, meanwhile, still unwilling to enter Rome during the outbreak, had taken up residence in the palatial Villa of the Quintilii just outside of Rome's southern boundary. The emperor had been kept unaware of the dire state of the city, maybe on purpose. A truly ferocious crisis needed to fester. Somehow, curiously, the mob knew exactly where to find the emperor. They surrounded his villa, pleading for the head of Cleander. The uproar that began in the Circus had now reached the ears of the emperor. Puzzled and terrified, Commodus turned to Marcia—his ambassador to the outside world while in quarantine.[57] Whether she acted as part of the conspiracy against Cleander will never be known, but her words to Commodus were likely the poison that brought the freedman down. We do not know what she said, but Herodian invented a speech for Commodus's surviving eldest sister Fadilla. These comments provide a reasonable impression of how Rome's "civil war" may have been relayed to Commodus in that desperate moment:

> Cleander has armed the people and the soldiers against you. Those who hate him because they hold differing opinions, the mob, and the entire imperial cavalry, who support him, are up in arms, killing each other and choking the city with blood. The fury of both factions will fall upon us unless you immediately hand over to them for execution this scoundrelly servant of yours, who already has been the cause of so much destruction for the people and who threatens to be the cause of so much destruction for us.[58]

Herodian believed that Cleander "desired the Empire," and so he crafted a speech to fit his narrative.[59] In reality, if the low-born freedman really harbored such unrealistic ambitions, he was a fool. But the accusation need not have been true; it just needed to be plausible enough to frighten Commodus into action.[60] The totality of the crisis—the epidemic, the grain shortage, the mob violence, the schemes and plots— may have washed over the emperor in one alarming moment. Commodus needed to immediately pacify the mob before all was lost.

The terrified emperor played the role offered to him. He had his "dagger man" swiftly executed. Cleander's corpse was then handed over to the crowd for further degradation and abuse. The emperor clearly gave some credence to the rumors of an attempted coup because Cleander's sons and associates were also killed—murders consistent with an effort to squash any claims from credible rivals for power.[61] Interestingly, however, the emperor also meted out justice to many of Cleander's enemies in short order, including Papirius. But by far the most consequential development was that Commodus ceased running the state through dependent, low-born intermediaries. Following the epidemic and subsequent crisis, Commodus took the reins of government himself. The Antonine plague was over; but now a new pestilence—the twisted, deranged, and megalomaniacal Commodus himself—was fully unleashed on the weakened city. In the words of Cassius Dio, Commodus became "a greater curse to the Romans than any plague."[62]

A Greater Curse

Even after the pandemic died out, the ghost of the Antonine plague haunted many, but perhaps no one more persistently than the emperor Commodus himself. Of course we cannot know for sure what drove Commodus's descent into madness, but that it immediately followed the epidemic of AD 190 seems no coincidence. The isolated emperor's final years are worth dwelling upon, as they are in some ways a microcosm of Rome's experience of the Antonine plague more generally. Apart from one known childhood bout with disease—and we do not know if he suffered from the Antonine plague disease itself—Commodus experienced the pandemic as a specter perhaps more than a sickness. Even if the infamous pestilence were responsible for the epidemic of 190, disease melded with other calamities—famine, migrations, and political violence. Commodus's fragile mind might have cracked anyway, but the chaos of disease, famine, and violence ripped a possible future across the threshold of reality, and into historicity. In body, Commodus survived the multifaceted crisis that was the Antonine plague. His identity, however—the essence of who he was—fundamentally and permanently changed. So too went the Roman Empire.

Like a frightened child, Commodus had hidden from an epidemic in the arms of his consort Marcia in his villa at Laurentum. But after emerging from quarantine, Commodus elected to rule Rome directly— the first time he had ever done so. His father and uncle were dead of disease. His mother too had also passed away. His sister had been executed (by his own order), as had numerous other advisors and former friends. And now, even his freedman confidant Cleander's headless body was rotting in some dark corner of Rome. Now alone, it was Commodus's moment to shine. Rome felt the unmediated heat of Marcus's divine son, and the city burned.

Literally, Rome burned. In what Cassius Dio saw as a "portent . . . that the evil would not be confined to the city but would extend over the entire civilized world," a ravenous fire ripped through Rome in early AD 192.[63] Accounts of earlier and more famous fires, such as the Great Fire under Nero, describe wood buildings bursting into flames, wailing women and children, and fire-surrounded streets like horrific mazes with no escape.[64] The blaze not only took out much of the imperial palace—including its important archive of state records—but destroyed warehouses of exotic goods. Many of Galen's books and notes too were lost.[65] A trove of these burned when the Temple of Pax—one of Rome's most beautiful monuments—succumbed to the flames. The loss of that temple was emblematic of the previous twenty-five years. Within a single generation, the Pax Romana itself was a smoldering ruin. And from the ashes rose Commodus's terrifying new persona.

For Commodus, as it was for Rome, the epidemic era was a turning point. Much like Hercules, who survived the trials given him by Apollo, Commodus had triumphed. After his father's generational war in Magna Germania, Commodus secured a decade of peace. He survived his sister's plots and betrayal. He humbled a hostile and petulant Senate by commissioning freedmen and other outsiders to bear the burdens of governance. He thwarted the riot (or insurrection, if it was such) associated with the deserter Maternus. He protected the grain supply after years of shortage. He pacified a riotous mob by giving them the head of his second-in-command Cleander. And now, the pestilence which had ravaged Rome for as long as he could remember had passed him over. Commodus had defied death again and again, and this last time in spectacular fashion—surviving perhaps the same devastating disease that had killed so many others, even possibly members of his own family. Following such miraculous endurance, a thought both awesome and terrible entered the emperor's wounded mind: Commodus was Rome's own Hercules—a new golden god for a new golden age.[66]

It is not a stretch to link Commodus's sense of invulnerability—even divine invincibility—to his survival of deadly epidemics. In fact, the same sentiments, albeit on a less grandiose scale, had cropped up among Athenians during the plague under Pericles. Thucydides records that those who recovered from the disease soon noticed that they did not catch the disease again, causing people to overestimate their invulnerability: "all men congratulated [the survivors], and they themselves, in the excess of their joy at the moment, had an innocent fancy that they could not die of any other sickness."[67] In a world absent germ theory

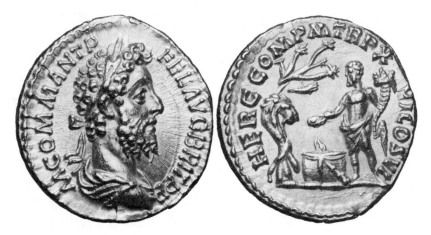

FIG. 7.2. A gold aureus minted in 190 showing Commodus as Hercules sacrificing and holding a cornucopia. RIC III 221d. Roma Numismatics Ltd, lot 492,
Commodus AV Aureus, www.numisbids.com.

and immunology, ideas about fate, luck, and the supernatural took hold.
If disease was brought about by impiety, then surviving disease was due
to divine favor. Besides, Commodus's father, Marcus, had been made a
god after death; Commodus was therefore the son of a god. It was no
logical leap for the emperor to believe that his endurance in the face of
so much death was robust evidence that he was specially chosen—that
his own godhood had arrived a little ahead of schedule.

Surviving evidence shows that Commodus's new persona emerged
and evolved speedily. In AD 190, Commodus's coin types feature the
normal titles and names. But on coin reverses, Hercules surges into
prominence.[68] The demi-god—who looked strikingly like Commodus
himself—held a cornucopia, representing prosperity, and poured a
drink offering from a sacrificial bowl.

The relevant text on these coin types—HERC COM—could be read
as *Herculi Commodiano* ("the Herculean Commodus").[69] And Cassius
Dio tells us: "Vast numbers of statues were erected representing him as
Hercules."[70] Indeed, one of the most well-preserved statues of the divine emperor—the Capitoline bust of Commodus as Hercules—shows
the emperor in full herculean garb, with club in hand and dressed in the
skin of the Nemean lion. The significance of the lion skin would not be

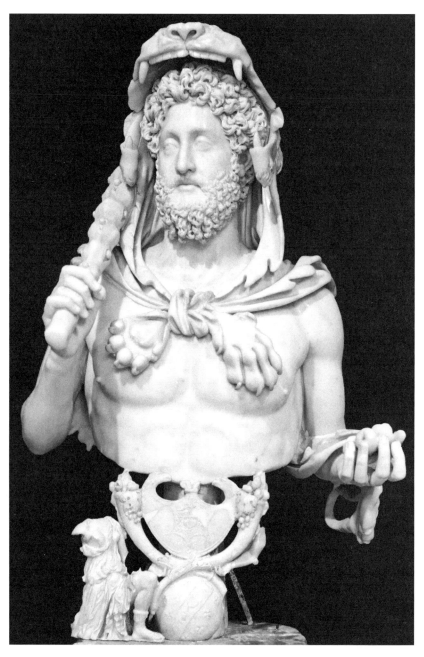
FIG. 7.3. Capitoline bust of Commodus as Hercules, likely dated to AD 190. Marie-Lan Nguyen.

lost upon ancient audiences. The first of Apollo's trials required Hercules to defeat the lion, whose skin was impervious to arrows. After strangling the lion to death, Hercules skinned the beast and fashioned a cloak of invulnerability. As with the coinage, cornucopia frame the bust. Commodus had supposedly secured lasting prosperity when the grain fleet finally arrived and the epidemic abated in the summer of 190.

Finally, the Capitoline bust shows Commodus in his philosopher's locks. But as the emperor's absurdities evolved, so too did his appearance. Shortly after the bust was commissioned, Commodus shaved his curls and adopted the clipped crop of a gladiator. Once a closely guarded secret, Commodus's gladiator bouts became public spectacle. The invulnerable emperor and survivor of Apollo's plague arrows proved his divinity under the gaze of tens of thousands of his countrymen in the arena. The god became a gladiator.

Both custom and law prohibited nobility from fighting in the arena, but Commodus would be restrained by no human institution.[71] The emperor's spectacles were unlike anything the city had ever seen. Or at least, this is what they were supposed to be. The emperor dressed in elaborate costumes; other times he fought nearly nude. At first, he murdered animals. Suspended from a bridge above the killing grounds, Commodus shot arrow after arrow into a sea of one hundred bears— massacring them all. As the emperor grew bolder, he took to the sands—slaughtering domesticated animals. As the tame beasts were brought to him, sometimes in nets, Commodus performed the work of a butcher, imagining it was something brave. He soon upgraded to more exotic victims—hippopotamuses, elephants, rhinoceroses, and a giraffe. Commodus demanded adulation for his bloody slayings. Cassius Dio says that the senators were required to routinely proclaim: "You are master and first and the most fortunate of all men! A victor now and forevermore you shall be! Amazonian, you are the conqueror!"[72] Under Commodus, "master" (*dominus*) surged into prominence as an imperial honorific.[73]

Eventually, Commodus fought real gladiators in staged battles, always with his prefect and bodyguard at his side. The unstated rules were similar to those when playing a wookie at chess: let the madman win.[74] At no time was Commodus ever in real danger. The contests were carefully controlled pantomimes. Commodus then turned to murdering his own subjects in public. The emperor's men rounded up some of Rome's disabled who had lost feet or legs due to accidents or disease. They were bound and dressed as serpents and given sponges as weapons. The Herculean Commodus then walked among them with his giant club, bludgeoning them to death as though he were destroying mythical monsters.[75] One very real monster walked the sands that day.

The divine gladiator's victims were also symbolic. The emperor seemingly left no public thing unmarred. Commodus had reinvented himself; why not reinvent his empire as well? The imperial palace became "the *Commodian* palace," the legions became "the *Commodian* legions," and, most distasteful, Commodus renamed the Roman Senate: "the *Commodian* Senate."[76] The emperor effectively flushed Rome's dignity down the toilet, renaming the thousand-year-old city "Commodiana" and refounding it as a colony "most immortal and fortunate of those of the whole earth."[77] Cowering senators played along, voting Commodus a series of unique titles and ostentatious names such as "Amazonius": an epithet referencing Hercules's victory over the Amazons; "Invictus": the invincible one; and "Exsuperatorius": the one who conquers all. These names and all of Commodus's others were then grafted onto the months of the year—sacrilegiously erasing the names of gods and emperors like Janus (January), Mars (March), Julius Caesar (July), and Augustus (August). Commodus also dropped from his own nomenclature the names associated with his father and grandfather—"Marcus" and "Antoninus." Commodus was a different person altogether. It was as though Commodus the guileless coward, the reclusive gladiator fanboy, the frightened hypochondriac who hid from disease and death had indeed perished in the pestilence.

For some elites, the damage done by Rome's cracked emperor dwarfed even the epidemic that seemingly spawned him. Unlike the contagion, however, there was no quarantine from the Roman Hercules. His divine presence was everywhere. Neither could elites defy the emperor and expect to live. Galen somehow survived the final years of Commodus's reign, writing afterward that "the crimes committed by

Commodus in a few years are worse than any in the whole of recorded history." As Commodus's childhood physician, Galen knew the young emperor better than most, and even he was aghast at the change that came over his former patient. Galen soon feared for his life and livelihood: "when I saw all of these things happening daily, I schooled my imagination to prepare for the total loss of everything that I had . . . like other innocent victims."[78]

For some elites, the same remedies that thwarted the pestilence also helped them survive Commodus. Cassius Dio recounts a day when Commodus decapitated an ostrich in the arena and shook its limp head at the senators in attendance. They took this gesture to mean that Commodus would do the same to them. But in that moment, the wagging head and Commodus's smirking face was not frightening; it was hilarious. And so:

> Many would indeed have perished by the sword on the spot, for laughing at him (for it was laughter rather than indignation that overcame us), if I had not chewed some laurel leaves, which I got from my garland, myself, and persuaded the others who were sitting near me to do the same, so that in the steady movement of our jaws we might conceal the fact that we were laughing.[79]

Commodus was a laughingstock, but he was also emperor—and he had already proved his limitless capacity for murder. So Cassius Dio and his senatorial companions mitigated the wrath of Commodus in the same way they mitigated pestilence—with laurel leaves. Instead of smelling the plant, however, the senators chewed the laurel—and in filling their mouths, they avoided the snickering that would have surely led to their deaths.

But the senators had the last laugh. In December of AD 192—after more than two wearisome years of Commodus's megalomaniacal post-plague turn—elite conspirators finally put together a serious plot to murder the invincible gladiator. The emperor himself gave them the proper motivation. Commodus allegedly planned an unprecedented New Year's Day massacre. The kill list included several senators, the praetorian prefect, both consuls, and many of his servants, perhaps even

Marcia, his trusted mistress. Marcia had protected Commodus while he cowered from disease at Laurentum. Now she embraced the executioner's role. As Commodus drank to the coming new year, she slipped poison into his food. But Commodus drank so excessively that evening that he voided his stomach before the poison took full effect. Swooning, the emperor went to recover in his baths. The opportunity to be rid of Commodus seemed lost. But an athlete named Narcissus rescued the plot. He crept into the baths and strangled Commodus with his own bare hands. Within minutes, the invulnerable gladiator was dead—another pestilence finally eradicated.[80]

Roman elites wanted neither a resurgent plague nor another Commodus. The former was out of their control. The latter threat they mitigated by condemning the emperor in the strongest possible terms. A record of the Senate's decrees upon Commodus's death seemingly survives in a fourth-century AD biography. The lengthy and damning invectives condemn not only the physical body and actions of Commodus but even his memory:

> Let the honours of the murderer be taken away; let the murderer be dragged in the dust. The foe of his fatherland, the murderer, the gladiator, in the charnel-house let him be mangled. He is foe to the gods, slayer of the senate. . . . Cast the gladiator into the charnel-house . . . he who slew the guiltless, let him be dragged with the hook. . . . On all sides are statues of the foe, on all sides are statues of the murderer, on all sides are statues of the gladiator. The statues of the murderer and gladiator, let them be cast down. . . . Let the memory of the murderer and the gladiator be utterly wiped away.[81]

In a sense, the Senate expiated Commodus in the same way that cities across the Empire had expiated disease. Commodus became the pandemic's final scapegoat. The troubles of the Antonine plague era—the epidemics to be sure but also so much more—were affixed to Commodus's name and purged with extreme prejudice. With his death, the terrors that had plagued a generation were seemingly at an end. But so too was the Pax Romana.

8

THE END OF
AN ERA

Whether slowly suffocated near the end of the 170s, or with a bang in 190, the Antonine plague pandemic disappeared. And the familiar forces that spread and sustained the pandemic also diminished or temporarily dissipated in the late second century. Epidemic aftershocks may have occurred, but these escaped the notice of ancient writers. In fact, pestilence itself nearly vanishes from Roman sources for the next half century. Why this silence? In part, the Empire's elite writers became captivated by the dramatic events of the post-Pax era. But the Roman Empire had also changed rapidly and permanently during the Antonine plague years. Challenges which were abnormal to the generations born and raised during the Pax Romana became routine to their descendants who knew little else but unreliable Egyptian grain, price instability, coin debasement, martial treachery, brigandage, and other depressing markers of a rusting age.

So now the final verdict. Did the Antonine plague cause all these problems? Hardly, but the pandemic was nevertheless a catalyst of change in several crucial ways. The pandemic represented a comprehensive emergency. The pandemic's demographic, economic, social, political, and even spiritual components fertilized the sprouting stresses that preceded it. These crises then flowered in the 160s and 170s. Over time, the pandemic's very real presence diffused into a looming ethereal threat, even as the disease itself died out. The world's first observed pandemic—even if lacked the mortality of subsequent plagues—left a lasting impact on the societies that carried it for so many years. Disease deaths marred the Empire's demography for generations, no doubt straining the tax base, suppressing military recruitment, and prolonging violence as the survivors fought over scarce resources. Economic inequality should have been reduced by drops in land prices, but the economic changes during and after the Antonine plague were complicated, to say the least. But one thing is clear: the enduring presence and pangs of the Antonine plague—both real and perceived—left an indelible mark on the course of Roman history, helping foster the birth of a new late antique age.

A Turning Point?

How much responsibility does the Antonine plague pandemic bear for the Pax Romana's end? Was the pandemic, as ancient historian Kyle Harper puts it, "a turning point, the end of a certain trajectory in the development of Roman state and society"?[1] As is expertly shown by Harper's book *The Fate of Rome* and the fruitful debate which has followed, the question of whether any pandemic was a true historical turning point depends not only on how historians assess the scope and severity of the pandemic itself but also on its political, economic, and environmental contexts, among other factors.[2] Historians are also pulled by preexisting frameworks.[3] If scholars believe, for example, that the structures and institutions of the second-century AD Roman Empire were robust and resilient—that the Antonine plague clawed at a highly integrated society, with healthy economic and social connectivity, high birth rates, and low child mortality compared to other preindustrial societies—then even millions of plague deaths could have been overcome with time. The Empire's recovery is also directly related to how many people the pandemic actually killed—a number historians will never know. If conservative guesses at the level of death—such as 1 or 2 percent of the Empire's population—are correct, then not much recovery may have been needed. If mortality was higher, then Roman institutions required impressive resilience to sustain and rebound from such demographic devastation.

Insurmountable challenges prevent historians from accurately estimating the Antonine plague's overall impact. At minimum, scholars would need to know: (1) how many people lived in the Roman Empire prior to the pandemic, (2) how long the outbreak lasted, (3) total mortality, and (4) at what rate the population recovered. We know none of these things. Even guessing at these figures produces its own wide set of variables. So historians must instead construct compelling narratives based largely on qualitative arguments and informed speculation. Readers now have my story of the Antonine plague. And I make no secret that my account rests on the notion that the Pax Romana may not have had far to fall in the first place. It is true that producers, transporters, and other economic actors during the Pax Romana had larger ships, better equipment, and improved technology compared to earlier or later periods.[4] But Roman elites were also excellent propagandists, and we should question their monumental claims about the greatness of their empire prior to the Antonine plague. Historians do not know, for example, whether overall capital stocks in the Empire as a whole, especially relative to the growing population prior to the Antonine plague, were much higher compared to previous centuries.[5] At best, the Pax Romana may have been but a little more prosperous than what came before or after—despite some evidence of a momentary economic effloresce in per capita economic growth.[6] To put it another way: the Antonine plague did not knock Rome off its pedestal because there was no pedestal. The most enduring changes stimulated by the pandemic were political, social, and cultural—the result of a perceived pandemic, as much as a real one. The pandemic obviously generated real and in some cases crippling economic effects, but these factors' long-term impact accompanied gradual ecological shifts and institutional innovations.

Broadly speaking, I agree with Harper's assessment that the Antonine plague was both a "turning point" and yet was no "fatal blow" to the Empire, but for different reasons. Harper sees a resilient Roman Empire withstanding around seven million plague deaths. That figure seems plausible if the pandemic indeed lasted a full twenty-five years. My view

of the evidence suggests a pandemic half that length at most, and therefore less deadly as well. But a far lower guess at total mortality—just one
or two million excess deaths from plague, for example—would nevertheless severely disrupt military recruitment, tax collection, food production, and a host of other fundamentals of Roman power and resilience. Whatever the correct death toll, the systemic damage, in my view,
was in many cases indirect. The pandemic exposed and accelerated inherent weaknesses in the tributary mechanisms of the Roman economy—a system fundamentally unsustainable from its outset.[7] State
intervention underwrote the Empire's connectivity and monumentality.
Free-flowing trade, surging capital stocks, technological innovation, and
dynamic labor markets seem to have been marginal phenomena under
the Antonine emperors, if not in the preindustrial world more broadly.
Even highly marketable luxury goods from Egypt, for example, made
their way to Rome on the back of the *annona* grain fleet. Much of the
Pax Romana coincided with favorable ecological conditions and one-off
fortuitous events (e.g., the conquest of Egypt, the procurement of mines
in Dacia, the collapse of the Parthian Empire, etc.) that were just sufficient to stave off fragmentation. The peace and prosperity of the Pax
Romana rested upon a house of cards even before the pandemic blew
through the Empire.

The pandemic's arrival activated what historians call a "catastrophe-
flip"—a situation in which smaller and even "invisible" changes accumulate in the structures of society, eventually passing a threshold
which ushers in a dramatic and sudden crisis.[8] The Antonine plague
was as much a catalyst of catastrophe as it was a catastrophe in its own
right. Against the fragile Pax Romana, the Antonine plague pressed
suddenly and unexpectedly, jolting Roman society into a new era that
had been silently prepared in prior decades. As a catastrophe-flip, the
pandemic's impact alone was less important than how it combined and
augmented other changes at work in key structures and systems. Nearly
two thousand years of hindsight and vastly improved knowledge, despite a dearth of surviving evidence, give modern historians insights
that the Romans lacked. Historians' long-term perspective helps them
see the transformation that occurred—how different Roman society

was in the third century as opposed to the second century. This hind-sight illuminates both the individual factors and key interactions among these factors which accelerated the foundational shifts that ended the Pax Romana.

The first issue of note is that the pandemic did indeed end, although it is true that we cannot say with full assurance when the Antonine plague wrapped up its terrorizing tour of the Roman world. On the one hand, the pandemic may have fizzled out way back in the 170s—and the epidemic of 190 was some local pestilence or other novel disease. On the other, the apparent reverberations in the sources—descriptions of pox outbreaks in the Roman Empire, China, and the Arabic world along with DNA-confirmed aVARV in Viking Age skeletons—may signal that the disease never truly abated; it just burned out or became semi-endemic in a few localities and thus no longer seemed worth mention-ing by ancient authors. But if military movements, food shortages, and climate change in key regions were essential elements in the Antonine plague's story, it is worth tracking these same factors as the pandemic faded into history. In the twenty-five years since the disease's initial in-cursion into Roman territory, much had in fact changed.

Commodus's reign—especially compared to his father's—lacked a major conflict that entangled massive armies—the preindustrial world's most effective disease vector. Under Marcus, the Empire fought large-scale, protracted back-to-back wars in Parthian territory (AD 161–166) and then along the border of Magna Germania (AD 166–180). Troop movements related to these major conflicts seem a significant factor in the Antonine plague's persistent presence in the Empire. But Commodus bought a respite from such conflicts and their requisite military mobiliza-tions and demobilizations. Instead, his reign was characterized by smaller-scale insurrections, revolts, and brigandage—activities perhaps sufficient to keep a communicable disease circulating (maybe to eventu-ally return to Rome in 190) but insufficient to sustain Empire-wide epi-demic waves of any but the most highly transmissible diseases.

Shortly after Commodus died, however, a period of civil wars fol-lowed from AD 193 to 197. If the disease responsible for the Antonine plague were still around—perhaps only on life support—we should expect to see a vengeful return. The eventual victor of those wars, the emperor Septimius Severus who reigned through AD 211, marched armies back and forth across the Empire—from Pannonia to Italy, then all the way to Syria and then back to Gaul in the west. Immediately following his victories against armies of fellow Romans, Septimius then took soldiers beyond Roman borders back into the Parthian Empire. Like Avidius Cassius thirty years prior, Septimius even sacked Ctesiphon. He ventured to Egypt as well. Cassius Dio recounts that Septimius went up the Nile and encountered a pestilence at the Ethiopian frontier.[9] All of this military activity, and yet, no renewed burst of the pandemic, or indeed any epidemic disease? But as we saw with the military movements prior to the Antonine plague, the Roman Empire was not intrinsically conducive to large-scale epidemics. Nor were roving armies the only factor. Military movements under Augustus and Trajan, for example, seemed especially prone to bring novel viruses into the Empire, and yet such never materialized. To prompt a pandemic in the loosely integrated preindustrial world, an entire set of conditions had to align with exactitude.

Perhaps waning immunity held new outbreaks at bay during the 190s? Back in the 160s, Lucius's vulnerable soldiers flooded into Parthian territory, wintered in plague-infested cities, and then marched back through the eastern Empire, becoming traveling petri dishes and shedding contamination wherever they went. And these returning soldiers traversed through populations which apparently also lacked immunity, even if the disease had already hit some cities in Asia Minor. It seems as though conditions in the mid-190s were different. Some of Septimius's soldiers—no small number of which hailed from the Danubian provinces—were either veterans of the Marcomannic Wars or were children in those areas when the pandemic burned at its hottest. Some, maybe even most of these men, either as children or adults, had probably gotten sick and survived. In the 190s, the territories through which those soldiers marched and the cities they besieged were undoubtedly populated with plague survivors as well. Did the cities of the eastern Mediterranean enjoy population immunity sufficient to stifle new epidemics before they could begin?

Other conditions also seem different. In the 160s and 170s, regional food shortages and climate changes exacerbated the Antonine plague's intensity. While these problems did not necessarily go away—indeed, both phenomena contextualize the 190 epidemic at Rome—conditions in various Mediterranean localities, as they were wont to do, continued to shift. Roman officials also finally got around to adjusting institutional arrangements. In the early 190s, for example, Commodus's administration mitigated the increasingly fickle Egyptian grain supply by returning to the less productive but now more reliable standby of North Africa. While Africa had always been an important supplier to Rome, Commodus set up a new "African fleet" of grain ships to provide for Rome in years when Egypt failed.[10] Coins in all imperial denominations—a message thus aimed at all classes of people—commemorate the attempt to stop the shortages, but the message was mixed. On the one hand, more grain would now arrive at Rome; on the other, the action was a tacit admission that the Egyptian breadbasket bonanza was over. It was a harbinger of things to come. By the end of the next century, the political center of the Empire moved eastward toward Constantinople. By the time of that transition, the province of Africa—not Egypt— became the main supplier of grain to Rome.[11]

Increased state intervention mitigated food shortages (temporarily, and largely in Rome) in other ways. Late in Commodus's reign, merchants were forced to use part of their shipping capacity to transport Rome's *annona* grain.[12] In the short term, more grain would have flowed into the capital. Maybe it was enough to keep malnutrition at bay during those critical years after 190? Nile floods appear to have been fair at best in the 180s and terrible in the 190s. Officials' tinkering with the system may have kept the Empire on life support during those hard years, but not for much longer. Irrigation systems in Egypt went unmaintained.[13] Instead of banditry, outright civil war flared up again and again. Unsurprisingly, a new pandemic—the Cyprianic plague—emerged at the same time.[14] Much of what occurred under the Antonine plague—from religious persecution to economic crises—also returned, but far, far worse.

How did Romans perceive the changes swirling around them? From their writings, it is clear that some were sounding the alarms. But in the

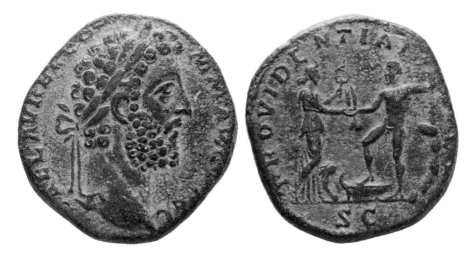

FIG. 8.1. Bronze sestertius of Commodus minted in Rome in AD 192. Hercules stands on the prow of a ship and receives grain from Africa. Classical Numismatic Group. Freiburg, Seminar für Alte Geschichte der Universität.

history of an empire that lasted centuries, the Antonine plague years were but a brief moment in time. In the lives of those who lived through the period, even changes which were at first alarming would have gradually accumulated into a new normal. The passivity of governing elites suggests they failed to react to changing realities until long after they had occurred. Hayek's knowledge problem reared its head: even if Roman officials could correctly identify the causes of change, and even sought to mitigate maleffects, they lacked essential knowledge to implement solutions free of negative consequences and knock-on effects.[15] As an example, let's return to Commodus's Alexandrian-styled fleet for transporting African grain to Rome during Egyptian shortages. Commodus's coins celebrated "the foresight (*providentiae*) of the emperor"— a distortion to put it mildly.[16] In reality, the intervention was decades too late. And there were both short- and long-term trade-offs. Diverting African grain did not increase overall grain supplies. Rather, the new arrangement merely *redirected existing grain* toward Rome, benefiting the city to be sure. But in the Roman Empire's zero-sum redistributive economy, less grain was then available to other cities; increased market prices of grain from the 190s onward (see below) likely reflect this situation. Rome's feast became the rest of the Empire's famine. The food shortages that had brought political instability in Rome were subsequently exported onto the cities and territories that formerly received African grain—likely some of the very same cities that erupted in civil war by the mid-third century. We see the same phenomenon, but even more clearly, with state-supplied olive oil. As political elites rapidly invested in African oil in the second century, production in Spain and Gaul subsequently nosedived.[17] Elites relocated in droves to Africa; they simply followed the money.[18]

We also see officials' late actions in surviving Egyptian grain prices. For more than a century, market prices of wheat in Egypt had been relatively stable at around 8 drachms per *artaba* (25–30 kg) of wheat.[19] In the decades following the Antonine plague, however, market prices fluctuated wildly between 12 and 24 drachms per *artaba*—about double the previous average price.[20] Grain was scarce, labor was expensive, and the quality of money had dropped. Prices never returned to the previous norm. And even as market prices increased to reflect Egypt's postplague volatility, state officials apparently failed to adjust their administrative "prices" for decades. The first state price above 8 drachms per *artaba* does not appear in the sources until the year 246!

Markets, where they existed, responded dynamically to structural changes; government officials and policy were far more rigid, even if the Pax Romana was relatively unbureaucratic compared to the late antique Empire. During the Pax Romana, gaming the system was absurdly simple. In Egypt, the grain tax could be paid in physical grain or taxpayers could substitute cash at the state rate for grain—and clearly the gap between the state rate and market prices widened following the Antonine plague.[21] In years of plenty, when market prices dropped below fixed state rates, sellers gladly sold the state their grain instead of taking the lower market rates. In years of scarcity, however, when market prices were high, sellers were free and clear to just pay a lower cash payment to the state and then take their physical grain to market, earning substantial profits. As the bad years increased, and market prices were more than double state prices, state granaries must have found their reserves diminishing. Even worse for Rome, the supply of *annona* grain would

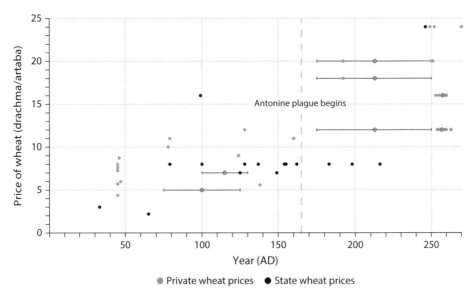

FIG. 8.2. Private and state wheat prices in Roman Egypt, AD 1–270.
For data, see Harper 2016b; Rathbone and von Reden 2015; Rathbone 1997.

have also been reduced, as the high profits available on markets incentivized tax dodging. Consistent with officials' passive administration and lack of preventative governance (see the first chapter of this book), no local or imperial official in Egypt thought to implement a simple legal fix to mitigate the situation. It took an imperial edict by the emperor Septimius Severus in the early third century to ban the substitute cash payments, forcing Egyptians to pay their grain taxes in physical grain no matter what the market price was.[22] By then, however, epidemics and food shortages over several decades had irrevocably damaged both Egypt and the Empire it fed.

For the remainder of the Roman period, land values in Egypt (if not elsewhere) never returned to their pre-pandemic highs. It is true that a group of ultra-rich estate owners was already on the rise prior to the Antonine plague—and would have taken over in good time anyway—but poor floods and then the pandemic ignited a fire sale in real estate. In the decades that followed, land consolidation and economic inequality accelerated dramatically.[23] By the fourth century, economic inequality in the Roman Empire reached an unsustainable pinnacle.[24] A painful leveling then followed.[25]

In theory, permanently cheaper land prices should have weakened the ultra-rich. Their main capital asset was real estate. Much of the Roman economy, however, operated on a different paradigm to theoretical free markets. Latent market forces in real estate did not have a chance to restore balance, as imperial elites swept in during the Antonine plague's aftermath and expanded their power and control over agriculturally productive land. In Asia Minor, for example, the imperial government bullied local elites into giving up control over the collection and expenditure of surplus resources.[26] Septimius Severus's warpath during the civil wars of the 190s led him through the region, where he confiscated numerous estates and looted the cities of his own empire. Emperors increased their use of secret police (*frumentarii*) to squeeze taxes and rents out of provincials. State officials had become used to certain levels of income and expenditure. In fact, military costs had ballooned. So rather than settle for reduced revenues in light of the pandemic and other calamities, officials plundered their own people at sword point to make up the difference. Herodian's account of the deeds of the emperor Maximinus Thrax (AD 235–238), for example, stand in stark contrast to Roman rule prior to the pandemic:

> After Maximinus had impoverished most of the distinguished men and confiscated their estates, which he considered small and insignificant and not sufficient for his purposes, he turned to the public treasuries; all the funds which had been collected for the citizens' welfare or for gifts, all the funds being held in reserve for shows or festivals, he transferred to his own personal fortune. The offerings which belonged to the temples, the statues of the gods, the tokens of honor of the heroes, the decorations on public buildings, the adornments of the city, in short, any material suitable for making coins, he handed over to the mints.[27]

The literary sources suggest that soldiers were major beneficiaries of the social and economic reorientation that followed the Antonine plague.[28] During the pandemic, neither Marcus nor Commodus increased legionary

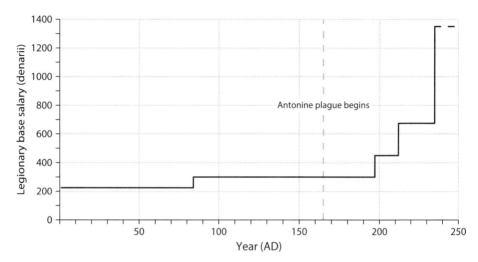

FIG. 8.3. Legionary base salaries, AD 1–250.
After Alston 1994. From AD 235, legionary base salaries are impossible to
calculate and the dashed line is meant to represent this uncertainty.

base salaries—constrained by tradition perhaps but certainly by the
lack of silver. But Septimius Severus made a splash by raising nominal
soldier base pay (exclusive of bonuses) from 300 to 450 denarii per year
in AD 197. Septimius's son Caracalla added a further 200 denarii to military salaries in 212. Finally, Maximinus Thrax took the booty looted
from his own citizens and doubled Caracalla's pay rise to a whopping
1,350 denarii per year.[29]

These ballooning salaries may in part reflect a direct effect of the Antonine plague: deaths among soldiers and the military recruitment base.
Fewer soldiers but greater demand (due to civil wars) would have put
upward pressure on salaries that even emperors could not ignore
forever—but other forces were also at work. Septimius dutifully rewarded
his legions for supporting him during his civil war for supremacy; he had
to, otherwise he risked the same fate of those he himself supplanted. Securing and sustaining power in this post–Pax Romana became a matter
of funneling as much money as possible to the soldiers. Hence, Septimius's son Caracalla probably passed out his salary increase from a need
for survival more than anything else, as did Maximinus Thrax.

But the overwhelming cause of rising soldier wages must have been the fact that the quality of imperial coinage went into freefall following the Antonine plague. Rome had no central bank to manipulate interest rates—no helicopter to litter city streets with freshly printed cash.[30] Instead of running the printing press at breakneck speed, the Roman mint diluted the silver coinage with base metal to fund emperors' scandalous spending spree on soldiers. If the silver mines had recovered from the Antonine plague and the concurrent outbreaks of violence, we would expect that the debasement would have been far less severe. Instead, as metallurgical analyses confirm, the mints simply recycled older coins—stretching existing silver supplies into more and more lower-quality coins. From the founding of the Empire until the Antonine plague—nearly two centuries—Roman coin standards show remarkable stability. The only sudden change in the denarius standard occurred under Nero.[31] Remarkably, the Antonine plague years show no substantial change in coin quality. Only as the pandemic wound down was monetary chaos unleashed. The freefall continued for several decades. By the mid-third century, the silver denarius—a denomination with a four-hundred-year history of reliability and high quality—was reduced to funny money.[32] It became, in essence, a copper coin with barely enough silver to pass muster. By the early AD 240s, denarius production ceased entirely. It was the end of one of human history's longest and most stable monetary regimes.

We would expect that such monetary mayhem would have generated skyrocketing inflation. The Antonine plague would have also put upward pressure on wages, as deaths reduced the supply of workers. Unfortunately, outside of military salaries, data on wages in the immediate aftermath of the pandemic are difficult to find. Surviving records from Egypt—ancient historians' meager statistics bank—produce some wage rates for unskilled laborers between the mid-second and mid-third centuries AD, but these are difficult to date. Scheidel's study of these sources and others shows that while wages indeed more than doubled in nominal terms following the Antonine plague, their real increase—due to offsetting changes in other areas of the economy—was far more moderate. He proposes two reasons for this unexpected situation: either

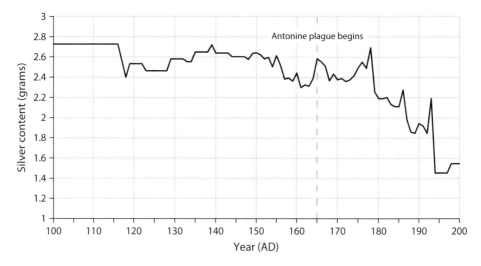

FIG. 8.4. Grams of silver in the Roman denarius, AD 100–200.
Target weight and fineness data for Trajan: Woytek et al. 2007. Fineness for
Hadrian through Commodus: Butcher and Ponting 2012. Fineness for Septimius: Gitler and Ponting 2003. Target weights for Hadrian through Septimius:
Duncan-Jones 1994. Fineness for years 145–146/7 is not known and so Butcher
and Ponting's figure for 144 was substituted for these years (an unfortunate
"fudging" for the sake of illustration but one unlikely to be misleading). Since
tribunician years run from December to December of the calendar year, the
latter year was used for the graph's data table. Unfortunately, metrological data
for third-century coinage still await revision, and I do not use the data found in
Walker 1978.

plague mortality was not as severe as that of subsequent pandemics,
such as the Black Death, or there were "institutional arrangements" that
prevented surviving workers from taking advantage of their improved
market position.[33] Both possibilities merit serious consideration.

To Scheidel's first point—that the Antonine plague was not as severe
as future pandemics—there now should be little debate. The Black
Death killed scores of millions. Bubonic plague's case fatality rate rose
as high as 50 percent in preindustrial cities—one of the deadliest figures
for any disease on record. And bubonic plague endured and spread even
into rural communities because of its animal reservoir. Wherever black
rats and/or carrier fleas could hitchhike via human transportation infrastructure, so too could bubonic plague. The disease responsible for

the Antonine plague, however, seemingly had a far lower case fatality rate. As a thought experiment, we might imagine for a moment that an orthopoxvirus not unlike aVARV was behind the Antonine plague—a virus that might have infected a wider range of host organisms compared to modern smallpox but also carried lower virulence.[34] From what we know of the demography and connectivity of the Roman Empire, such a disease would have quickly burned through cities—perhaps more than once. And even if the new disease did not kill at rates comparable to history's deadliest pathogens, elites across the Empire would soon come to recognize its symptoms, and to fear them.

But let's imagine a worst-case scenario as well: that the Antonine plague pathogen killed at rates witnessed in early modern smallpox pandemics (around 30 percent of cases). Let's also imagine that this highly lethal disease infected all 10–15 million or so of the Empire's urbanites and soldiers. Even in such an extreme counterfactual, a maximum of around 3–5 million would have died, plus some smaller number of rural inhabitants. But in reality, not everyone in the cities caught whatever disease was in fact behind the Antonine plague—even if it hit some population centers more than once, as appears to be the case in Rome and perhaps other major cities. The total mortality from epidemics during the Antonine plague, therefore, especially if the pandemic lasted only a decade or so, could have easily been as low as one or two million deaths—less than 5 percent of the Empire's population. Although that hypothetical number is "minimalist" compared to estimates and models, one or two million excess deaths would hardly be insignificant—especially as mortality from other routine causes pushed gross mortality during the Antonine plague much higher. And the longer the pandemic lasted, the higher its death toll and demographic impact—especially if the disease lingered long enough to generate relapses in cities once population immunity dissipated. In my view, therefore, Harper's estimate of around 10 percent aggregate mortality for a much longer twenty-five-year pandemic (with higher death rates in the cities and military, lower rates in the hinterlands) is also not outside the realm of possibility. Harper and I disagree about the length of the pandemic, perhaps less so its severity. Even then, as Harper rightly points out, the Antonine plague was still "the worst disease event in human history up to that time."[35] And more frightening in the long term, even with the pandemic's unprecedented body count, the outbreak was but a prelude to the deadlier outbreaks still to come as the era of pandemics ascended.

Scheidel's second point—that institutional arrangements thwarted workers' market power—also rings true in the evidence assembled in this book. First, general inflationary pressures, no doubt driven by changes in coin quality and quantity, ensured that nominal prices across the board rose—keeping increases in real wages low.[36] Price clearance during and after inflationary periods lags even in modern economies, and disparities between the real values of wages and commodities must have persisted for some time in Egypt. After all, how would Egyptian workers, or workers in any other part of the Empire, know that they even had the market power to demand higher wages during economic distortions? There were no empire-wide or even local wage statistics available to them, or anyone else for that matter. There were certainly no labor unions as such among agricultural workers to fight for the suddenly available extra money. Furthermore, as this book has shown, cooperating with the Antonine plague were grain shortages, violence, inflation, and other era-specific problems as well as broader constraints like predation, limited technological innovation, and a dominant cultural obsession with status.[37] Under such conditions, market clearance would have been slow, stilted, and heavily distorted by cultural mores, overriding social customs, and capricious state power. In a more free-market economy by contrast, population reductions during the Antonine plague would have given workers more bargaining power almost instantly. But the prevailing economic and social paradigms of the age survived the pandemic. Estate owners kept wages low because *they could*. They had overwhelmingly superior economic knowledge and power. The Roman system was constructed by and for patrimonial elites. The cultural, social, and economic power that gave elites their privileged place in various hierarchies also kept them there in the aftermath of the Antonine plague. Elite dominance, I suppose, is one thing that even pandemics cannot altogether eliminate.

The Antonine plague's accelerating effect was, therefore, both real and powerful—a result of both its own pathology and the unique historical world in which it ran rampant for a time. Slowly emerging but nevertheless serious stresses combined into an emergency once the disease arrived in the 160s and 170s—and this before the causes and effects could be recognized and mitigated. Instead of reflective countermeasures and dynamic institutional adjustments—where trade-offs and opportunity costs could be judiciously considered, or at least reflected in economic outputs—the Roman state's clumsy and often late interventions failed to solve existing problems and sowed the seeds of further crises down the road. Edicts commissioning cargo space in ship holds, for example, mitigated food supply problems in the short term but had devastating long-term consequences. Long-distance sea trade was risky, and therefore costly. Such high risk needed to be offset by high profits. Even small spaces on ships, therefore, were valuable. But transporting state grain at fixed prices—which as we saw were lower than market prices—was a burden rather than a boon for shippers. Transportation along the Nile became more controlled and coercive from the late second century.[38] As the machinery of the state increasingly and myopically fed the grain system, the grain system devoured the economic capacity of the Roman Empire. Overall shipping profits diminished, causing marginal enterprises to fail, their capital capacity and resources lost forever. Goods of all kinds—luxury goods but also oil, wine, and, yes, grain—made fewer long-distance journeys and became more expensive compared to a counterfactual world without such mandates.[39] Sharp declines in amphorae finds and other markers of trade from around the time of the Antonine plague, and just after, are evidence of such general forces—although, again, there were multiple and sometimes local reasons for these shifts.[40] The sad fortunes of our Puteolian traders from chapter 6, for example, were but a local foretaste of the kinds of shortages and supply chain disruptions that multiplied in the third century AD. It is no surprise that those mandated to ship state grain soon sought to escape their profession and obligations. Did Roman officials reflect upon how their own policies had contributed to the crisis? No, of course not. Instead they pressed forward into the folly of command economics—doubling down on destructive authoritarianism. The emperors soon made it illegal to switch professions, and subsequently even bound sons to take up the professions of their fathers.[41]

The pandemic—as both a demographic shock in its own right and a companion to other crises—compressed into a few decades changes that likely would have occurred in the much longer term. Food shortages, for example, were to be Rome's destiny from the mid-second century, plague or not, save some inventor somewhere harnessing steam power (it may surprise readers to learn that the necessary ingredients were in fact available during the Pax Romana).[42] But Rome's economy was simply too fragile, and its surpluses too marginal, to allow for any other trajectory in its preindustrial context. But in a counterfactual world without the Antonine plague, and its unpredictable epidemic bursts, the Empire might have dedicated more resources to mitigating changing realities in other spheres. We can see what might have been if we look to the years after the Antonine plague. To entertain just one counterfactual: had a ban on cash payments for grain taxes in Egypt been enacted even a decade or two earlier in an empire not dealing with plague-hampered protracted wars, grain supplies would have been higher and demand far lower. More soldiers would have been demobilized; and instead of killing Germanic peoples, and consuming state-expropriated food, those men might have instead produced grain in the fields, satiating both themselves and the wider Mediterranean grain market. The Pax Romana, fragile though it was, might have continued its miracle run into the third century AD. Instead, nature, but also the Romans themselves, chose a different path. And that path dead-ended with the Antonine plague.

Violence Once Again

The Antonine plague was a serious and deadly pandemic event, but its effects varied wildly in the Roman Empire. As hard hit as the armies and cities must have been, some regions barely noticed the pandemic or the accompanying crises of the age. But crises need not be "total" to still have widespread and even transformative effects. Disparities in eco-

nomic resources and resilience in the eastern and western parts of the
Roman world, for example, predated the Antonine plague—but disease
outbreaks clearly sped along the west's decline at a more rapid pace.[43]
Empire-wide pottery distributions following the Antonine plague show
a reduction in east-west commerce, suggesting that supply networks
gradually reduced in scale.[44] Market connectivity disintegrated. The
hallmarks of a command economy emerged. Less than a decade after
the AD 190 epidemic, for example, the emperor Septimius Severus in-
stituted a "temporary" tax—the *annona militaris*—to pilfer wine, meat,
oil, bread, and other necessities for his army directly from the population. This army then used those resources to murder fellow Romans.
Unsurprisingly, the tax became permanent. The violence endemic to so
many of Rome's institutions—at times veiled during the Pax Romana—
also enjoyed a robust and long-lasting resurgence.

The new economic realities that emerged during the Antonine plague
anticipated the political disintegration that followed. In the year after
Commodus's death, five different men claimed to be emperor. Their
wars for dominance crisscrossed the Roman world for several years,
leaving even more devastation and death in their wake. The victor in
those wars, Septimius Severus, established a new dynasty—although
he audaciously adopted himself into the family line of Marcus Aurelius
retroactively. Yet violence remained endemic, and competing factions
fought over the scraps of a diminishing empire. The short-lived Severan
dynasty gave way to outright rule by warlords. Then a separatist "Gallic
Empire" made up of provinces in Gaul, Britain, and Iberia divided from
the central Roman authority. Shortly thereafter, a second split, this time
in the east, pulled provinces in eastern Asia Minor, Syria, Palestine, and
Egypt under the authority of newly minted monarchs in the Syrian city
of Palmyra. The economic fragmentation that seems to have begun just
prior to the Antonine plague blossomed into permanent political bal-
kanization. Even when the Empire was "reunified" for a time in the
fourth century, it was ruled by multiple emperors in a highly regionalized and often antagonistic conglomeration.

After the Pax Romana, brutish emperors attempted to arrest decline
through the only means they understood: naked violence and coercion.[45]

By the early fourth century AD, maximum prices were set on many goods throughout the Roman world. The policy obviously ushered in shortages, misery, and death. The veil of the Pax Romana had been snatched away. But whether via the gladius, the bayonet, or presidential pen, capricious state power brings neither prosperity nor sustainability. And violence and coercion cannot mitigate pandemics and their broader effects either; indeed, totalitarian mitigations often have the opposite effect, and compound and extend diseases' intrinsic suffering. The Roman Empire failed to understand this lesson. For subsequent world powers, the jury is still out.

THE SPIRIT OF PANDEMIC

Madness is something rare in individuals—but in groups, parties, peoples, ages it is the rule.

—FRIEDRICH NIETZSCHE

Even the survivors of the Antonine plague were now long dead; well, most of them anyway. It was the middle of the third century AD. The Antonine plague's final curtain fell some sixty years prior. Now a second pandemic—the plague of Cyprian—swept through a shattered, divided, and war-beleaguered Roman Empire. The bygone Pax Romana gave way to an era of permanent emergency. For some, it seemed the world hurled toward apparent dissolution. Meager harvests, dead livestock, burning cities, civil wars, and now once again empire-wide pestilence carried on unabated. Surviving inscriptions from the period reflect the desperation of the times: "save the imperial system!" the stones cry to various gods.[1] But the same deities that failed during the Antonine plague continued to ignore Romans' pleas for a miracle.

It was not as if the Romans grew lax in religious fervor in the decades following the Antonine plague. If anything, they had gone to ever more extravagant extremes to satisfy their gods' enduring fury. To note just one indicator: over the previous half century, thousands of Christians had been slaughtered for their lack of deference to Roman gods and emperors alike. But evidently such ghastly levels of human sacrifice were still not enough to waylay whatever deities still tortured and pummeled the earth. The local rituals of cleansing, expiation, and scapegoating that had not worked during the Antonine plague were expanded. Roman officials and the useful idiots that followed them responded like most would during a moral panic—concluding that their irrational mitigations had failed not because their entire frame of reference was intrinsically flawed but because they had not pursued their mad butchery with sufficient devotion, unity, and totality. A sadly familiar outcome followed, as punishing and persecuting the noncompliant somehow evolved into an essential article of faith. What we might call the spirit of pandemic—a new global conception of disease, and especially its causes, effects, and remedies—had broken containment and now ran free in the Roman Empire.

As the spirit of pandemic infected those at the top of Rome's political apparatus, a new proclamation inaugurated the next phase of sanctifying atrocities.[2] The emperor Trajan Decius (AD 249–251) enacted a grand mandate. Every single inhabitant within Roman territory must contribute to collective inoculation through ritual worship of traditional gods. There were to be no religious exemptions. In fact, officials even forced some to carry a unique "passport" as such: a certificate verifying that an individual had duly sacrificed and was, therefore, immune from blame for the woes of an evil age. Failing to produce this official proof of obeisance not only brought social and economic marginalization, but not sacrificing was a capital offense. The civic supplications to Apollo during the Antonine plague had failed—but here was the same mitigation strategy once again, only writ large.[3] Undoubtedly many hoped the universal sacrifices would arrest the Empire's unraveling. For the ruling elite, however, it was crucial that someone else take the blame—the insufficiently pious, the gods themselves even. It did not matter how tenuous the connection, so long as those in charge never be held responsible.[4]

Aurelius Diogenes—aged seventy-two years—complied with the emperor's edict in Upper Egypt on June 26, AD 250. We have his official papers to prove it. Aurelius was one of a select few individuals still alive who had lived through the Antonine plague. And yet he, like everyone else, was required to submit to the whims of a regime that had abandoned itself to ignorance, madness, and folly. His signed certificate includes a litany: "I have always sacrificed regularly to the gods, and now, in your presence, in accordance with the edict, I have done sacrifice, and poured the drink offering, and tasted of the sacrifices."[5] We do not know if the old man bore his sacrifice certificate gleefully or reluctantly, or whether he might have even been a Christian collaborating in his own persecution in the vain hope that his abusers would relent if they saw sufficient abasement in their victims. Either way, Aurelius lived out his final years in a dark period in Roman history. How did things go so unimaginably wrong?

Variations on the paradoxical mainstream extremism that blossomed in the century following the Antonine plague have in fact appeared often in human history. Famines, plagues, and wars place demands upon prevailing beliefs, ideologies, and practices that they cannot meet.[6] Disasters, therefore, tend to motivate rapid cultural evolution. Established Roman religion could neither explain nor arrest the accelerating crises that emerged with the Antonine plague. Asclepius, for example, for all he was during the Antonine plague—patron deity of Galen and visitor to Marcus Aurelius's dreams—was never again sought out by Roman officials to ward off plague.[7] Statues of Mercury were systematically mutilated, stripped of all divine attributes, and buried in Londinium near the end of the second century—a sign of disillusionment and even rage against the old gods.[8] Inscriptions from villagers in Asia Minor confess individual acts of impiety against various gods and detail the punishments dished out by the vengeful deities.[9] But the Antonine plague and its fallout not only undermined public trust in specific deities but threatened the religious establishment itself.[10] Rives called the Decian mandate "the culmination of earlier concerns with religious impropriety."[11] Later, when the dust had settled following Christianity's eventual triumph, Augustine of Hippo said as much in his *City of God*: "Where, then, were those gods who are supposed to be justly worshipped for the slender and delusive prosperity of this world, when the Romans, who were seduced to their service by lying wiles, were harassed by such calamities?"[12] It was an "I told you so" hundreds of years in the making.

The Antonine plague pandemic arrived during an age of angst—a time of growing unease in an otherwise prosperous period. In the middle of the third century, however, full-blown terror reigned in many corners of the Empire. As a new pandemic pestilence exploded onto the scene, things got ugly quickly. The African bishop Cyprian—the plague's namesake, and key witness to its effects—was thrust into the middle of the fray. Anti-Christian sentiment in his area was at a fever pitch, and the African governor Demetrianus was railing for blood. In reply, Cyprian published an open letter, detailing the claims of Demetrianus and his fellow agitators: "you say that very many are complaining and are blaming us because wars are arising more frequently, because the plague, famines are raging, and because long droughts are suspending the rains and showers . . . because your gods are not worshipped by us."[13] Interestingly, the bishop's reply confirms the basic facts in his accuser's now lost missive. "The world has now grown old," Cyprian writes, before listing a body of evidence eerily familiar to readers of this book:

> In the winter the supply of rain is not so plentiful for the nourishment of seeds; there is not the accustomed heat in the summer for ripening the harvest; neither are the corn fields so joyous in the spring nor are the autumn seasons so fecund in their leafy products. To a less extent are slabs of marble dug out of the disemboweled and wearied mountains; to a less extent do the mines already exhausted produce quantities of silver and gold, and the impoverished veins are lessened day by day. The farmer is vanishing and disappearing in the fields, the sailor on the sea, the soldier in the camp, innocence in the market, justice in the courts, harmony among friendships, skill among the arts, discipline in morals. . . . wars continue with greater frequency, that barrenness and famine accumulate anxiety, that health is broken by raging diseases, that the human race is laid waste by ravages of pestilence.[14]

Many of the same signs of distress that accompanied the Antonine plague had remerged, but now with more ferocity. Cyprian prepared an alternative explanation for these calamities: the one true God was accelerating the world he created toward a final judgment. Demetrianus and his ilk were not saving the world by persecuting Christians, they were unwittingly destroying it. In a sense, it was Demetrianus's own argument and evidence thrown back in his face. Except Cyprian had a major advantage. From the days of the Antonine plague to his own time more than half a century later, appeals to the traditional gods had been met with silence.

By contrast, Cyprian's argument was both compelling and urgent. The true God was in fact speaking, as he had been for ages past, but only his chosen people heard his voice. Old Testament prophecies (Cyprian quotes Haggai, Habakkuk, Malachi, Amos, and Hosea, among others) reframed the evidence cited by the church's enemies into a coherent case for a long-announced apocalypse.[15] Disasters compounded in the age so that "the wrath of God may be known."[16]

And God spoke through other witnesses too. Running parallel to the legacy of failure of traditional religion and ritualism, an army of Christians had endured martyrdom. As God poured out his wrath in increasing measure, Cyprian could prove that Christians withstood the crisis with stoic devotion—outdoing even the most principled philosophers of the age. The rewards God promised his faithful soldiers would come not so much in this life, but the risen Christ himself, the lamb become the lion, would distribute unmeasured blessings from his white throne in the heavenly kingdom yet to come.[17] And so the Christian framework offered triumph in the face of trial, and even joy in the midst of suffering. Cyprian made sure to point this out to the church's critics:

We are not prostrated by adversities, nor are we broken down, nor do we grieve, nor do we murmur in any catastrophe of events or in sickness of body. Living by the spirit rather than by the flesh we overcome the weakness of the body by the strength of the soul. By those very things that torture and weary us we know and are confident that we are proved and strengthened. Do you think that we endure adversities equally with you, when you see that the same adversities are not sustained equally by us and by you? With you there is always a

clamorous and querulous impatience; with us there is a strong and
religious patience always quiet and always grateful to God.[18]

In fact, the tribulations of the mid-third century represented the merciful interventions of a loving God. They were a means by which he pa-
tiently warned those outside the fold of an inescapable, inevitable, and
imminent judgment. In the epidemics, famines, and wars, God was offering the Roman Empire a lengthy (yet not indefinite) opportunity to
turn from idolatry and repent, before it was too late.[19]

Cyprian's letter and the criticisms to which it responded illustrate the
centralizing spirit that had swept the Empire—in the words of Rives: "a
shift in focus from actual local communities to the imagined community of the empire as a whole."[20] Both Christians and non-Christians
were drawing upon expanded thinking about both the natural and spiritual realms. Not long after the bishop's death, imperial authorities would
come to exercise almost totalitarian control over inhabitants of the
Roman world—believing they should and could regulate employment,
private religion, and even the prices paid for basic goods.

The Antonine plague seems a crucial waypoint along the path toward
the new normal of the late Roman Empire. The pandemic's real effects
mattered, as this book has shown, although in some localities more than
others. But did the categorical novelty of the pandemic wield enduring
conceptual power in the universalizing age that followed the Pax Romana? Once diseases were perceived as global, it may have been simply
a matter of time before appropriately grandiose and totalizing remedies
were implemented.

The power of pandemic perceptions is evident in the ease with which
Cyprian as well as his critics spoke in such grand and globalizing terms.
The problems cited were total: climate, pandemics, the gods—causes
that afflicted "the whole world," at least as ancient peoples understood.
How many in the mid-third century remembered those killed in the
Antonine plague? The total number of victims was, of course, never
known. But even by then, the mythology of "the great pestilence" may
have mattered more than its already embellished reality. Tales of its scale
and scope and its associated trauma were what survived. These echoes

evidence the way in which the Antonine plague shaped views of crises, as well as their remedies.

The arrival of pandemics like the one witnessed during the Antonine plague—diseases of such virulence and transmission sufficient to strike whole empires—seems a key development in an evolving late antique zeitgeist. The Antonine plague was the first of these, but hardly the last. The evidence of Cyprian's letter, the empire-wide mandate to sacrifice, and the monumental religious shifts that accompanied Late Antiquity's arrival—all of these seem to have emerged from perceptions, even if vaguely defined, that had formed and imbibed amid crisis. They signify reaction rather than reflection.[21] Many discourses of the age, whatever their source or audience—Christian, pagan, local, or imperial—are totalizing and universalizing. They reflect a notion of global catastrophe which memories of the Antonine plague must have helped shape.

In spiritual terms, it may not have much mattered that the disease's real effects were highly regionalized, varied, and sometimes even nonexistent. That it was a disease with the potential to strike anyone anywhere—features shared by subsequent pandemics—nevertheless gave its terror a historical novelty. Later pandemics—the Justinianic plague, the Black Death, and the smallpox pandemics of the early modern period—would overshadow the Antonine plague in terms of total mortality, quality and quantity of source material, and ongoing popular and scholarly interest. But that first pandemic, because it was first but also because it struck ascendant empires connected across three continents—empires which subsequently birthed nations and peoples, many of which still exist—exerted a disproportionate influence on how our very species conceived of and responded to global disease in the ages that followed.

History's turns are ever strange. The zeitgeists of ages past leave clear ripples across cultures, economies, and political systems long after their catalysts have sunk beneath the dark, unrecoverable depths. The Antonine plague—whether it splashed like a stone, or crashed like a cannonball—slammed into the societies of Eurasia. This first pandemic set in motion actions, reactions, patterns, and proclivities. Variants of Antonine Age responses would reemerge again in other periods, including our own. And pandemics are written into our world's future fate. Whatever the pathology of these forthcoming scourges—their mortality, their transmission, and, hopefully, their cures—we must now ask: will all-too-familiar patterns of angst, panic, and persecution return again and again? If human societies are to endure or even thrive amid such inevitable stresses, contemporary medical interventions and scientific knowledge alone will not prompt necessary social evolution. To learn to live with pandemics and their deadly realities, we must all become historians, and sound the depths in search of the embedded echoes of pandemics past.

ACKNOWLEDGMENTS

Many people made this book possible—so many that I worry that I might forget a few. Paul Erdkamp and Kyle Harper read the entire manuscript—more than once—and offered detailed, critical, and invaluable feedback as part of a book workshop held at Indiana University in the spring of 2022. Brandon McDonald generously and thoroughly critiqued a late version of the manuscript while it was in press; I incorporated as many of his interventions and references as I could before production deadlines forced me to stop. Ann Carmichael read and commented on the earliest version of the book and kindly kept me informed of new publications in the years following. My colleague Peter Guardino also read the manuscript and offered advice to improve the book's accessibility to a wider audience. Other Indiana University colleagues Dan Caner, Rich Holdeman and Jeremy Schott looked over chapters or sections of texts which were in dire need of outside specialists. Bill Beck and Matthew Christ helped me translate some of Galen's most puzzling Greek. Daniel Gaines kindly checked over my graphs and also ran a change-point analysis on the lead emissions data in chapter 6. Véronique Boudon-Millot, Werner Eck, Mischa Meier, Vivian Nutton, Niki Papavramidou, Caitlin Pepperell, Nichole Sheldrick, Robin Symonds, and John Wilkins provided expertise, insights, translation help, and/or access to their work. Sadie Elliott acted as a beta reader. My colleagues Deborah Deliyannis and Eric Robinson provided encouragement and mentorship. Three excellent department chairs have supported my work on the Antonine plague: Eric Sandweiss, Wendy Gamber, and Michael McGerr. Finally, I wish to thank my many inspiring students at Indiana University.

This book would not exist without Barry Strauss, who offered helpful advice on the proposal and manuscript, and I suspect sparked the relationship between myself and Princeton University Press. Princeton's team has been a delight to work with, especially Rob Tempio. Rob helped me craft my existing research on the Antonine plague and its context into a book I am truly proud of. Besides his advice, ideas, and practical help, Rob also found fantastic anonymous referees who offered thoughtful, critical, clear, but also constructive and encouraging feedback. In addition to the many others who guided the book through the production process, I would like to thank Jenn Backer for her meticulous copyediting. Any errors that remain are my own.

The book is dedicated to my grandparents, all of whom are now gone. I thank my mother and brother for support both past and present. To my children, Eva, Lily, and Roo: you are my treasures, for whom I would give anything. Thank you for motivating me to work diligently, while also being the reason for my work. Thank you Sadie, my love. Your worth is greater than precious stones, and nothing I could desire compares to you.

NOTES

All translations of ancient sources are quoted or adapted from the Loeb Classical Library unless noted otherwise. Biblical passages come from the English Standard Version. *IGRR* 4.1498 adapted from Parke 1985, 150–51.

Introduction: A Furious Beginning

1. Pliny claims Seleucia's population was 600,000; see Plin. *HN* 6.122.

2. Hom. *Il.* 1.33–53.

3. Amm. Marc. 23.6.24; SHA *Verus* 8.1–4.

4. Mayor 2020, 156–78, 215.

5. Toner 2013, 180–82.

6. See, for example, Niebuhr 1875, 241, 246–47; Seeck 1897, 398–405.

7. Gilliam 1961; Salmon 1974, 134–39.

8. Littman and Littman 1973; Zelener 2003.

9. Duncan-Jones 1996, 2018.

10. Flemming 2019; Bruun 2007, 201.

11. Suggesting caution is Newfield, Duggan, and Poinar 2022.

12. A discussion I take up in chapters 3 and 4. For now, no doubt to some readers' great annoyance, I will use the term "pandemic" in anticipation of this discussion.

13. Toner 2013, 52.

14. As is the case with the Cyprianic and Justinianic plagues; see Harper 2018, 3.

15. Duncan-Jones 1996, 121.

16. Elliott 2016.

17. Such as Grunewald 2004, 17–18.

18. Tac. *Agr.* 30.4. Translation after Morley 2010, 38.

19. Noreña 2021; Davidde 2018.

20. Dio Cass. 72.36.4.

21. Millar 1964, 122–23.

22. More on the nature of "complexity" in Ross and Steadman 2017, 1–5; Tainter 1988, 22–38.

23. Scheffer 2009, 101–3.

24. Sheldrick 2021.

25. Haldon et al. 2014.

26. Bang 2008.

27. Cleary 2013, 464–66.

28. This book will avoid treating the Antonine plague as a "plague concept"—an almost mythological assumption that makes an outbreak, epidemic, or pandemic an agent of historical change by default. See Eisenberg and Mordechai 2020.

Chapter 1. Rome's Fragile Peace

1. Aristid. *Or.* 26.11–18, as translated in Lewis and Reinhold 1990, 123.

2. *HDF* 1.78.

3. A case eloquently argued throughout his *The Imperial Order*, but especially at Wesson 1967, 242–43.

4. Aristid. *Or.* 26.70.

5. Tac. *Hist.* 1.4.

6. Bowes 2020a, 2020b.

7. After Walker et al. 2004. For a discussion of resilience in the Roman Empire, see Erdkamp 2019.

8. Scheffer 2009, 103.

9. I borrow this language from Harper 2016a, 109.

10. Hayek 1988, 33.

11. Scheidel 2019.

12. See, for example, Amm. Marc. 14.6.24.

13. Ellis 2000, 1–5.

14. And far more common in the Vesuvian cities; see Wallace-Hadrill 1994, 72–82.

15. Israelowich 2015, 118.

16. Laes 2011, 38–39.

17. McGinn 2004, 295–302.

18. Ibid., 55–71.

19. Sen. *Controv.* 10.4.8. On the invention of Pax Romana, see Sen. *Clem.* 1.4.2 and the commentary in Braund 2009, 215–16.

20. Sen. *Ep.* 104.6.

21. Mattern 2013, 116–17.

22. Juvenal 3.247.

23. Aldrete 2018, 373–74.

24. Many examples (including those following) provided and translated in Varone 2015.

25. *CIL* 4.7714, 7715.

26. Platts 2019, 263–64n134.

27. *CIL* 4.6641.

28. *CIL* 4.7038.

29. *CIL* 6.31615, 4.3872, 3832, 4586; Koloski-Ostrow 2015, 111–12.

30. Scobie 1986, 413.

31. *Dig.* 9.3.1, 43.10.1.

32. As described in Aldrete 2014, 46–48; Koloski-Ostrow 2015, 81.

33. Aldrete 2007, 142.

34. SHA *M. Ant.* 8.4–5.

35. Koloski-Ostrow 2015, 64–66.

36. Smith and Kahila 1992.

37. Carroll 2018, 24–25.

38. Or at least attempts were made; see Suet. *Heliog.* 17.1–2.

39. Koloski-Ostrow 2015, 68.

40. See the rough calculations in Bodel 2000, 129. Malaria, however, probably drove the death rate even higher; see Scheidel 2003, 174–75.

41. Graham 2006; Bodel 2000, 131–34; Varro *Ling.* 5.25.

42. Suet. *Claud.* 25.2.

43. Philo *Spec.* 3.114–15.

44. MacKinnon 2013, 126–27.

45. Mart. *Ep.* 10.5.

46. Suet. *Vesp.* 5.4.

47. Gal. *Hipp. Epid. IV* 4.10.

48. Scheidel 2012b, 276.

49. Koloski-Ostrow 2015, 73.

50. Frontin. *Aq.* 16.

51. On fluorine and lead in skeletal remains, see Killgrove 2018, 2017.

52. Gal. *SMT* 1.7.

53. Tan 2017, 25–26.

54. Evans 1994, 140–41.

55. On these categories, see commentary in ibid., 8–12.

56. On benefits of Roman aqueducts, see Kron 2012, 218–20.

57. Such as lice; see ibid., 234.

58. M. Aur. *Med* 8.24.

59. See the discussion in Fagan 1999, 183–84.

60. Mattern 2013, 118. And this without the chlorine to kill bacteria.

61. Fagan 1999, 182–83.

62. SHA *Had.* 22.7.

63. Celsus *Med.* 5.26.28d.

64. We do not need the frequent references in SHA *Heliog.* to tell us this.

65. McGinn 2004, 23–26.

66. Plin. *HN* 11.99.

67. Mitchell 2017, 54.

68. Mitchell 2017; Ledger et al. 2018.

69. Gal. *Purg. Med. Fac.* 2 11.328K.

70. Genetic samples are suggestive but still unclear; see Marciniak et al. 2016.

71. Sallares 2002, 221–30.

72. Scheidel 2007a, 327.

73. I.e., death; see Horace, *Epist.* 1.7.8–9.

74. Sallares 2002, 283. And now see Browning 2021.

75. Jongman, Jacobs, and Klein Goldewijk 2019. For more on measures of "biological standard of living," see Komlos 1994, 1995. On the problems with using stature as a proxy for economic performance, see Gowland and Walther 2018; Flohr 2018; Scheidel 2012a.

76. All cited in Kron 2012, 204.

77. Martyn et al. 2018; Rowan 2017, 2016.

78. Jongman, Jacobs, and Klein Goldewijk 2019, 146. Malnutrition must have also played a role, as the following chapter discusses; see also Garnsey 1999; Harper 2021a, 192.

79. Differences were not statistically significant, but they were noted by Killgrove (2018). See also some criticisms in Saller 2022, 20–21.

80. Scheidel 2012b, 267–69.

81. Kertzer and Barbagli 2001, 167.

82. Frier 2001, 150.

83. Hin 2013, 104.

84. Sallares 2002, 277; Scheidel 2013, 55–56.

85. Antonio et al. 2019.

86. Harper 2021b, 22.

87. The topic is much debated, but see at least Goldsmith 1984; Lo Cascio 1994; Scheidel 2001b; Frier 2001; Scheidel 2008; de Ligt 2012. On probabilities for population, see Lavan 2019.

88. For example: *OGIS* 484, *AE* 1936, 128, *Dig.* 1.3.38.

89. Suet. *Tit.* 8.4.

90. Dio Cass. 72.18.5.

91. Toner 2013, 91–99.

92. See examples in Livy 3.7.6–8, 4.25.3, 5.31.5. Discussion in Szabó 2020, 807.

93. The low estimate is 7–9 million people; see Scheidel 2007b, 80. A higher and perhaps more reliable estimate of 14–15 million has more recently been offered by Hanson and Ortman (2017). See also Temin 2013, 251–52.

94. Plin. *Ep.* 10.37.

95. Plin. *Ep.* 10.38.

96. Morley 2010, 17.

97. Plin. *Ep.* 10.47. The Apameans claimed to be willing for Pliny to inspect their accounts but also noted that "it was their long-established custom and privilege to manage their internal affairs in their own way."

98. Lewis and Reinhold 1990, 251.

99. Such as *FIRA* 1.80.

100. *SEG* 14.479.

101. Toner 2013, 186.

102. Erdkamp 2002, 107–10.

103. Philostr. *VA* 1.15.

104. Amm. Marc. 26.3.6.

105. Erdkamp 2002, 102.

106. Plin. *Ep.* 10.43. This and other excepts from Pliny's letters are modified from the translation of Munro 1904.

107. Amm. Marc. 14.7.5–6.

108. Jongman 2003; Scheidel 2003; Morley 1996.

109. Segre 1947.

110. After Erdkamp 2018, 304; Kron 2012, 208–10; Sallares 1991, 203–93.

111. Estimates such as those in Wilson 2011. On migration in Italy, see Isayev 2017.

112. Lib. *Orat.* 19.59.

113. Garnsey and de Ligt 2016.

114. Bernard 2016.

115. For more on seasonal labor, see Erdkamp 2016; Hawkins 2016, 23–65.

116. Tacoma 2016, 196.

Chapter 2. The Dry Tinder of Disease

1. Birley 2002, 120.

2. Dio Cass. 71.1.1.

3. Fronto *ad Ant.* 4.1.

4. For this date, rather than autumn of AD 161, see Aldrete 2007, 30.

5. For a lucid description of the maladies listed in this paragraph, see ibid., 143–50. On flood frequency, see ibid., 72–74.

6. Dio Cass. 53.33.5.

7. Plin. *Ep.* 8.17.

8. Dio Cass. 54.1.2.

9. Sigl et al. 2015; Baillie and McAneney 2015; Rossignol and Durost 2007.

10. McConnell et al. 2020.

11. Fell et al. 2020.

12. McDonald 2021, 381–84, 393; Sigl et al. 2015.

13. Elliott 2016; Newfield and Labuhn 2017.

14. Büntgen et al. 2011; Ahmed et al. 2013; Haldon 2016, 220–24; Margaritelli et al. 2020.

15. Most emblematically Horden and Purcell 2000.

16. Erdkamp 2021b.

17. Büntgen et al. 2011; Ahmed et al. 2013.

18. Austrian Alps: Mangini, Spötl, and Verdes 2005. The Spanish cave data have been less clear. A study initially suggested no anomaly but was later called into question: Martín-Chivelet et al. 2011; Domínguez-Villar 2013. New data taken from sites throughout the Iberian Peninsula suggest microregional variability: Thatcher et al. 2020; Domínguez-Villar et al. 2017. On the general picture of speleothems and Roman climate, see Harper and McCormick 2019, 26–30.

19. Erdkamp 2021a, 10–12.

20. Labuhn et al. 2016.

21. To borrow language from Toner 2013, 158.

22. Bowman 1986, 37.

23. On Egypt as the main source of Roman *annona* grain, see Erdkamp 2019, 441–42; Erdkamp 2005, 226–37. Erdkamp estimates that two-thirds of Rome's grain came via state-managed channels. Contra Temin 2006, 137–38.

24. See a more thorough discussion of these factors, rather than my crude summary, in Erdkamp 2005. On the involvement of the state in Nile grain transport, see Adams 2017.

25. Blouin 2016.

26. Elliott 2016. Greater detail and precision in McDonald 2021.

27. Bernhardt, Horton, and Stanley 2012.

28. Bagnall 1993, 16.

29. Strab. 17.1.48.

30. Sen. *QNat.* 41a.2.2.

31. Plin. *HN* 5.58.

32. Ibid.

33. Dio Cass. 51.21.4.

34. Zanker 1990, 180–81.

35. Dio Cass. 51.17.1.

36. Suet. *Claud.* 18.2; Tac. *Ann.* 12.43.2–4.

37. Sen. *Brev. vit.* 18.5–6.

38. Tac. *Ann.* 12.43.4.

39. Suet. *Claud.* 18.2.

40. Suet. *Claud.* 19.1; Gai. *Inst.* 1.32C. See also the excellent summary in Levick 2001, 109–10.

41. Tac. *Ann.* 15.18.2. The grain was probably spoiled.

42. Plin. *Pan.* 31.6. For more on the interplay between ecology, culture, and monetization in Roman Egypt, see Elliott 2021.

43. Plin. *Pan.* 31.5.

44. As conditions during and following the Antonine plague make abundantly clear; see especially chapter 8.

45. McCormick 2013. The Fayyum seems to have been spared until the third century AD, perhaps because of its reservoir. On the Fayyum, see Huebner 2020.

46. *P. Berlin* 372.

47. Ritner 1998, 16–17.

48. Bonneau 1971, 133–35.

49. Numerous errors are shown by Huebner 2020, 507–11, for example.

50. Hassan 2007.

51. Siler et al. 2017.

52. Brunstein and Yamaguchi 1992.

53. Routson, Woodhouse, and Overpeck 2011.

54. Zaroug, Eltahir, and Giorgi 2014.

55. Nash et al. 2016.

56. Harper 2018, 2.

57. On these non-ENSO phenomena and Ethiopia, see Viste and Sorteberg 2013.

58. Gebregiorgis, Rayner, and Linderholm 2019.

59. Wils et al., n.d.

60. Dubache et al. 2019; Choi et al. 2015.

61. Woodson et al. 2017; Woodson 2014.

62. On the connection between sea surface temperature and the monsoon, see Black 2005; Song et al. 2012.

63. Ferdière 2020, 457–58.

64. SHA *Comm.* 17.7.

65. Spurr 1986, 21.

66. Kehoe 2020, 500–501.

67. Symm. Ep. 2.6–7; Amm. Marc. 19.10.

68. For additional proxies, see McDonald 2021.

69. Garnsey 1999, 50.

70. With acknowledgment of the challenges of these terms; see Heinrich 2018, 102–3.

71. Much in this paragraph, crude summary that it is, comes with much gratitude from Heinrich and Hansen 2021.

72. Ps-Josh. *Chron.* 38. Translation is Wright 1882.

73. Ps-Josh. *Chron.* 42.

74. Stathakopoulos 2012, 108. On the confirmed presence of an ancestral orthopoxvirus across Europe in the seventh century AD, see Mühlemann et al. 2020.

75. Ps-Josh. *Chron.* 26.

76. Jutikkala and Kauppinen 1971.

77. Scheidel 2007b, 61.

78. Scrimshaw, Taylor, and Gordon 1968.

79. McMillen 2015, 15–56; Jones 2003.

80. Gal. *Diff. Febr.* 1.4.

81. Brown 1971, 12.

82. On "endemic" malnutrition, see especially the introduction of Garnsey 1999.

83. Heinrich and Erdkamp 2018, 1019.

84. Heinrich 2018, 108–12.

85. Gourevitch 2013, 40.

86. Gal. *Alim. Fac.* 1.37.

87. Gal. *Nat. Fac.* 1.14.56.

88. Garnsey 1999, 56–57. See also Killgrove 2017.

89. Buccellato and Catalano 2003.

90. Jongman 2007b, 607–9. Studies of skeletal remains elsewhere, including Egypt, show similar nutrient deficiencies; see Scheidel 2001a; Scheidel 2012b, 272–75.

91. Scheidel 2012b, 273.

92. Harper 2017, 78. And no doubt inequality as well; see Scheidel 2012a.

93. See the aforementioned study by Jongman, Jacobs, and Klein Goldewijk 2019.

94. Killgrove and Tykot 2013.

95. Stathakopoulos 2004, 55.

96. Here I summarize the excellent outline in Stathakopoulos 2012, 107.

97. Garnsey 1998, 240–41.

98. See the concise discussion of Holleran 2012, 133–36. Prices in Plin. *HN* 18.90. Commentary in Elliott 2022.

99. Gal. *Vict. Att.* 22.

100. Gal. *Alim. Fac.* 1.7.

101. As suggests Tchernia 2016, 214–15.

102. Toner 2013, 158.

103. Orib. 1.14.1, 15.4.

104. A good summary is found in Gourevitch 2013, 32–36.

105. Euseb. *Hist. eccl.* 9.8.6. All Eusebius texts follow Schott 2019.

106. On markets, social cooperation, and resilience in food systems, both ancient and modern, see especially Heinrich and Hansen 2021, 64–67.

107. Bang 2008, 84–93.

108. Toner 2013, 91.

109. Gal. *De Prob. et Prav. Alim. Succ.* 1. As translated in Wilkins 2015.

110. Using this language is Patterson, Witcher, and Di Giuseppe 2020, 207.

111. Plin. *Pan.* 30–31; *CIG* 2927. See also Erdkamp 2018, 299; Erdkamp 2005, 233–34; Garnsey and Saller 2014, 122–23.

112. Figures discussed in Garnsey 1989, 211–14. On making the dole more exclusive, see Bernard 2016, 55–59.

113. Erdkamp 2005, 242.

114. Quenemoen 2013, 68.

115. Hayek 2014, 371. See also Hayek 1945, 1937.

116. A good summary of such sources (and their theoretical ignorance!) is found in Erdkamp 2005, 262–65.

117. *CIL* 3, pp. 2208–9.

118. Erdkamp 2018, 300.

119. Euseb. *Hist. eccl.* 9.8.9.

120. Calculations after Tchernia 2016, 214–15. A lower figure of 150,000,000 kilograms is given in Erdkamp 2013, 263.

121. Broekaert and Zuiderhoek 2020, 110–11.

122. Beresford 2012; Horden and Purcell 2000, 142.

123. Brandt 2006, 34.

124. Greene 1990, 28–29; Rickman 2002.

125. *BGU* 1.27.

126. On the matter of a "convoy," historians tend to follow the language of Sen. *Ep. 77.1–3;* see, for example: Bagnall 2021, 60; Alcock 2006, 228; Garnsey 1989, 235; Rickman 1980. The exact operational mechanisms of the convoy, however, are unknown. See also Tac. *Hist.* 4.38 and perhaps even Cic. *Off.* 3.50–53, although the latter is a hypothetical case. Convoys of ships were common in Roman-era trade; see Adams 2017, 186–87; Lo Cascio 2018, 128–29; Schneider 2007, 163. Questioning the notion of a convoy is Geraci 2018, 229–30.

127. *Cod. Theod.* 13.5.6.

128. *AE* 1955, 184.

129. *Cod. Theod.* 14.22.1. See extended commentary in Tran 2020.

130. Brandt 2006, 37.

131. Calculated using *ORBIS* (https://orbis.stanford.edu/).

132. Tchernia 2016, 215.

133. Sen. *Ep.* 77.1–3. Also Erdkamp 2013, 271–72. For estimates of Roman food consumption, see Tchernia 2016, 214.

134. Plin. *Pan.* 32-1-3.

135. *Dig.* 50.5.3, 6.6. See also Broekaert and Zuiderhoek 2020, 111–12.

136. As clear connections between numbers of senatorial elites and regional agricultural product show; see Weisweiler 2021.

137. McNeill 1998, 130.

138. Heather 2017.

Chapter 3. Rumors of Death

1. Sallares 2007, 37.

2. SHA *M. Ant.* 9.3–5.

3. Robin 1992, 222.

4. See especially Harper 2017, 98–99.

5. Davidde 2018; Sedov and Salles 2010; Young 2001, 30–31.

6. Davidde 2018, 583.

7. Robin 1992, 231–32.

8. A comprehensive survey of scholarship on trade in the western Indian Ocean is provided in Seland 2014.

9. On the emergence of these longer journeys, see Cobb 2018a.

10. *Periplus* 57. Writing in the early first century AD, Strabo (17.1.13) corroborates the emergence of long-haul Indian Ocean voyages: "In earlier times, at least, not so many as twenty vessels would dare to traverse the Arabian Gulf far enough to get a peep outside the straits, but at the present time even large fleets are dispatched as far as India and the extremities of Ethiopia, from which the most valuable cargoes are brought to Egypt, and thence sent forth again to the other regions; so that double duties are collected, on both imports and exports."

11. On the size and construction of Roman Indian Ocean and Red Sea ships, see Sidebotham 2019, 195–205.

12. Evers 2017, 83–116; Cobb 2018b, 84–86.

13. Fitzpatrick 2011, 40–41.

14. Ptol. *Geog.* 1.11, 17.

15. Young 2001, 29.

16. *Hou Hanshu* 88.12. As translated in Hill 2009.

17. Benjamin 2018, 170–74.

18. Ibid., 101.

19. Yeh et al. 2016.

20. Rossignol 2012, 91–95.

21. De Crespigny 2007, 514.

22. Bivar 1970.

23. As we see in the Muziris Papyrus (*SB* 18.13167). See commentary in Evers 2017, 105–6.

24. Most of these ships carried under 75 tonnes of cargo; see Broekaert and Zuiderhoek 2020, 111–12. On Alexandria, see Strab. 17.1.13.

25. Dio Chrys. *Ad Alexandr.* 40.

26. See the helpful description and images found in McKenzie 2007, 173–220.

27. A helpful discussion of Egypt's limited entry points is found in Alston 1995, 18–19. The "artery of communication" phrase comes from Scheidel 2002, 98.

28. Rathbone 2007, 706.

29. Scheidel 2001a, 57–61.

30. Ibid., 76.

31. *P. Edwin Smith.* Nunn 2002, 106.

32. Plin. *HN* 26.3.

33. See most recently the survey by Huebner and McDonald, forthcoming.

34. Although how significant these routes were during the Roman period remains a matter of controversy; see Benjamin 2018, 131–33.

35. Strab. 16.2.30. See also the discussion in Millar 2006, 282–83.

36. Bowersock 1983, 83–84.

37. Bang 2008, 204.

38. Such as Eck 2012b, 104.

39. Ivleva 2016, 162–64.

40. Bowman 1998, 72, 78.

41. James 2019, 254.

42. Retsö 2003; Marek 1993.

43. Strab. 16.4.24.

44. Ibid.

45. On the existence of a "fleet" in the Red Sea, see Nappo 2015, 57–62.

46. Terpstra 2015, 74.

47. Although Cassius Dio discusses unsanitary conditions in the military camps; see Dio Cass. 68.31.4.

48. Ivleva 2016.

49. *P. Vindob.* G. 40822. See additional commentary in De Romanis 2020, 287–89. On the Roman approach to protecting existing trade as opposed to directing or creating trade routes, see the helpful commentary of Young 2001, 193.

50. Al-Talhi and Al-Daire 2005.

51. Young 2001, 94–96.

52. Costa 1977.

53. Nappo 2015, 67.

54. de Procé and Phillips 2010; Phillips, Villeneuve, and Facey 2004.

55. Plin. *HN* 6.176; Strab. 16.4.18; Aristid. *Or.* 26.70.

56. Mathew 2017, 90–94.

57. Alston 1995, 98–99.

58. Detachments such as the Cohors I Flavia Cilicia, which constructed a monument to Lucius and Marcus at Egypt's southern border. See *AE* 664.

59. These movements are attested in several inscriptions. See *ILS* 1097–8, 2311.

60. For a succinct list, see Birley 2002, 125.

61. Luc. *Hist. Conscr.* 15.

62. Pollard 2000, 58–59.

63. Gregoratti 2020, 463–64.

64. Baird 2018, 87–122.

65. James 2019, 265.

66. Leriche 1986.

67. Kennedy 1983.

68. Edwell 2007, 116.

69. Amm. Marc. 23.6.24.

70. Rossignol 2012, 92.

71. *MAMA* 4.275a. Commentary in Miller 1985, 50–52.

72. Haldon et al. 2018, 4.

73. Graf 2008, 74–77.

74. Paus. 1.3.4.

75. Aristid. *ST* 2.38.

76. *CIG* 3165.

77. Flemming 2019, 222–23.

Chapter 4. Plague Unleashed

1. Nutton 2020, 31–32.

2. Gal. *Praen.* 4.6 also speaks of high profits for physicians in Rome during Galen's time.

3. Plin. *HN* 29.8.18, 21. As translated in Healey 1991.

4. Gal. *MM* 9.8.

5. Boudon-Millot 2001, 41.

6. Gal. *Hipp. Prog.* 7.850 K.

7. Assuming smallpox and running such models is Zelener 2003. See also Zelener 2012.

8. *De theriaca ad Pisonem* 16. On translating this source, and also its disputed authorship, see Leigh 2016.

9. Harper 2021a, 192.

10. Measles' reproduction number (R0) is between 12 and 18; see Guerra et al. 2017; Russell et al. 2019.

11. Pezzullo et al. 2023; Blackburn et al. 2020.

12. Balows et al. 2012, 413. No doubt some of these deaths were caused by indirect effects; see Sabraa and Borsch 2016.

13. Fenner et al. 1988.

14. According to Gal. *Lib. Prop.* 3. Dio Cass. 73.14.3 links the plague with events in mid-spring.

15. McDonald 2021, 374; Rossignol 2012.

16. Krylova and Earn 2020; Scott and Duncan 1998, 181–83; Fenn 2002, 156–57.

17. Huq 1976.

18. Public health interventions were crucial; see Krylova and Earn 2020.

19. Dio Cass. 71.2.4.

20. *CIG* 1495.

21. Dodd 1911, 235–38.

22. Millar 1993, 112.

23. Alföldy and Halfmann 1979, 206.

24. Fronto *ad. Am.* 1.6.

25. Birley 2002, 144–45.

26. *AE* 1913, 170. See commentary in Roth 1999, 239–40.

27. Kulikowski 2016, 49.

28. Hankinson 2008, 13–14.

29. Nutton 2020, 36.

30. Gal. *Lib. Prop.* 1.15.

31. Nutton 1973, 159.

32. Andorlini 2012, 19n15.

33. Harper 2015a; Scheidel 2013, 45–49.

34. Harper 2017, 81–84.

35. For troop arrival in late August, see Singer 2014, 78n6.

36. On street traders, see Holleran 2012, 194–231.

37. SHA *Verus* 13.1–3.

38. Toner 2013, 72.

39. For example, John of Ephesus's account of the Justinianic plague in Constantinople, e.g., *Incerti auctoris* 2.

40. SHA *Verus* 13.4.

41. Bruun 2012, 138–43.

42. Procop. *Bell.* 2.23.3.

43. Blanchard et al. 2007; Castex et al. 2009; Kacki et al. 2013; Salesse et al. 2014.

44. McDonald 2020, 123.

45. Mitrofan 2014, 10.

46. Jer. *Chron.* 270h (Helm); Suet. *Tit.* 8.3–4. Other rooms yielded third-century coins, perhaps connecting those burials to the Cyprianic plague, but such a conclusion is disputed. See Harper 2015b, 226; contra Huebner 2021, 168.

47. For more detail on these burials, see McDonald 2020, 122–28.

48. SHA *Verus* 13.5–6.

49. Procop. *Bell.* 2.23.18.

50. Euseb. *Hist. eccl.* 9.8.6–11.

51. Similar stoppages occurred during the Black Death; see More et al. 2017.

52. The case that Fronto died near the end of 166 or beginning of 167 is convincingly made in Champlin 1980, 139–42.

53. See especially M. Aur. *Med.* 1.8.

54. Fronto *ad Ver.* 2.3.

55. SHA *M. Ant.* 2.5.

56. Gal. *Ind.* 35. As translated by Nutton in Singer 2014.

57. Case in point: Viking-era smallpox material; see Mühlemann et al. 2020.

58. Littman and Littman 1973; Gourevitch 2013; Lo Cascio 2012.

59. Carmichael and Silverstein 1987.

60. Duggan et al. 2016.

61. The age of smallpox continues to be a matter of controversy. See, for example, Thèves, Crubézy, and Biagini 2016.

62. Newfield, Duggan, and Poinar 2022; Mühlemann et al. 2020.

63. Mühlemann et al. 2020. See also the sources in Needham 2000, 124–27.

64. Shchelkunov 2011.

65. The most comprehensive summary of symptoms is still found in Littman and Littman 1973. Also see Cunha and Cunha 2008, 9–13.

66. Gal. *MM* 5.12. Galen uses similar language ("like scales") in Gal. *At. Bil.* I should thank Kyle Harper for pressing me to investigate Galen's comments on scarring more thoroughly and my Indiana University colleague Bill Beck for his comments on Galen's Greek, which were invaluable.

67. Mulhall 2019, 175–76.

68. Cunha and Cunha 2008, 12.

69. Mulhall 2021.

70. Gal. *MM* 5.12.

71. Helpful comparisons recently in Harper 2021b, 26–28; Harper 2017, 104–7.

72. Flemming 2019, 233–34.

73. Vlach 2022, 91–92.

74. Mühlemann et al. 2020.

75. Harper 2021a, 195–96. See also now Huebner and McDonald, forthcoming.

76. Eisenberg and Mordechai 2019; Mordechai et al. 2019; Mordechai and Eisenberg 2019; Eisenberg and Mordechai 2020; Newfield 2022.

77. Gilliam 1961; Littman and Littman 1973.

78. Duncan-Jones 1996; Scheidel 2002; Zelener 2003; Paine and Storey 2012. A recent moderating view between maximalist and minimalist positions on plague mortality at around 10–20 percent is offered in Harper 2017, 115. Skepticism of the highest estimates appears in Bagnall 2002; Greenberg 2003; Bruun 2003, 2012.

79. Bailey 2013; Scheidel 1996.

80. Dio Cass. 72.14.3.

81. Varlik 2015, 253–75.

82. *Incerti auctoris* 2.14–15.

83. Toner 2013, 149–50.

84. Jer. *Chron.* 270h (Helm). It is unclear if this is the same plague mentioned in Suet. *Tit.* 8.3–4.

85. The discussion here of the *sodales Antoniniani* rests on the discussion in Bruun 2012, 125–26.

86. On population densities in the Roman Empire, see especially Bowman and Wilson 2011; Wilson 2011.

87. Eichner and Dietz 2003.

88. Hays 2006, 46; Fenner et al. 1988, 196; Anderson and May 1982.

89. Cooper 1965, 86.

90. Vlach 2022, 91. Since the Antonine plague *was not* smallpox, we must see such models as heuristic.

91. Silk and Fefferman 2021.

92. See the estimates in Wilson 2011.

93. Sallares 1991, 230.

94. Fenn 2002, 28.

95. Hopkins 2002, 8–9.

96. Amm. Marc. 23.6.24.

97. Harper 2021a, 193.

98. Wilson 2011, 188; Hanson 2011, 249; Woolf 2000, 137–38.

99. Wilson 2011, 188; Audin 1970. Revised figure in Audin 1986, 11.

100. As may have happened in AD 177; see chapter 5.

101. Dossey 2010, 43–45.

102. Marzano 2013, 151.

103. *ILS* 3230.

104. Birley 1974.

105. Hor. *Carm.* 1.21.13–16.

106. Jones 2005, 299.

107. SHA *M. Ant.* 13.1, 21.6.

108. Fentress et al. 1991, 226–27.

109. Jones 2006.

110. Fentress 2003, 63–66.

111. Dio Cass. 78.15.2–7.

112. Rowan 2012, 115–26.

113. Bruun 2012, 132–36.

114. Simmonds, Marquez-Grant, and Loe 2008.

115. Ibid., 141.

116. Ibid., 33, 41. Small numbers in other categories (e.g., neonate, older adult, etc.) make up the remaining percentage.

117. Duncan, Scott, and Duncan 1994, 256.

118. Davenport, Schwarz, and Boulton 2011, 1295.

119. Morris 1992, 42.

120. Chenery et al. 2010.

121. The excavators wonder whether the burials were for transients and impoverished peoples but still prefer an epidemic-related interpretation; see Simmonds, Marquez-Grant, and Loe 2008, 139–40.

122. Beck 1986, 340.

123. *ZZTJ* 54.1757.A; *HHS* 107/17.3351. See also De Crespigny 2018, 60.

124. *HHS* 65/55.2133; *ZZTJ* 55.1761.B.

125. *ZZTJ* 55.1792.

126. De Crespigny 2016, 404.

127. *ZZTJ* 56.1826.

128. McNeill 1998, 298; De Crespigny 2007, 514. For AD 166, see *ZZTJ* 55.1792.

129. Hanson 2012, 5–6.

130. De Crespigny 2007, 1058; Twitchett and Loewe, 1986, 876.

131. The date and even authorship of the source are in some dispute; see Conrad and Wujas-tyk 2017, 23–24.

132. Ko Hung, Chouhou Beiji Fang (肘後備急方) 2.13.81. As translated in De Crespigny 2016, 405n105. Tao Hongjing edited the work in the early sixth century, and it is not always clear which parts are original to Ge Hong. See Needham 2000, 125–26.

133. Eighteenth-century British figures and analysis in Davenport 2020.

134. *Incerti auctoris* 2.100–106. See commentary in Morony 2006, 74–75.

135. Gal. *Hipp. Ep. IV et G. comm.* 1.29.

136. A variation on the pithy comments of Paine and Storey 2012, 189.

137. Heather 2012, 96–107; Goffart 2010, 242.

138. The chronology of the siege of Aquileia is unclear, and a matter of controversy.

139. Roselaar 2016, 146.

140. Echoing the idea that "the geographical shift of power away from Rome and Italy" was "already apparent in embryo in the second century" in Heather 2007, 66.

141. *CIL* 5.1874. Commentary in Mrozek 1994, 98.

142. As discussed in Erdkamp 2005, 266, 286–87.

143. Dio Cass. 54.1.1.

144. Hankinson 2008, 15.

145. Gal. *Lib. Prop.* 1.18.

146. Gal. *Praen.* 9.6.

147. Aur. Vict. *Caes.* 16.5.

148. Gal. *De praes. ex puls.* 3.3–5.

Chapter 5. The Age of Angst

1. Ael. fr. 206; Eutr. 8.10.

2. Dodds 1965; Downie 2013, 25.

3. E.g., MacMullen 1983, 64, 122–24.

4. Petit 1976, 117.

5. Martin 2013, 438.

6. Thuc. 2.53.4.

7. Toner 2013, 77.

8. Gal. *Lib. Prop.* 1.19.

9. Miller 2020, 106–7.

10. M. Aur. *Med.* 1.17.9. All excerpts from the *Meditations* are as translated by Hard (2011) unless otherwise noted.

11. Nutton 2002, 1983.

12. Hippocrates, *Nature of Man*, 5.16–19 notes, "Whenever many men are attacked by one disease at the same time, the cause should be assigned to that which is most common, and which we all use most. This it is which we breathe in."

13. Gal. *Diff. Febr.* 1.3.

14. SHA *M. Ant.* 28.8.

15. Thuc. 2.51.4.

16. Harris 2021, 239–40.

17. See examples from the Justinianic plague in Mordechai and Eisenberg 2019, 34–35.

18. Sen. *Ep.* 104.1.

19. Gal. *MM* 5.13.

20. Herodian 1.12.1–2.

21. Oliver and Clinton 1989, 376–77.

22. As pointed out in Bruun 2012, 126. See also Oliver 1970, 74–75.

23. Gourevitch 2013, 96.

24. Harris 2021.

25. See the summary in Israelowich 2015, 99–105.

26. Panagiotidou 2016, 91.

27. Lucr. 6.1272–74.

28. *SB* 16.12816.

29. Lucr. 6.1274.

30. These were adult males; children and women were not counted in censuses. For figures, see Duncan-Jones 1996, 120–21.

31. On the depopulation trend prior to the Antonine plague, see Bagnall 2002; Bagnall and Frier 1994, 169.

32. Scheidel 2001a, 115–16. The number in Butzer 1976, 74–75 (172.3) is lower.

33. Wilson 2011, 185–87.

34. Rathbone 2007, 706.

35. Duncan-Jones 2018, 45; Duncan-Jones 1996, 121–24.

36. Bagnall 2000, 292.

37. *P. Thmouis* 1, 104.9–21; see Blouin 2014, 271.

38. Dio Cass. 72.4.2.

39. Ibid.

40. See the excellent analyses of Blouin 2014, 267–97; Alston 1999.

41. Lewis 1993, 101–2; Lewis 1982, 70–79.

42. Philo *De spec. leg.* 3.30.159–62.

43. Dio Cass. 72.4.1.

44. Capponi 2010.

45. Grunewald 2004, 29–30. See also Strab. 17.1.19.

46. Gal. *Opt. med. cogn.* 1.4.

47. Or perhaps "A Hypochondriac and His God," as put by Phillips (1952).

48. Aristid. *ST* 2.38.

49. *MAMA* 4.275a.

50. Gourevitch 2013, 64–65.

51. At worst, he had malaria (*P. vivax*); see Browning 2021.

52. *CIL* 2.6278; Oliver and Palmer 1955, 340.

53. Gal. *SMT* 9.246; *Opera Omnia* 12.190ff.

54. Gal. *SMT* 9.1. Translation kindly provided by John Wilkins.

55. Fabbri 2007, 255–57.

56. *Ther. Pamph.* 1.14299 K.

57. Assuming it was indeed Galen who wrote *Ther. Pis.* 280–81, but this may be doubtful; see Leigh 2016, 19–61.

58. Herodian 1.12.2. As translated in Echols 1961.

59. Gal. *SMT* 10.15.

60. Nutton 2016, 275; Keyser 1997, 189.

61. Gal. *De praes. ex puls.* 3.4.

62. Nutton 2004, 162.

63. Panagiotidou 2016, 96.

64. On the idea that this verse may not have originated with Alexander's Glycon, see Thonemann 2021, 118–19.

65. Luc. *Alex.* 36.

66. Faraone 2018, 117.

67. Jones 2005, 297.

68. Parke 1985, 152–54.

69. Nutton 2004, 288–90.

70. Jones 2016.

71. The case is compellingly made in ibid., 471–72. The kissing reference also connects it to the Antonine plague and Alexander; see Thonemann 2021, 126–27.

72. Perring 2011, 273–80.

73. Irby-Massie 2018, 143–44.

74. Merrifield 1996, 111.

75. Perring 2011, 269–73.

76. Alexander himself petitioned for these coin designs, according to Luc. *Alex.* 58.

77. Luc. *Alex.* 48.

78. *IGR* 590.

79. Luc. *Alex.* 36.

80. Janssen 1994.

81. Kirkup 2013.

82. Nutton 2004, 288.

83. Nutton 1990, 253–54.

84. Furedi 2019, 111.

85. Johnston 2009, 35–36.

86. Serv. *Ad Aen.* 3.57.

87. Bremmer 1983.

88. Philostr. *VA* 4.10.

89. Graf 2015, 514–15.

90. Ibid., 514; Parke 1985, 152.

91. Gordon et al. 1993, 150; Nutton 2004, 289.

92. Graf 1992.

93. The epicureans were the other group.

94. On Christian faith, see Gal. *Diff. Puls.* 2.4. Galen's praise of Christians comes from a somewhat murky transmission history of Galen's lost summary of Plato's *Republic*; see Walzer 1949, 15–16.

95. Stark 1996, 6–13; Hopkins 1998.

96. Plin. *Ep.* 10.96. See also Tert. *Apol.* 1. All excepts from the *Apology* as translated in Roberts and Donaldson 1868.

97. Euseb. *Hist. eccl.* 5.20.5; Irenaeus *Adv. Haer.* 4.30.1.

98. After Schott 2019, 172–73.

99. de Ste. Croix 1963.

100. Rives 2007, 198.

101. Janssen 1979.

102. Aristid. *Or.* 49.38. See commentary in Jones 2018a.

103. Jones 2018b, 338. Eusebius names two different authors to the rescript: Antoninus Pius and then Marcus Aurelius. In my view, this slightly confusing (to the modern reader) situation may be due to the fact that while Antoninus Pius was Augustus, Marcus was his Caesar and could thus be expected to execute Antoninus's orders. The interpolated rescript survives as a likely appendage of the *Apology* of Melito; see Schott 2019, 189–90.

104. *Dig.* 48.19.30.

105. Oliver and Palmer 1955, 327.

106. Rives 2011, 209–10. See the epilogue for thoughts on the connection between Antonine plague–era persecution and these later systemic persecutions.

107. Tert. *Apol.* 40.

108. Euseb. *Hist. eccl.* 4.26.5–6.

109. *Acta Justini* (A). A brief yet helpful discussion of the authenticity of the various versions of the *Acta* is found in Moss 2012, 89–90.

110. Euseb. *Hist. eccl.* 5.1.

111. As discussed in chapter 6.

112. Amm. Marc. 23.6.24.

113. Min. Fel. *Oct.* 9.5–6.

114. Tert. *Apol.* 8.7.

115. Rives 2011, 200–201.

116. Plin. *Ep.* 10.96.

117. M. Aur. *Med.* 11.3. As translated in Clark 2004, 43.

118. Acts 1:8.

119. Tert. *Apol.* 22. See also Reff 2004, 67–69.

120. Revelation 21:4.

121. Philippians 3:8–10.

122. Cypr. *De mort.* 15–16.

123. M. Aur. *Med.* 4.39, as translated in Hays 2002.

124. Euseb. *Hist. eccl.* 5.21.1 notes that under Commodus, "things became easier for us, when with divine grace, peace spread to the churches throughout the whole inhabited world."

125. John 15:12. See also 1 John 4:7–21.

126. 1 John 4:19.

127. Ferngren 2016, 99–104.

128. Julian *Ep.* 22.430D. On whether such charity extended to outsiders in earlier periods, see now Caner 2021, 39–48.

129. Stark 1996, 86.

130. Euseb. *Hist. eccl.* 7.22.7–8.

131. Miller 1997, 21.

132. Aristides *Apol.* 15. As translated in Harris 1891.

133. Justin *Apol.* 1.67.6–7.

134. Euseb. *Hist. eccl.* 4.23.10.

135. Clem. Alex. 33.2–6. See discussion in Caner 2021, 44.

136. Tert. *Apol.* 39.

137. *Apostolic Tradition* 35.

138. Euseb. *Hist. eccl.* 7.22.9.

139. Hope 2002, 108–10.

140. See examples, admittedly from slightly later periods, in Rebillard 2009, 93–95.

141. Thuc. 2.51.5.

142. Cypr. *De mort.* 15–6. As translated in Deferrari 1958.

143. Euseb. *Hist. eccl.* 7.22.10.

144. M. Aur. *Med.* 3.8.

145. On reading Galen's *On Avoiding Distress* in light of the Antonine plague, see Flemming 2019, 219.

146. *CIL* 2.6278. Translated in Mahoney 2001, 96.

Chapter 6. An Empire Exhausted

1. Echoing Jongman 2007a, 199.

2. Heather 2012, 96–107. For a different view, see Drinkwater 2007, 28–30.

3. SHA *M. Ant.* 22.7, 21.1.

4. I repurpose Ken Adelman's famous (and misguided) claim in 2002 that American military intervention in Iraq would be a "cakewalk."

5. Gal. *Praen.* 9.7.

6. SHA *M. Ant.* 17.2.

7. Eutr. 8.12. He also claims "whole armies had been lost" because of the plague and fighting.

8. Jer. *Chron.* 287f, 288h (Helm).

9. Language I borrow from Talty 2009.

10. Raoult et al. 2006.

11. Cirillo 2008.

12. Kaniewski and Marriner 2020.

13. Vlach 2020, 29.

14. Ivleva 2016, 162–64.

15. Examples of the kind of "civilizing" work performed by soldiers can be found in Hassall 2000, 342–43.

16. McGinn 2003, 127–29; Phang 2001, 52–61.

17. James 2019, 252–53.

18. On Roman soldiers being more likely to die of sickness than their wounds, see Boudon-Millot 2022, 129–30.

19. Oros. *Hist.* 7.15.5–6. Translated in Raymond 1936.

20. *CIL* 3.14507. Commentary in Wilkes 1999.

21. On diplomas, see the exhaustive summary in Phang 2001, 53–85.

22. Roxan 1986, 266–68. On the diversity and disparities of privileges, see Waebens 2012, 270–72.

23. As posited in Duncan-Jones 2018, 53; Duncan-Jones 1996, 124; Eck 2012a.

24. Greenberg 2003, 414–15.

25. Waebens 2012, 275–76.

26. Also noted in Duncan-Jones 2018, 53.

27. SHA *M. Ant.* 21.6–8. Such recruitment crises had occurred several times in the Roman past; see, for example, Livy 40.19.7.

28. *CIL* 3.6580.

29. See, for example, *AE* 1969–70.

30. Duncan-Jones 2018, 52.

31. Jones 2012.

32. Alston 1994, 115. The same rates appear in Duncan-Jones 1994, 34. See also Speidel 2014.

33. SHA *M. Ant.* 7.9.

34. After Duncan-Jones 1994, 89.

35. Ibid., 14.

36. SHA *M. Ant.* 21.9; Zonar. 12.1.

37. Dio Cass. 72.3.3.

38. Holleran 2016.

39. Hirt 2010, 169–201.

40. Ţentea 2003.

41. Wilson 2002, 28.

42. Tab.Cer.D.20. Commentary in Mitrofan 2014, 11.

43. McDonald 2021, 395–96; Wilson 2007, 115; Duncan-Jones 1996, 121.

44. Pavlyshyn, Johnstone, and Saller 2020.

45. Fant 1989, 62–66.

46. Ibid., 213–17; Russell 2013, 195.

47. This paragraph summarizes evidence and arguments found in Perring 2022, 279–95.

48. Erdkamp 2005, 246–47.

49. Fant 1989, 213n44.

50. Plin. *HN* 33.31.97. On state-supplied labor, see the remark in Holleran 2016, 104.

51. Greenberg 2003, 419. On the limits of Roman water-lifting technology to dewater completely flooded mine galleries, see Wilson 2009, 78.

52. McDonald, forthcoming; Tomber 2018, 532–34.

53. McDonald 2021, 394.

54. Rizzo 2018; Weisweiler 2021, 20–21.

55. Elliott 2016.

56. Elliott 2020a.

57. The sources, however, are of uncertain dates and may have been influenced by the Cyprianic plague. See Scheidel 2002, 104–6; Harper 2016c; Harper 2015b.

58. Silver 2011.

59. *IRCPacen* 121.

60. See discussion of the slave population in Bruun 2007, 215–17.

61. App. *Gall.* 1.2. See also now Roymans 2019.

62. Saller 2012, 81.

63. *CIL* 2.6278, 3.7106.

64. Carter 2003, 87.

65. *CIL* 2.6278, 3.7106.

66. According to the inscriptions themselves (*Itaque facessat sive illut ducentiens annum seu trecenties est*).

67. Birley 2002, 200–204.

68. Birley 2012, 167.

69. Euseb. *Hist. eccl.* 5.1.40.

70. *OGIS* 595.

71. On the enduring potential for Puteoli to receive Egyptian grain even after the improvements at Portus and Ostia, see Brandt 2006, 36–37. On declining trade in general as a cause, see Lewis and Reinhold 1990, 109.

72. For this rendering, see the convincing argument of Terpstra 2013, 70–84.

73. Although those three "low" prices are all of uncertain dates, so I urge caution.

74. See discussion in chapter 5.

75. On the spring date, see the evidence in Birley 2002, 186.

76. M. Aur. *Med.* 2.2. See further discussion in Birley 2002, 185.

77. Dio Cass. 72.22.3.

78. Dio Cass. 72.6.3–4.

79. Dio Cass. 72.24.

80. The details of which are noted in Heather 2012, 98.

81. Gal. *De praes. ex puls.* 3.3–5.

82. Gal. *MM* 5.12; see commentary in Gourevitch 2013, 59–61.

83. Gal. *Praen.* 12.

84. Gal. *MM Glauc.* 1.3.

85. Levick 2014, 84. For a more skeptical view, see Nutton 1979, 221.

86. SHA *Comm.* 13.1.

87. Gal. *Praen.* 9.

88. Kovács 2009, 239.

89. Dio Cass. 72.29.

90. The measures are summarized in Birley 2002, 191.

91. SHA *M. Ant.* 26.3.

92. *SB* 16.12816.

93. And even farther afield—in Han China—sources for the Han period record the rise of "religious bandits" at exactly the same time (AD 172–177). Source and translation in Ebrey 2009, 84.

94. Birley 2002, 198.

95. SHA *Did. Iul.* 1.9.

96. Cartledge and Spawforth 2002, 106.

97. *TAM* 2.291.

98. Grunewald 2004, 50–51.

99. Polyb. 6.39; Webster 1998, 264–68.

100. Jones 1986, 31.

101. Luke 3:14.

102. At least according to surviving sources; see Duncan-Jones 1994, 14.

103. Dio Cass. 72.32.3. The senator, however, defended the emperor by claiming Marcus "never avoided a single necessary expenditure."

104. Dio Cass. 77.15.2.

105. Suet. *Claud.* 25.

106. M. Aur. *Med.* 10.25.

107. *Dig.* 11.4.1.

108. *Dig.* 11.4.2.

109. Dio Cass. 73.14.5.

110. *AE* 1979, 624.

111. The story is told in Herodian 1.10.

112. Łuć 2020, 75.

113. *AE* 1959, 141. Alföldy 1971; Drinkwater 1983, 80; Okamura 1988, 289.

114. Łuć 2020, 76–78.

115. Hassall 2000, 336.

116. Duncan-Jones 1994, 89–90.

117. Ibid., 104, 118, 124.

118. Butcher and Ponting 2012, 75–76.

119. Kehoe 2012, 127.

120. Although the event described in Dio Cass. 74.11 was not exactly an auction as such; see Appelbaum 2007.

121. Elliott 2020c, 161–67.

122. Grunewald 2004, 128–32; Okamura 1988, 289.

123. Horden and Purcell 2000, 382.

124. Marzano 2021, 520–21.

125. Graziani 2010.

126. Patterson, Witcher, and Di Giuseppe 2020, 218–19.

127. Prowse et al. 2007. See, however, caveats noted in Bruun 2010.

128. Speculative, I know, but not unreasonable considering other periods; see Noy 2018, 160.

129. Weisweiler 2021, 26–27.

130. Emery et al. 2018.

Chapter 7. Redux?

1. For example, Kulikowski 2016, 60; Birley 2002, 209–10; Grant 1996, 63.

2. SHA *M. Ant.* 28.3.

3. Dio Cass. 72.33.1.

4. M. Aur. *Med.* 9.2.

5. Philostr. *VS* 2.561.

6. Not merely an ancient phenomenon; see Lukianoff and Haidt 2018.

7. Neatly summarized in Levick 2014, 174n28; see also Whitehorne 1977.

8. Dio Cass. 73.1.1. On Dio's Senate membership, see Millar 1964, 15.

9. Laes 2011, 169–71.

10. Herodian 1.3.1–2, 1.4.4.

11. Herodian 1.6.9.

12. According to Dio Cass. 73.2.3: "he obtained some arms from them and soldiers as well, thirteen thousand from the Quadi and a smaller number from the Marcomanni."

13. These numbers are all given in Dio Cass. 73.2–3.

14. *CIL* 3.5567.

15. Gilliam 1961, 236; Duncan-Jones 1996, 117; Duncan-Jones 2018, 54.

16. Hameter 2000, 43. Hameter's translation of the inscription is: "To the spirits of the departed. Iulius Victor, the son of Martial, died aged 55. His wife Bessa, daughter of Iuvenis died aged 45. Novella, the daughter of Essibnus died aged 18. Victorinus had (this monument) made for his parents, his wife and his daughter Victorina, who died through the plague in the year of the consuls Mamertinus and Rufus. And for Aurelius Iustinus, his brother, soldier of the second legion Italica, who having served for 10 years, died age 30."

17. *AE* 1994, 1334.

18. Beck 1998.

19. P. Oxy. 66.4527. Commentary in van Minnen 2001. See also Bagnall 2000. For approximating *artabas* to kilograms, I use Duncan-Jones 1976.

20. On these aspects of the Roman triumph, and the challenge of interpreting the sources, see Beard 2009, 85–92, 225–33.

21. Herodian 1.7.5.

22. Grant 1996, 70.

23. A handy list is found in Birley 2000, 186–87.

24. Dio Cass. 73.1.1.

25. Dio Cass. 73.17.1–2.

26. Examples of which are noted in Duncan-Jones 1994, 14–15.

27. Dio Cass. 73.7.4.

28. *CIL* 6.41118.

29. Hekster 2002, 75–76.

30. Ibid., 68.

31. Hekster 2012, 237.

32. Hawkins 2016, 37–42.

33. Herodian 1.12.1.

34. Zelener 2003, 2012.

35. Herodian 1.12.1–3.

36. Dio Cass. 73.14.3–4.

37. Parkin 2003, 175; Parkin 1992, 35–38; Hopkins 1983, 209n9; Sánchez-Moreno Ellart 2009, 224–25. Contra Virlouvet 1997. See also chapter 4.

38. Aristid. *ST* 2.38.

39. McDonald 2021, 387–91; Harper 2021a, 194–96.

40. Hom. *Il.* 1.33–67. An excellent exposition of plague and famine in Thucydides is found in Kallet 2013.

41. These and others discussed in Flemming 2019, 234–35.

42. Gourevitch 2013, 74–75.

43. Cuvigny 2018.

44. On the grain supply to Eastern Desert quarries, see Hirt 2010, 216–17.

45. Ironically, the doctors were also exposing Commodus to "one of the most malarial places on earth" according to Sallares 2002, 269.

46. Alföldy 1989, 105–6.

47. Herodian 1.12.4.

48. Dio Cass. 73.13.2.

49. Talbert 1987, 341–45.

50. Futrell 2010, 45–47.

51. Entertainment venues became a breeding ground for unrest and riots in the Principate. See Africa 1971; Whittaker 1964, 362ff.

52. Dio Cass. 73.13.3–4; Herodian 1.12.5.

53. SHA *Pert.* 4.2–3.

54. Dio Cass. 73.13.5. For the case that the soldiers in the crowd were praetorians, see Alföldy 1989, 111.

55. Herodian 1.13.1.

56. Hekster 2002, 78.

57. Alföldy 1989, 113.

58. Herodian 1.13.3.

59. Herodian 1.12.3.

60. See the careful reading of Whittaker 1964, 352.

61. Dio Cass. 73.13.6; Herodian 1.13.6.

62. Dio Cass. 73.15.1.

63. For the date, see Nicholls 2019, 247.

64. Tac. Ann. 15.38. See also now Barrett 2020.

65. Gal. *Ind.* 3–9; Gal. *Lib. Prop.* 1.21, 41; Tucci 2008; Nutton 2020, 38–39.

66. Birley 2000, 190–91.

67. Thuc. 21.51.6.

68. Only a single coin type of Commodus (RIC III Commodus 162) had referenced Hercules in its legend prior to AD 190.

69. Hekster 2003, 31–32.

70. Dio Cass. 73.15.6.

71. Kyle 2012, 90.

72. Dio Cass. 73.20.2.

73. Noreña 2011, 283–97.

74. These exploits are recounted in Dio Cass. 73.19.

75. According to Dio Cass. 73.20.3.

76. After language in Toner 2015, 28. See also Dio Cass. 73.15.2.

77. Dio Cass. 73.15.2.

78. Gal. *Ind.* 54–55.

79. Dio Cass. 73.21.2.

80. Dio Cass. 73.22–23; Herodian 1.16–17.

81. Abridged from SHA *Comm.* 18.1–19.9. Such decrees are referenced in Dio Cass. 74.2. Even if the text is fabricated, it surely represents sentiments held by many senators.

Chapter 8. The End of an Era

1. Harper 2017, 115.

2. Haldon et al. 2018; Harper 2018.

3. Newfield 2022; Eisenberg and Mordechai 2020.

4. Erdkamp, Verboven, and Zuiderhoek 2020, 22.

5. Garnsey and Saller 2014, 71–90; Temin 2006.

6. As argued in Scheidel 2007b, 74–75. On a lack of sustained economic growth in the Pax Romana, see now Saller 2022.

7. For Harper's rough estimate, see Harper 2017, 18.

8. The concept is elucidated in Wickham 2005, 13ff.

9. Dio Cass. 76.13.1.

10. SHA *Comm.* 17.7.

11. Euseb. *Hist. eccl.* 8.14.6 and also Stathakopoulos 2004, 51–52, 178–79.

12. Lo Cascio 2007, 641.

13. Huebner 2020.

14. Harper 2015b.

15. See chapter 2 and also Hayek 2014.

16. Commentary on this coin is found in Yarrow 2012, 447–48.

17. Fentress et al. 2004.

18. Weisweiler 2021. The archaeology of African prosperity even during the worst years of the Antonine plague could not be more clear; see Sheldrick 2021.

19. On Egyptian measurements, see Rathbone 1983; Duncan-Jones 1976.

20. Harper 2016c; Elliott 2020b.

21. Criscuolo 2011, 171–72.

22. *P. Col.* 6.123.

23. Rathbone 2006, 112–13.

24. Moorhead 2013, 27.

25. Scheidel 2017, 78–79.

26. Zuiderhoek 2009.

27. Herodian 7.3.5.

28. Alston 1994.

29. It is possible that salary increases were even greater; see Speidel 1992, 2014.

30. As former Federal Reserve chairman Ben Bernanke once jokingly claimed he would do to fight deflation; see Bernanke 2002.

31. Trajan's "debasement" was merely a reification of the Neronian standard, following experimentation in the intervening years. See Butcher and Ponting 2015.

32. Elliott 2014.

33. Scheidel 2012b, 285.

34. Mühlemann et al. 2020. On lower lethality, see comments in Gorman 2020.

35. Harper 2017, 115.

36. Elliott 2020c, 110–57; Elliott 2020a; Scheidel 2010.

37. Garnsey and Saller 2014, 71–72.

38. Adams 2017. Adams describes this process as "devolved," and in a sense it is, in that the use of liturgies for "the mechanics of the transport of tax in kind" was carried out through liturgies, some of them voluntary. Nevertheless, Adams emphasizes state dominance of infrastructure and supervisory aspects.

39. For different but complementary views on the usefulness of counterfactuals in Roman history, see Elliott 2020c; Scheidel 2019.

40. Patterson, Witcher, and Di Giuseppe 2020, 193–207; Callataÿ 2005; Parker 1992. Shipping routes changed over the course of Roman history as did the material used to contain goods; so not all evidence of "declining trade" is actually such. See, for example, Erdkamp 2019, 426–27; Tchernia 2016, 117–21.

41. See, for example, *Cod. Theod.* 7.22.1, 8.5.1, 13.5.2; see also Bond 2016, 160.

42. Morley 2000.

43. Erdkamp 2020, 46–47.

44. Reynolds 2017.

45. Giardina 2007, 761.

Epilogue: The Spirit of Pandemic

1. Eck 2007, 33–34.

2. The chronology of the plague and Decian edict are uncertain. Decius decreed the edict late in 249, and the Cyprianic plague may have entered the eastern Empire that same year according to Harper 2017, 137, 153–54. A revised view, however, suggests Harper's chronology is a year or so too early: Huebner 2021.

3. Or "scaled up," as described in Harper 2017, 154.

4. Toner 2013, 287.

5. *P. Wilcken* 124.

6. Stark 1996, 77.

7. Renberg 2006, 90.

8. Merrifield 1996, 111.

9. Chaniotis 1995.

10. Rives 1999.

11. Rives 2007, 199.

12. August. *De civ. D.* 3.17.

13. Cyp. *Dem.* 2–3. As translated in Deferrari 1958.

14. Cyp. *Dem.* 3–5.

15. For an excellent summary of apocalyptic literature as it relates to plagues, see Sessa 2019, 237–44. See also Carmichael 2006, 14–15.

16. Cyp. *Dem.* 22.

17. Williams 2020, 264.

18. Cyp. *Dem.* 18–19.

19. Toner 2013, 264.

20. Rives 2011, 211.

21. On the new ideological weight of sacrifice for both Christians and their persecutors, see especially Rives 2020. On the possibility of Decius's decree and sacrifice certifications being adopted "on a whim," see Rives 1999, 151.

BIBLIOGRAPHY

Adams, C. 2017. "Nile River Transport under the Romans." In *Trade, Commerce, and the State in the Roman World*, ed. A. Wilson and A. K. Bowman, 175–208. Oxford: Oxford University Press.

Adelman, K. 2002. "Cakewalk in Iraq." *Washington Post*, February 13.

Africa, T. W. 1971. "Urban Violence in Imperial Rome." *Journal of Interdisciplinary History* 2 (1): 3–21.

Ahmed, M., K. J. Anchukaitis, A. Asrat, H. P. Borgaonkar, M. Braida, B. M. Buckley, U. Büntgen, et al. 2013. "Continental-Scale Temperature Variability during the Past Two Millennia." *Nature Geoscience* 6 (5): 339–46.

Alcock, J. P. 2006. *Food in the Ancient World*. Westport, CT: Greenwood Publishing Group.

Aldrete, G. S. 2018. "Hazards of Life in Ancient Rome." In *A Companion to the City of Rome*, ed. C. Holleran and A. Claridge, 363–81. New York: John Wiley & Sons.

———. 2014. "Urban Sensations: Opulence and Ordure." In *A Cultural History of the Senses in Antiquity*, ed. J. Toner, 45–68. London: Bloomsbury Publishing.

———. 2007. *Floods of the Tiber in Ancient Rome*. Ancient Society and History. Baltimore: Johns Hopkins University Press.

Alföldy, G. 1989. "Cleanders Sturz und die antike Überlieferung." In *Die Krise des Römischen Reiches: Geschichte, Geschichtsschreibung und Geschichtsbetrachtung*, 81–126. Stuttgart: Franz Steiner Verlag.

———. 1971. "Bellum Desertorum." *Bonner Jahrbücher* 171: 367–76.

Alföldy, G., and H. Halfmann. 1979. "Iunius Maximus und die victoria Parthica." *Zeitschrift für Papyrologie und Epigraphik* 35: 195–212.

Alston, R. 1999. "The Revolt of the Boukoloi: Geography, History and Myth." In *Organised Crime in the Ancient World*, ed. K. Hopwood, 129–53. London: Duckworth.

———. 1995. *Soldier and Society in Roman Egypt: A Social History*. London: Routledge.

———. 1994. "Roman Military Pay from Caesar to Diocletian." *Journal of Roman Studies* 84: 113–23.

Al-Talhi, D., and M. Al-Daire. 2005. "Roman Presence in the Desert: A New Inscription from Hegra." *Chiron* 35: 205–17.

Anderson, R. M., and R. M. May. 1982. "Coevolution of Hosts and Parasites." *Parasitology* 85 (Pt. 2): 411–26.

Andorlini, I. 2012. "Considerazioni sulla 'peste antonina' in Egitto alla luce delle testimonianze papirologiche." In *L'Impatto della peste antonina*, ed. E. Lo Cascio, 15–28. Bari: Edipuglia.

Antonio, M. L., Z. Gao, H. M. Moots, M. Lucci, F. Candilio, S. Sawyer, V. Oberreiter, et al. 2019. "Ancient Rome: A Genetic Crossroads of Europe and the Mediterranean." *Science* 366 (6466): 708–14.

Appelbaum, A. 2007. "Another Look at the Assassination of Pertinax and the Accession of Julianus." *Classical Philology* 102: 198–207.

Audin, A. 1986. *Gens de Lugdunum*. Brussels: Revue d'études latines.

———. 1970. "La population de Lugdunum au IIᵉ siècle." *Cahiers d'Histoire* 15: 7–14.

Bagnall, R. S., ed. 2021. *Roman Egypt: A History*. Cambridge: Cambridge University Press.

———. 2002. "The Effects of Plague: Model and Evidence." *Journal of Roman Archaeology* 15: 114–20.

———. 2000. "P. Oxy 4527 and the Antonine Plague in Egypt: Death or Flight?" *Journal of Roman Archaeology* 13: 288–92.

———. 1993. *Egypt in Late Antiquity*. Princeton: Princeton University Press.

Bagnall, R. S., and B. W. Frier. 1994. *The Demography of Roman Egypt*. Cambridge: Cambridge University Press.

Bailey, M. 2013. "Roman Money and Numerical Practice." *Revue Belge de Philologie et d'Histoire* 91 (1): 153–86.

Baillie, M., and J. McAneney. 2015. "Tree Ring Effects and Ice Core Acidities Clarify the Volcanic Record of the First Millennium." *Climate of the Past* 11: 105–14.

Baird, J. 2018. *Dura-Europos*. New York: Bloomsbury Publishing.

Balows, A., W.J.J. Hausler, M. Ohashi, and A. Turano. 2012. *Laboratory Diagnosis of Infectious Diseases: Principles and Practice*. New York: Springer Science & Business Media.

Bang, P. F. 2008. *The Roman Bazaar: A Comparative Study of Trade and Markets in a Tributary Empire*. Cambridge: Cambridge University Press.

Barrett, A. A. 2020. *Rome Is Burning: Nero and the Fire That Ended a Dynasty*. Princeton: Princeton University Press.

Beard, M. 2009. *The Roman Triumph*. Cambridge, MA: Harvard University Press.

Beck, B.J.M. 1986. "The Fall of Han." In *The Cambridge History of China*. Vol. 1: *The Ch'in and Han Empires, 221 BC–AD 220*, ed. D. Twitchett and M. Loewe, 317–76. Cambridge: Cambridge University Press.

Beck, R. 1998. "'Qui Mortalitatis Causa Convenerunt': The Meeting of the Virunum Mithraists on June 26, A.D. 184." *Phoenix* 52 (3/4): 335–44.

Benjamin, C. 2018. *Empires of Ancient Eurasia: The First Silk Roads Era, 100 BCE–250 CE*. Cambridge: Cambridge University Press.

Beresford, J. 2012. *The Ancient Sailing Season*. Leiden: Brill.

Bernanke, B. 2002. "Deflation: Making Sure 'It' Doesn't Happen Here." Presented at the National Economists Club, Washington, DC.

Bernard, S. 2016. "Food Distributions and Immigration in Imperial Rome." In *Migration and Mobility in the Early Roman Empire*, ed. L. de Ligt and L. E. Tacoma, 50–71. Leiden: Brill.

Bernhardt, C. E., B. P. Horton, and J.-D. Stanley. 2012. "Nile Delta Vegetation Response to Holocene Climate Variability." *Geology* 40 (7): 615–18.

Birley, A. R. 2012. "Marcus' Life as Emperor." In *A Companion to Marcus Aurelius*, ed. M. van Ackeren, 155–70. Chichester: John Wiley & Sons.

———. 2002. *Marcus Aurelius: A Biography*. 2nd ed. London: Taylor & Francis.

———. 2000. "Hadrian to the Antonines." In *The Cambridge Ancient History*, ed. A. K. Bowman, P. Garnsey, and D. W. Rathbone, 11:132–94. Cambridge: Cambridge University Press.

Birley, E. 1974. "Cohors I Tungrorum and the Oracle of Clarian Apollo." *Chiron* 4: 511–13.

Bivar, A.D.H. 1970. "Hāritī and the Chronology of the Kuṣāṇas." *Bulletin of the School of Oriental and African Studies, University of London* 33 (1): 10–21.

Black, E. 2005. "The Relationship between Indian Ocean Sea-Surface Temperature and East African Rainfall." *Philosophical Transactions: Series A, Mathematical, Physical, and Engineering Sciences* 363 (1826): 43–47.

Blackburn, J., C. T. Yiannoutsos, A. E. Carroll, P. K. Halverson, and N. Menachemi. 2020. "Infection Fatality Ratios for COVID-19 among Noninstitutionalized Persons 12 and Older: Results of a Random-Sample Prevalence Study." *Annals of Internal Medicine* 174 (1): 135–36.

Blanchard, P., D. Castex, M. Coquerelle, R. Giuliani, and M. Ricciardi. 2007. "A Mass Grave from the Catacomb of Saints Peter and Marcellinus in Rome, Second–Third Century AD." *Antiquity* 81: 989–98.

Blouin, K. 2016. "A Breadbasket, Mais Encore? The Socio-Economics of Food Production in the Nile Delta from Antiquity Onwards." In *A History of Water*. Vol. 3: *Water and Food: From Hunter-Gatherers to Global Production in Africa*, ed. T. Tvedt and T. Oestigaard, 101–20. London: I. B. Tauris.

———. 2014. *Triangular Landscapes: Environment, Society, and the State in the Nile Delta under Roman Rule*. Oxford: Oxford University Press.

Bodel, J. 2000. "Dealing with the Dead: Undertakers, Executioners and Potter's Fields in Ancient Rome." In *Death and Disease in the Ancient City*, ed. V. M. Hope and E. Marshall, 128–51. London: Routledge.

Bond, S. 2016. *Trade and Taboo: Disreputable Professions in the Roman Mediterranean*. Ann Arbor: University of Michigan Press.

Bonneau, D. 1971. *Le fisc et le Nil: Incidences des irrégularités de la crue du Nil sur la fiscalité foncière dans l'Égypte grecque et romaine*. Publications de l'Institut de droit romain de l'Université de Paris no 2. Paris: Cujas.

Boudon-Millot, V. 2022. "Galien à Aquilée, ou les derniers jours de Lucius Vérus." In *Altino 169 d.C. : Intorno alla morte dell'imperatore Lucio Vero*, ed. Giovannella Cresci Marrone, François Chausson, and Benoît Rossignol, 115–41. Venezia: Istituto veneto di scienze.

———. 2001. "Galien face à la 'peste antonine,' ou comment penser l'invisible." In *Air, miasmes et contagion: Les epidémies dans l'Antiquité et au Moyen Age*, 29–54. Langres: Dominique Guéniot.

Bowersock, G. W. 1983. *Roman Arabia*. Cambridge, MA: Harvard University Press.

Bowes, K., ed. 2020a. *The Roman Peasant Project, 2009–2014: Excavating the Roman Rural Poor*. Vol. 1. Philadelphia: University of Pennsylvania Press.

———, ed. 2020b. *The Roman Peasant Project, 2009–2014: Excavating the Roman Rural Poor*. Vol. 2. Philadelphia: University of Pennsylvania Press.

Bowman, A. K. 1998. *Life and Letters on the Roman Frontier: Vindolanda and Its People*. London: Psychology Press.

Bowman, A. K. 1986. *Egypt after the Pharaohs, 332 BC–AD 642: From Alexander to the Arab Conquest*. Berkeley: University of California Press.

Bowman, A., and A. Wilson. 2011. *Settlement, Urbanization, and Population*. Oxford: Oxford University Press.

Brandt, J. R. 2006. "'The Warehouse of the World': A Comment on Rome's Supply Chain during the Empire." *Orizzonti—Rassegna di Archeologia* 6: 25–47.

Braund, S. 2009. *Seneca: De Clementia*. Oxford: Oxford University Press.

Bremmer, J. 1983. "Scapegoat Rituals in Ancient Greece." *Harvard Studies in Classical Philology* 87: 299–320.

Broekaert, W., and A. Zuiderhoek. 2020. "Capital Goods in the Roman Economy." In *Capital, Investment, and Innovation in the Roman World*, ed. P. Erdkamp, K. Verboven, and A. Zuiderhoek, 99–146. Oxford: Oxford University Press.

Broux, Y., and W. Clarysee. 2009. "Two Greek Funerary Stelae from Lydia and the Antonine Plague." *Tyche* 24 (1): 27–33.

Brown, P. 1971. *The World of Late Antiquity: AD 150–750*. Ed. G. Barraclough. New York: W. W. Norton.

Browning, D. C., Jr. 2021. "All Roads Lead to Risk: Malaria Threat to Travellers in the Roman World." *Cartographica: The International Journal for Geographic Information and Geovisualization* 56 (1): 64–86.

Brunstein, F. C., and D. K. Yamaguchi. 1992. "The Oldest Known Rocky Mountain Bristlecone Pines (Pinus Aristata Engelm)." *Arctic and Alpine Research* 24 (3): 253–56.

Bruun, C. 2012. "La mancanza di prove di un effetto catastrofico della 'peste antonina' (dal 166 d.C. in poi)." In *L'Impatto della peste antonina*, ed. E. Lo Cascio, 123–65. Bari: Edipuglia.

———. 2010. "Water, Oxygen Isotopes, and Immigration to Ostia-Portus." *Journal of Roman Archaeology* 23: 109.

———. 2007. "The Antonine Plague and the 'Third Century Crisis.'" In *Crises and the Roman Empire*, ed. O. Hekster, G. de Kleijn, and D. Slootjes, 201–18. Leiden: Brill.

———. 2003. "The Antonine Plague in Rome and Ostia." *Journal of Roman Archaeology* 16: 426–34.

Buccellato, A., and P. Catalano. 2003. "Il comprensorio della necropoli di via Basiliano (Roma): Un'indagine multidisciplinare." *Mélanges de l'école française de Rome* 115 (1): 311–76.

Büntgen, U., W. Tegel, K. Nicolussi, M. McCormick, D. Frank, V. Trouet, J. O. Kaplan, et al. 2011. "2500 Years of European Climate Variability and Human Susceptibility." *Science* 331 (6017): 578–82.

Butcher, K., and M. Ponting. 2015. *The Metallurgy of Roman Silver Coinage: From the Reform of Nero to the Reform of Trajan*. Cambridge: Cambridge University Press.

———. 2012. "The Beginning of the End? The Denarius in the Second Century." *Numismatic Chronicle* 172: 63–83.

Butzer, K. W. 1976. *Early Hydraulic Civilization in Egypt: A Study in Cultural Ecology*. Chicago: University of Chicago Press.

Callataÿ, F. de. 2005. "The Graeco-Roman Economy in the Super Long-Run: Lead, Copper, and Shipwrecks." *Journal of Roman Archaeology* 18: 361–72.

Caner, D. 2021. *The Rich and the Pure: Philanthropy and the Making of Christian Society in Early Byzantium*. Berkeley: University of California Press.

Capponi, L. 2010. "Serapis, Boukoloi and Christians from Hadrian to Marcus Aurelius." In *Hadrian and the Christians*, ed. M. Rizzi, 121–40. Millennium-Studien. Berlin: De Gruyter.

Carmichael, A. 2006. "Infectious Diseases and Human Agency: An Historical Overview." In *Interactions between Global Change and Human Health*, ed. M. Andreae, 3–46. Vatican City: Pontificia Academia Scientiarum.

Carmichael, A. G., and A. M. Silverstein. 1987. "Smallpox in Europe before the Seventeenth Century: Virulent Killer or Benign Disease?" *Journal of the History of Medicine and Allied Sciences* 42 (2): 147–68.

Carroll, M. 2018. *Infancy and Earliest Childhood in the Roman World: "A Fragment of Time."* Illustrated edition. Oxford: Oxford University Press.

Carter, M. 2003. "Gladiatorial Ranking and the 'SC de Pretiis Gladiatorum Minuendis' (CIL II 6278 = ILS 5163)." *Phoenix* 57 (1/2): 83–114.

Cartledge, P., and A. Spawforth. 2002. *Hellenistic and Roman Sparta: A Tale of Two Cities*. New York: Psychology Press.

Castex, D., P. Blanchard, H. Réveillas, S. Kacki, and R. Giuliani. 2009. "Les sépultures du secteur central de la catacombe des Saints Pierre-et-Marcellin (Rome): État des analyses bio-archéologique et perspectives." *Mélanges de l'école française de Rome* 121 (1): 287–97.

Champlin, E. 1980. *Fronto and Antonine Rome*. Cambridge, MA: Harvard University Press.

Chaniotis, A. 1995. "Illness and Cures in the Greek Propitiatory Inscriptions and Dedications of Lydia and Phrygia." In *Ancient Medicine in Its Socio-Cultural Context*, vol. 2, ed. H.F.J. Horstmanshoff, Philip J. van der Eijk, and P. H. Schrijvers, 323–44. Leiden: Brill.

Chenery, C., G. Müldner, J. Evans, H. Eckardt, and M. Lewis. 2010. "Strontium and Stable Isotope Evidence for Diet and Mobility in Roman Gloucester, UK." *Journal of Archaeological Science* 37 (1): 150–63.

Choi, K.-S., Y.-M. Cha, S.-D. Kang, and H.-D. Kim. 2015. "Relationship between SST in the Equatorial Eastern Pacific and TC Frequency That Affects Korea." *Theoretical and Applied Climatology* 121 (1): 243–52.

Cirillo, V. J. 2008. "Two Faces of Death: Fatalities from Disease and Combat in America's Principal Wars, 1775 to Present." *Perspectives in Biology and Medicine* 51 (1): 121–33.

Clark, G. 2004. *Christianity and Roman Society*. Cambridge: Cambridge University Press.

Cleary, S. E. 2013. *The Roman West, AD 200–500: An Archaeological Study*. Cambridge: Cambridge University Press.

Cobb, M. A. 2018a. "From the Ptolemies to Augustus: Mediterranean Integration into the Indian Ocean Trade." In *The Indian Ocean Trade in Antiquity: Political, Cultural and Economic Impacts*, ed. M. A. Cobb, 17–51. London: Routledge.

———. 2018b. *Rome and the Indian Ocean Trade from Augustus to the Early Third Century CE*. Leiden: Brill.

Conrad, L. I., and D. Wujastyk. 2017. *Contagion: Perspectives from Pre-Modern Societies*. New York: Taylor & Francis.

Cooper, D. B. 1965. *Epidemic Disease in Mexico City, 1761–1813: An Administrative, Social, and Medical Study*. Austin: University of Texas Press.

Costa, P. M. 1977. "A Latin-Greek Inscription from the Jawf of the Yemen." *Proceedings of the Seminar for Arabian Studies* 7: 69–72.

Criscuolo, L. 2011. "Observations on the Economy in Kind in Ptolemaic Egypt." In *The Economies of Hellenistic Societies, Third to First Centuries BC*, ed. Z. Archibald, J. K. Davies, and V. Gabrielsen, 166–76. Oxford: Oxford University Press.

Cunha, C. B., and B. A. Cunha. 2008. "Great Plagues of the Past and Remaining Questions." In *Paleomicrobiology: Past Human Infections*, ed. D. Raoult and M. Drancourt, 1–21. Berlin: Springer Science & Business Media.

Cuvigny, H. 2018. "A Survey of Place-Names in the Egyptian Eastern Desert during the Principate According to the Ostraca and the Inscriptions." In *The Eastern Desert of Egypt during the Greco-Roman Period: Archaeological Reports*, ed. J.-P. Brun, T. Faucher, B. Redon, and S. Sidebotham. Institut des civilisations. Paris: Collège de France.

Davenport, R. 2020. "Cultures of Contagion and Containment? The Geography of Smallpox in Britain in the Pre-Vaccination Era." In *The Anthropological Demography of Health*, ed. V. Petit, K. Qureshi, Y. Charbit, and P. Kreager, 61–84. Oxford: Oxford University Press.

Davenport, R., L. Schwarz, and J. Boulton. 2011. "The Decline of Adult Smallpox in Eighteenth-Century London." *Economic History Review* 64 (4): 1289–1314.

Davidde, B. 2018. "The Port of Qana', a Junction between the Indian Ocean and the Mediterranean Sea." In *Trade, Commerce, and the State in the Roman World*, ed. A. K. Bowman and A. Wilson, 579–97. Oxford: Oxford University Press.

De Crespigny, R. 2018. *Emperor Huan and Emperor Ling: Being the Chronicle of Later Han for the Years 157 to 189 AD as Recorded in Chapter 54 to 59 of the Zizhi Tongjian of Sima Guang*. Internet edition. Canberra: Asian Studies Monographs.

———. 2016. *Fire over Luoyang: A History of the Later Han Dynasty, 23–220 AD*. Leiden: Brill.

———. 2007. *A Biographical Dictionary of Later Han to the Three Kingdoms (23–220 AD)*. Leiden: Brill.

de Ligt, L. 2012. *Peasants, Citizens and Soldiers: Studies in the Demographic History of Roman Italy, 225 BC–AD 100*. Cambridge: Cambridge University Press.

de Procé, S. M., and C. Phillips. 2010. South Arabian Inscriptions from the Farasān Islands (Saudi Arabia) (Poster). *Proceedings of the Seminar for Arabian Studies* 40: 277–82.

De Romanis, F. 2020. *The Indo-Roman Pepper Trade and the Muziris Papyrus*. Oxford: Oxford University Press.

de Ste. Croix, G.E.M. 1963. "Why Were the Early Christians Persecuted?" *Past & Present* 26 (1): 6–38.

Deferrari, R. J., trans. 1958. *Saint Cyprian: Treatises*. The Fathers of the Church. New York: Catholic University Press.

Demiéville, P. 1986. "Philosophy and Religion from Han to Sui." In *The Cambridge History of China*. Vol. 1: *The Ch'in and Han Empires, 221 BC–AD 220*, ed. D. Twitchett and M. Loewe, 1:808–72. Cambridge: Cambridge University Press.

Dodd, C. H. 1911. "Chronology of the Eastern Campaigns of the Emperor Lucius Verus." *Numismatic Chronicle* 11: 209–67.

Dodds, E. R. 1965. *Pagan and Christian in an Age of Anxiety: Some Aspects of Religious Experience from Marcus Aurelius to Constantine*. Cambridge: Cambridge University Press.

Domínguez-Villar, D. 2013. Comment on "Land Surface Temperature Changes in Northern Iberia since 4000 Yr BP, Based on Δ13C of Speleothems." *Global and Planetary Change* 100: 291–94.

Domínguez-Villar, D., X. Wang, K. Krklec, H. Cheng, and R. L. Edwards. 2017. "The Control of the Tropical North Atlantic on Holocene Millennial Climate Oscillations." *Geology* 45: 303–6.

Dossey, L. 2010. *Peasant and Empire in Christian North Africa*. Berkeley: University of California Press.

Downie, J. 2013. *At the Limits of Art: A Literary Study of Aelius Aristides' Hieroi Logoi*. Oxford: Oxford University Press.

Drinkwater, J. F. 2007. *The Alamanni and Rome, 213–496: Caracalla to Clovis*. Oxford: Oxford University Press.

———. 1983. *Roman Gaul: The Three Provinces, 58 BC–AD 260*. New York: Routledge.

Dubache, G., B. A. Ogwang, V. Ongoma, and A. R. Md. Towfiqul Islam. 2019. "The Effect of Indian Ocean on Ethiopian Seasonal Rainfall." *Meteorology and Atmospheric Physics* 131 (6): 1753–61.

Duggan, A. T., M. F. Perdomo, D. Piombino-Mascali, S. Marciniak, D. Poinar, M. V. Emery, J. P. Buchmann, et al. 2016. "17th Century Variola Virus Reveals the Recent History of Smallpox." *Current Biology* 26 (24): 3407–12.

Duncan, S. R., S. Scott, and C. J. Duncan. 1994. "Smallpox Epidemics in Cities in Britain." *Journal of Interdisciplinary History* 25 (2): 255–71.

Duncan-Jones, R. 2018. "The Antonine Plague Revisited." *Arctos—Acta Philologica Fennica* 52: 41–72.

———. 1996. "The Impact of the Antonine Plague." *Journal of Roman Archaeology* 9: 108–36.

———. 1994. *Money and Government in the Roman Empire*. Cambridge: Cambridge University Press.

———. 1976. "The Choenix, the Artaba and the Modius." *Zeitschrift für Papyrologie und Epigraphik* 21: 43–52.

Ebrey, P. B. 2009. *Chinese Civilization: A Sourcebook*. 2nd ed. New York: Simon and Schuster.

Echols, E. C., trans. 1961. *Herodian of Antioch's History of the Roman Empire*. Berkeley: University of California Press.

Eck, W. 2012a. "Die Seuche unter Mark Aurel: Ihre Auswirkungen auf das Heer." In *L'Impatto della peste antonina*, ed. E. Lo Cascio, 63–78. Bari: Edipuglia.

———. 2012b. "The Political State of the Roman Empire." In *A Companion to Marcus Aurelius*, ed. M. van Ackeren, 95–109. Chichester: John Wiley & Sons.

———. 2007. "Krise oder Nichtkrise—Das ist hier die Frage. Köln und sein Territorium in der 2. Hälfte des 3. Jahrhunderts." In *Crises and the Roman Empire*, ed. O. Hekster, D. Slootjes, and G. Kleijn, 21–44. Leiden: Brill.

Edwell, P. 2007. *Between Rome and Persia: The Middle Euphrates, Mesopotamia and Palmyra under Roman Control*. London: Routledge.

Eichner, M., and K. Dietz. 2003. "Transmission Potential of Smallpox: Estimates Based on Detailed Data from an Outbreak." *American Journal of Epidemiology* 158 (2): 110–17.

Eisenberg, M., and L. Mordechai. 2020. "The Justinianic Plague and Global Pandemics: The Making of the Plague Concept." *American Historical Review* 125 (5): 1632–67.

Eisenberg, M., and L. Mordechai. 2019. "The Justinianic Plague: An Interdisciplinary Review." *Byzantine and Modern Greek Studies* 43 (2): 156–80.

Elliott, C. P. 2022. "Money, Capital and Inequality in the Age of Augustus." In *Capital in Classical Antiquity*, ed. N. Morley and M. Koedijk, 243–60. Palgrave Studies in Ancient Economics. Cham: Palgrave Macmillan.

———. 2021. "The Ecology of Exchange: The Monetization of Roman Egypt." *American Historical Review* 126 (3): 900–921.

———. 2020a. "Coin Debasement, Climate and Contagion in Second-Century Egypt: Some Intersections." In *Debasement: Manipulation of Coin Standards in Pre-Modern Monetary Systems*, ed. K. Butcher, 63–72. Oxford: Oxbow.

———. 2020b. "Disease Proxies and the Diagnosis of the Late Antonine Economy." In *Complexity Economics: Building a New Approach to Ancient Economic History*, ed. K. Verboven. New York: Palgrave Macmillan.

———. 2020c. *Economic Theory and the Roman Monetary Economy*. Cambridge: Cambridge University Press.

———. 2016. "Climate Change, Plague and Local Violence in Roman Egypt." *Past & Present* 230 (2): 3–31.

———. 2014. "The Acceptance and Value of Roman Silver Coinage in the Second and Third Centuries AD." *Numismatic Chronicle* 174: 129–52.

Ellis, S. P. 2000. *Roman Housing*. London: Duckworth.

Emery, M. V., R. J. Stark, T. J. Murchie, S. Elford, H. P. Schwarcz, and T. L. Prowse. 2018. "Mapping the Origins of Imperial Roman Workers (1st–4th Century CE) at Vagnari, Southern Italy, Using 87Sr/86Sr and Δ18O Variability." *American Journal of Physical Anthropology* 166 (4): 837–50.

Erdkamp, P. 2021a. "A Historian's Introduction to Paleoclimatology." In *Climate Change and Ancient Societies in Europe and the Near East: Diversity in Collapse and Resilience*, ed. P. Erdkamp, J. G. Manning, and K. Verboven, 1–24. Palgrave Studies in Ancient Economies. Cham: Palgrave Macmillan.

———. 2021b. "Climate Change and the Productive Landscape in the Mediterranean Region in the Roman Period." In *Climate Change and Ancient Societies in Europe and the Near East: Diversity in Collapse and Resilience*, ed. P. Erdkamp, J. G. Manning, and K. Verboven, 411–42. Palgrave Studies in Ancient Economies. Cham: Palgrave Macmillan.

———. 2020. "Population, Technology, and Economic Growth in the Roman World." In *Capital, Investment, and Innovation in the Roman World*, ed. P. Erdkamp, K. Verboven, and A. Zuiderhoek, 39–66. Oxford: Oxford University Press.

———. 2019. "War, Food, Climate Change, and the Decline of the Roman Empire." *Journal of Late Antiquity* 12 (2): 422–65.

———. 2018. "Famine and Hunger in the Roman World." In *The Routledge Handbook of Diet and Nutrition in the Roman World*, ed. P. Erdkamp and C. Holleran, 296–307. London: Routledge.

———. 2016. "Seasonal Labour and Rural–Urban Migration in Roman Italy." In *Migration and Mobility in the Early Roman Empire*, ed. L. de Ligt and L. E. Tacoma, 33–49. Leiden: Brill.

———. 2013. "The Food Supply of the Capital." In *The Cambridge Companion to Ancient Rome*, ed. P. Erdkamp, 262–77. Cambridge Companions to the Ancient World. Cambridge: Cambridge University Press.

———. 2005. *The Grain Market in the Roman Empire: A Social, Political and Economic Study.* Cambridge: Cambridge University Press.

———. 2002. "'A Starving Mob Has No Respect': Urban Markets and Food Riots in the Roman World, 100 B.C.–400 A.D." In *The Transformation of Economic Life under the Roman Empire,* ed. L. de Blois and J. Rich, 93–115. Leiden: Brill.

Erdkamp, P., K. Verboven, and A. Zuiderhoek. 2020. Introduction to *Capital, Investment, and Innovation in the Roman World,* ed. P. Erdkamp, K. Verboven, and A. Zuiderhoek, 1–38. Oxford: Oxford University Press.

Evans, H. B. 1994. *Water Distribution in Ancient Rome: The Evidence of Frontinus.* Ann Arbor: University of Michigan Press.

Evers, K. G. 2017. *Worlds Apart Trading Together: The Organisation of Long-Distance Trade between Rome and India in Antiquity.* Oxford: Archaeopress.

Fabbri, C. N. 2007. "Treating Medieval Plague: The Wonderful Virtues of Theriac." *Early Science and Medicine* 12 (3): 247–83.

Fagan, G. G. 1999. *Bathing in Public in the Roman World.* Ann Arbor: University of Michigan Press.

Fant, J. C. 1989. *Cavum Antrum Phrygiae: The Organization and Operations of the Roman Imperial Marble Quarries in Phrygia.* Oxford: British Archaeological Reports.

Faraone, C. A. 2018. *The Transformation of Greek Amulets in Roman Imperial Times.* Philadelphia: University of Pennsylvania Press.

Fell, H. G., J.U.L. Baldini, B. Dodds, and G. J. Sharples. 2020. "Volcanism and Global Plague Pandemics: Towards an Interdisciplinary Synthesis." *Journal of Historical Geography* 70: 36–46.

Fenn, E. A. 2002. *Pox Americana: The Great Smallpox Epidemic of 1775–82.* New York: Macmillan.

Fenner, F., D. A. Henderson, I. Arita, Z. Jezek, and I. D. Ladnyi. 1988. *Smallpox and Its Eradication.* Geneva: World Health Organization.

Fentress, E. 2003. "Settlement between the Third and Fifth Centuries A.D." In *Cosa V: An Intermittent Town, Excavations 1991–1997,* ed. E. Fentress, J. Bodel, T. V. Buttrey, S. Camaiani, F. Cavari, L. Cerri, E. Cirelli, et al., 2:i–400. Ann Arbor: University of Michigan Press.

Fentress, E., T. Clay, M. Hobart, and M. Webb. 1991. "Late Roman and Medieval Cosa I: The Arx and the Structure Near the Eastern Height." *Papers of the British School at Rome* 59: 197–230.

Fentress, E., S. Fontana, R. B. Hitchner, and P. Perkins. 2004. "Accounting for ARS: Fineware and Sites in Sicily and Africa." In *Side-by-Side Survey: Comparative Regional Studies in the Mediterranean World,* ed. S. E. Alcock and J. F. Cherry, 147–62. Oxford: Oxbow.

Ferdière, A. 2020. "Agriculture in Roman Gaul." In *A Companion to Ancient Agriculture,* ed. D. Hollander and T. Howe, 447–77. New York: John Wiley & Sons.

Ferngren, G. B. 2016. *Medicine and Health Care in Early Christianity.* Baltimore: Johns Hopkins University Press.

Fitzpatrick, M. P. 2011. "Provincializing Rome: The Indian Ocean Trade Network and Roman Imperialism." *Journal of World History* 22 (1): 27–54.

Flemming, R. 2019. "Galen and the Plague." In *Galen's Treatise Περὶ Ἀλυπίας (De Indolentia) in Context,* ed. C. Petit, 219–44. Leiden: Brill.

Flohr, M. 2018. "Skeletons in the Cupboard?: Femurs and Food Regimes in the Roman World." In *The Routledge Handbook of Diet and Nutrition in the Roman World*, ed. P. Erdkamp and C. Holleran, 273–80. London: Routledge.

Frier, B. W. 2001. "More Is Worse: Observations on the Population of the Roman Empire." In *Debating Roman Demography*, ed. W. Scheidel, 139–59. Leiden: Brill.

Furedi, F. 2019. *How Fear Works: Culture of Fear in the Twenty-First Century*. London: Bloomsbury Continuum.

Futrell, A. 2010. *Blood in the Arena: The Spectacle of Roman Power*. Austin: University of Texas Press.

Garnsey, P. 1999. *Food and Society in Classical Antiquity*. Cambridge: Cambridge University Press.

———. 1998. "Mass Diet and Nutrition in the City of Rome." In *Cities, Peasants and Food in Classical Antiquity: Essays in Social and Economic History*, ed. W. Scheidel, 226–52. Cambridge: Cambridge University Press.

———. 1989. *Famine and Food Supply in the Graeco-Roman World: Responses to Risk and Crisis*. Cambridge: Cambridge University Press.

Garnsey, P., and L. de Ligt. 2016. "Migration in Early-Imperial Italy: Herculaneum and Rome Compared." In *Migration and Mobility in the Early Roman Empire*, ed. L. de Ligt and L. E. Tacoma, 72–94. Leiden: Brill.

Garnsey, P., and R. P. Saller. 2014. *The Roman Empire: Economy, Society, and Culture*. 2nd ed. London: Bloomsbury.

Gebregiorgis, D., D. Rayner, and H. W. Linderholm. 2019. "Does the IOD Independently Influence Seasonal Monsoon Patterns in Northern Ethiopia?" *Atmosphere* 10 (8): 432.

Geraci, G. 2018. "Feeding Rome: The Grain Supply." In *A Companion to the City of Rome*, ed. C. Holleran and A. Claridge, trans. Claire Holleran, 219–46. London: John Wiley & Sons.

Giardina, A. 2007. "The Transition to Late Antiquity." In *The Cambridge Economic History of the Greco-Roman World*, ed. I. Morris, R. P. Saller, and W. Scheidel, 741–68. Cambridge: Cambridge University Press.

Gilliam, J. F. 1961. "The Plague under Marcus Aurelius." *American Journal of Philology* 82 (3): 225–51.

Gitler, H., and M. Ponting. 2003. *The Silver Coinage of Septimius Severus and His Family, 193–211 AD: A Study of the Chemical Composition of the Roman and Eastern Issues*. Milan: Ed. Ennerre.

Goffart, W. 2010. *Barbarian Tides: The Migration Age and the Later Roman Empire*. Philadelphia: University of Pennsylvania Press.

Goldsmith, R. W. 1984. "An Estimate of the Size and Structure of the National Product of the Early Roman Empire." *Review of Income and Wealth* 30 (3): 263–88.

Gordon, R., M. Beard, J. Reynolds, and C. Roueché. 1993. "Roman Inscriptions, 1986–90." *Journal of Roman Studies* 83: 131–58.

Gorman, J. 2020. "Viking Age Smallpox Complicates Story of Viral Evolution." *New York Times*, July 23, sec. Science.

Gourevitch, D. 2013. *Limos Kai Loimos: A Study of the Galenic Plague*. Paris: Editions de Boccard.

Gowland, R., and L. Walther. 2018. "Human Growth and Stature." In *The Science of Roman History: Biology, Climate, and the Future of the Past*, ed. W. Scheidel, 174–204. Princeton: Princeton University Press.

Graf, F. 2015. "Healing." In *The Oxford Handbook of Ancient Greek Religion*, ed. E. Eidinow and J. Kindt, 505–18. Oxford: Oxford University Press.

———. 2008. *Apollo*. London: Routledge.

———. 1992. "An Oracle against Pestilence from a Western Anatolian Town." *Zeitschrift für Papyrologie und Epigraphik* 92: 267–79.

Graham, E.-J. 2006. *The Burial of the Urban Poor in Italy in the Late Roman Republic and Early Empire*. Oxford: British Archaeological Reports.

Grant, M. 1996. *The Antonines: The Roman Empire in Transition*. New York: Psychology Press.

Graziani, S. 2010. "Abitare in città nella Romagna romana." In *Cultura abitativa nella Cisalpina Romana: 1. Forum Popilii*, ed. A. Coralini, 25–99. Florence: All'Insegna del Giglio.

Greenberg, J. 2003. "Plagued by Doubt: Reconsidering the Impact of a Mortality Crisis in the 2nd c. A.D." *Journal of Roman Archaeology* 16: 413–25.

Greene, K. 1990. *The Archaeology of the Roman Economy*. Berkeley: University of California Press.

Gregoratti, L. 2020. "Temples and Traders in Palmyra." In *Capital Investment and Innovation in the Roman World*, ed. P. Erdkamp, K. Verboven, and A. Zuiderhoek, 461–80. Oxford: Oxford University Press.

Gregory, H., trans. 2002. *Marcus Aurelius: Meditations: A New Translation*. New York: Random House.

Grunewald, T. 2004. *Bandits in the Roman Empire: Myth and Reality*. Trans. J. Drinkwater. London: Routledge.

Guerra, F. M., S. Bolotin, G. Lim, J. Heffernan, S. L. Deeks, Y. Li, and N. S. Crowcroft. 2017. "The Basic Reproduction Number (R0) of Measles: A Systematic Review." *Lancet Infectious Diseases* 17 (12): e420–e428.

Haklai-Rotenberg, M. 2011. "Aurelian's Monetary Reform: Between Debasement and Public Trust." *Chiron* 41: 1–39.

Haldon, J. 2016. *The Empire That Would Not Die: The Paradox of Eastern Roman Survival, 640–740*. Cambridge, MA: Harvard University Press.

Haldon, J., H. Elton, S. R. Huebner, A. Izdebski, L. Mordechai, and T. P. Newfield. 2018. "Plagues, Climate Change, and the End of an Empire. A Response to Kyle Harper's The Fate of Rome (2): Plagues and a Crisis of Empire." *History Compass* 16 (12): e12506.

Haldon, J., N. Roberts, A. Izdebski, D. Fleitmann, M. McCormick, M. Cassis, O. Doonan, et al. 2014. "The Climate and Environment of Byzantine Anatolia: Integrating Science, History, and Archaeology." *Journal of Interdisciplinary History* 45 (2): 113–61.

Hameter, W. 2000. "The Afterlife of Some Inscriptions from Noricum: Modifications and Falsifications." *Bulletin of the Institute of Classical Studies*, Supplement, no. 75: 37–46.

Hankinson, R. J. 2008. "The Man and His Work." In *The Cambridge Companion to Galen*, ed. R. J. Hankinson, 1–33. Cambridge Companions to Philosophy. Cambridge: Cambridge University Press.

Hanson, J. W. 2011. "The Urban System of Roman Asia Minor and Wider Urban Connectivity." In *Settlement, Urbanization, and Population*, ed. A. K. Bowman and A. Wilson, 229–75. Oxford: Oxford University Press.

Hanson, J. W., and S. G. Ortman. 2017. "A Systematic Method for Estimating the Populations of Greek and Roman Settlements." *Journal of Roman Archaeology* 30: 301–24.

Hanson, M. 2012. *Speaking of Epidemics in Chinese Medicine: Disease and the Geographic Imagination in Late Imperial China*. London: Routledge.

Hard, R., trans. 2011. *Meditations: With Selected Correspondence*. Oxford: Oxford University Press.

Harper, K. 2021a. *Plagues upon the Earth: Disease and the Course of Human History*. Princeton: Princeton University Press.

———. 2021b. "Germs and Empire: The Agency of the Microscopic." In *Empire and Religion in the Roman World*, ed. H. I. Flower, 13–34. Cambridge: Cambridge University Press.

———. 2018. "Integrating the Natural Sciences and Roman History: Challenges and Prospects." *History Compass* 16 (12): e12520.

———. 2017. *The Fate of Rome: Climate, Disease, and the End of an Empire*. Princeton: Princeton University Press.

———. 2016a. "The Environmental Fall of the Roman Empire." *Daedalus* 145 (2): 101–11.

———. 2016b. "Database of Prices, Wages, and Rents for Roman Egypt from the First through Seventh Centuries AD." DARMC Scholarly Data Series 2016–5, Center for Geographic Analysis, Harvard University.

———. 2016c. "People, Plagues, and Prices in the Roman World: The Evidence from Egypt." *Journal of Economic History* 76 (3): 803–39.

———. 2015a. "A Time to Die: Preliminary Notes on Seasonal Mortality in Late Antique Rome." In *Children and Family in Late Antiquity: Life, Death and Interaction*, ed. C. Laes, K. Mustakallio, and V. Vuolanto, 15–34. Leuven: Peeters.

———. 2015b. "Pandemics and Passages to Late Antiquity: Rethinking the Plague of c. 249–270." *Journal of Roman Archaeology* 28: 223–60.

Harper, K., and M. McCormick. 2019. "Reconstructing the Roman Climate." In *The Science of Roman History*, ed. W. Scheidel, 11–52. Princeton: Princeton University Press.

Harris, J. R. 1891. *The Apology of Aristides on Behalf of the Christians: From a Syriac Ms. Preserved on Mount Sinai*. Cambridge: Cambridge University Press.

Harris, W. V. 2021. "Three Questions about the Ancient Hospital." In *Late-Antique Studies in Memory of Alan Cameron*, ed. W. V. Harris and A. H. Chen, 233–46. Leiden: Brill.

Hassall, M. 2000. "The Army." In *The Cambridge Ancient History*, ed. A. K. Bowman, P. Garnsey, and D. W. Rathbone, 11:320–43. Cambridge: Cambridge University Press.

Hassan, F. A. 2007. "Extreme Nile Floods and Famines in Medieval Egypt (AD 930–1500) and Their Climatic Implications." *Quaternary International* 173–74: 101–12.

Hawkins, C. 2016. *Roman Artisans and the Urban Economy*. Cambridge: Cambridge University Press.

Hayek, F. A. 2014. "The Pretence of Knowledge." In *The Collected Works of F. A. Hayek: The Market and Other Orders*, ed. B. Caldwell, 15:362–72. Chicago: University of Chicago Press.

———. 1988. *The Fatal Conceit: The Errors of Socialism*. Ed. W. W. Bartley. New York: Routledge.

———. 1945. "The Use of Knowledge in Society." *American Economic Review* 35 (4): 519–30.

———. 1937. "Economics and Knowledge." *Economica* 4 (13): 33–54.

Hays, J. N. 2002. "Historians and Epidemics: Simple Questions." In *Plague and the End of Antiquity: The Pandemic of 541–750*, 33–56. Cambridge: Cambridge University Press.

Healey, J. F., trans. 1991. *Natural History: A Selection*. London: Penguin Classics.

Heather, P. J. 2017. "Refugees and the Roman Empire." *Journal of Refugee Studies* 30 (2): 221–42.

———. 2012. *Empires and Barbarians: The Fall of Rome and the Birth of Europe*. Oxford: Oxford University Press.

———. 2007. *The Fall of the Roman Empire: A New History of Rome and the Barbarians*. Oxford: Oxford University Press.

Heinrich, F. 2018. "Cereals and Bread." In *The Routledge Handbook of Diet and Nutrition in the Roman World*, ed. P. Erdkamp and C. Holleran, 101–15. London: Routledge.

Heinrich, F., and P. Erdkamp. 2018. "The Role of Modern Malnutrition in Modelling Roman Malnutrition: Aid or Anachronism?" *Journal of Archaeological Science: Reports* 19: 1016–22.

Heinrich, F., and A. M. Hansen. 2021. "A Hard Row to Hoe: Ancient Climate Change from the Crop Perspective." In *Climate Change and Ancient Societies in Europe and the Near East: Diversity in Collapse and Resilience*, ed. P. Erdkamp, J. G. Manning, and K. Verboven, 25–80. Palgrave Studies in Ancient Economies. Cham: Palgrave Macmillan.

Hekster, O. 2012. "The Roman Empire after His Death." In *A Companion to Marcus Aurelius*, ed. M. van Ackeren, 234–48. Chichester: John Wiley & Sons.

———. 2003. "Coins and Messages: Audience Targeting on Coins of Different Denominations." In *The Representation and Perception of Roman Imperial Power*, ed. P. Erdkamp, O. Hekster, G. de Kleijn, S.T.A.M. Mols, and L. de Blois, 20–35. Leiden: Brill.

———. 2002. *Commodus: An Emperor at the Crossroads*. Amsterdam: Gieben.

Hekster, O., G. de Kleijn, and D. Slootjes, eds. 2007. *Crises and the Roman Empire: Proceedings of the Seventh Workshop of the International Network Impact of Empire, Nijmegen, June 20–24, 2006*. Leiden: Brill.

Hill, J. E. 2009. *Through the Jade Gate to Rome: A Study of the Silk Routes during the Later Han Dynasty 1st to 2nd Centuries CE*. Charleston, SC: BookSurge.

Hin, S. 2013. *The Demography of Roman Italy: Population Dynamics in an Ancient Conquest Society, 201 BCE–14 CE*. Cambridge: Cambridge University Press.

Hirt, A. M. 2010. *Imperial Mines and Quarries in the Roman World: Organizational Aspects, 27 BC–AD 235*. Oxford: Oxford University Press.

Holder, P. 2006. *Roman Military Diplomas V*. London: Institute of Classical Studies.

Holleran, C. 2016. "Labour Mobility in the Roman World: A Case Study of Mines in Iberia." In *Migration and Mobility in the Early Roman Empire*, ed. L. de Ligt and L. E. Tacoma, 95–137. Leiden: Brill.

———. 2012. *Shopping in Ancient Rome: The Retail Trade in the Late Republic and the Principate*. Oxford: Oxford University Press.

Hope, V. M. 2002. "Contempt and Respect: The Treatment of the Corpses in Ancient Rome." In *Death and Disease in the Ancient City*, ed. V. M. Hope and E. Marshall, 104–27. London: Routledge.

Hopkins, D. R. 2002. *The Greatest Killer: Smallpox in History*. Chicago: University of Chicago Press.

Hopkins, K. 1998. "Christian Number and Its Implications." *Journal of Early Christian Studies* 6 (2): 185–226.

Hopkins, K. 1983. *Death and Renewal: Sociological Studies in Roman History*. Vol. 2. Cambridge: Cambridge University Press.

Horden, P., and N. Purcell. 2000. *The Corrupting Sea: A Study of Mediterranean History*. Oxford: Wiley-Blackwell.

Howgego, C., K. Butcher, and M. Ponting. Forthcoming. "Coinage and the Roman Economy in the Antonine Period: The View from Egypt." In *Mining, Metal Supply and Coinage in the Roman Empire*, ed. A. K. Bowman and A. Wilson. Oxford: Oxford University Press.

Huebner, S. R. 2021. "The 'Plague of Cyprian': A Revised View of the Origin and Spread of a 3rd-c. CE Pandemic." *Journal of Roman Archaeology* 34 (1): 151–74.

———. 2020. "Climate Change in the Breadbasket of the Roman Empire: Explaining the Decline of the Fayum Villages in the Third Century CE." *Studies in Late Antiquity* 4 (4): 486–518.

Huebner, S. R., and B. T. McDonald. Forthcoming. "Egypt as a Gateway for the Passage of Ancient Pathogens into the Mediterranean." *Journal of Interdisciplinary History*.

Huq, F. 1976. "Effect of Temperature and Relative Humidity on Variola Virus in Crusts." *Bulletin of the World Health Organization* 54 (6): 710–12.

Irby-Massie, G. 2018. *Military Religion in Roman Britain*. Leiden: Brill.

Isayev, E. 2017. *Migration, Mobility and Place in Ancient Italy*. Cambridge: Cambridge University Press.

Israelowich, I. 2015. *Patients and Healers in the High Roman Empire*. Baltimore: Johns Hopkins University Press.

Ivleva, T. 2016. "Peasants into Soldiers: Recruitment and Military Mobility in the Early Roman Empire." In *Migration and Mobility in the Early Roman Empire*, ed. L. de Ligt and L. E. Tacoma, 158–75. Leiden: Brill.

James, S. 2019. *The Roman Military Base at Dura-Europos, Syria: An Archaeological Visualization*. Oxford: Oxford University Press.

Janssen, L. F. 1979. "'Superstitio' and the Persecution of the Christians." *Vigiliae Christianae* 33 (2): 131–59.

Janssen, W. 1994. "Seat-Belt Wearing and Driving Behavior: An Instrumented-Vehicle Study." *Accident Analysis & Prevention* 26 (2): 249–61.

Johnston, S. I. 2009. *Ancient Religions*. Cambridge, MA: Harvard University Press.

Jones, A.H.M. 1986. *The Later Roman Empire, 284–602: A Social, Economic and Administrative Survey*. Baltimore: Johns Hopkins University Press.

Jones, C. P. 2018a. "A Letter of Antoninus Pius and an Antonine Rescript Concerning Christians." *Greek, Roman, and Byzantine Studies* 58 (1): 67–76.

———. 2018b. "Christian Apologists and the Antonine Emperors." *Arys* 16: 333–45.

———. 2016. "An Amulet from London and Events Surrounding the Antonine Plague." *Journal of Roman Archaeology* 29: 469–72.

———. 2012. "Recruitment in the Time of Plague: The Case of Thespiae." In *L'Impatto della peste antonina*, ed. E. Lo Cascio, 79–85. Bari: Edipuglia.

———. 2006. "Addendum to JRA 18 (2005): Cosa and the Antonine Plague?" *Journal of Roman Archaeology* 19: 368–69.

———. 2005. "Ten Dedications 'To the Gods and Goddesses' and the Antonine Plague." *Journal of Roman Archaeology* 18 (1): 293–301.

Jones, D. S. 2003. "Virgin Soils Revisited." *William and Mary Quarterly* 60 (4): 703–42.

Jongman, W. M. 2007a. "Gibbon Was Right: The Decline and Fall of the Roman Economy." In *Crises and the Roman Empire*, ed. O. Hekster, G. de Kleijn, and D. Slootjes, 183–200. Leiden: Brill.

———. 2007b. "The Early Roman Empire: Consumption." In *The Cambridge Economic History of the Greco-Roman World*, ed. W. Scheidel, I. Morris, and R. P. Saller, 592–618. Cambridge: Cambridge University Press.

———. 2003. "Slavery and the Growth of Rome: The Transformation of Italy in the Second and First Centuries B.C.E." In *Rome the Cosmopolis*, ed. C. Edwards and G. Woolf, 100–122. Cambridge: Cambridge University Press.

Jongman, W. M., J.P.A.M. Jacobs, and G. M. Klein Goldewijk. 2019. "Health and Wealth in the Roman Empire." *Economics and Human Biology* 34: 138–50.

Jutikkala, E., and M. Kauppinen. 1971. "The Structure of Mortality during Catastrophic Years in a Pre-Industrial Society." *Population Studies* 25 (2): 283–85.

Kacki, S., D. Castex, P. Blanchard, M. Bessou, R. Giuliani, and O. Dutour. 2013. "Differential Diagnosis of Carpal and Tarsal Ankylosis on Dry Bones: Example from the Catacomb of Saints Peter and Marcellinus (Rome, 1st–3rd Century AD)." *International Journal of Paleopathology* 3 (4): 274–81.

Kallet, L. 2013. "Thucydides, Apollo, the Plague, and the War." *American Journal of Philology* 134 (3): 355–82.

Kaniewski, D., and N. Marriner. 2020. "Conflicts and the Spread of Plagues in Pre-Industrial Europe." *Humanities and Social Sciences Communications* 7 (1): 1–10.

Kehoe, D. P. 2020. "Agriculture in Roman North Africa." In *A Companion to Ancient Agriculture*, ed. D. Hollander and T. Howe, 499–516. London: John Wiley & Sons.

———. 2012. "Contract Labor." In *The Cambridge Companion to the Roman Economy*, ed. W. Scheidel, 114–30. Cambridge: Cambridge University Press.

Kennedy, D. L. 1983. "Cohors XX Palmyrenorum: An Alternative Explanation of the Numeral." *Zeitschrift für Papyrologie und Epigraphik* 53: 214–16.

Kertzer, D. I., and M. Barbagli. 2001. *The History of the European Family: Family Life in Early Modern Times (1500–1789)*. New Haven: Yale University Press.

Keyser, P. 1997. "Science and Magic in Galen's Recipes (Sympathy and Efficacy)." In *Galen on Pharmacology*, ed. A. Debru, 175–98. Leiden: Brill.

Killgrove, K. 2018. "Using Skeletal Remains as a Proxy for Roman Lifestyles: The Potential and Problems with Osteological Reconstructions of Health, Diet, and Stature in Imperial Rome." In *The Routledge Handbook of Diet and Nutrition in the Roman World*, ed. P. Erdkamp and C. Holleran, 245–58. London: Routledge.

———. 2017. "Imperialism and Physiological Stress in Rome, First to Third Centuries A.D." In *Colonized Bodies, Worlds Transformed*, 247–77. Gainesville: University Press of Florida.

Killgrove, K., and R. H. Tykot. 2013. "Food for Rome: A Stable Isotope Investigation of Diet in the Imperial Period (1st–3rd Centuries AD)." *Journal of Anthropological Archaeology* 32 (1): 28–38.

Kirkup, A. 2013. "Poynton Town Centre." *Institution of Civil Engineers (ICE)*, July 18.

Koloski-Ostrow, A. O. 2015. *The Archaeology of Sanitation in Roman Italy: Toilets, Sewers, and Water Systems*. Chapel Hill: University of North Carolina Press.

Komlos, J. 1995. *The Biological Standard of Living on Three Continents: Further Explorations in Anthropometric History*. Boulder, CO: Westview Press.

———. 1994. *Stature, Living Standards, and Economic Development: Essays in Anthropometric History*. Chicago: University of Chicago Press.

Kovács, P. 2009. *Marcus Aurelius' Rain Miracle and the Marcomannic Wars*. Leiden: Brill.

Kron, G. 2012. "Nutrition, Hygiene and Mortality: Setting Parameters for Roman Health and Life Expectancy Consistent with Our Comparative Evidence." In *L'Impatto della peste antonina*, ed. E. Lo Cascio, 193–252. Bari: Edipuglia.

Krylova, O., and D.J.D. Earn. 2020. "Patterns of Smallpox Mortality in London, England, over Three Centuries." *PLOS Biology* 18 (12): e3000506.

Kulikowski, M. 2016. *The Triumph of Empire: The Roman World from Hadrian to Constantine*. Cambridge, MA: Harvard University Press.

Kyle, D. G. 2012. *Spectacles of Death in Ancient Rome*. London: Routledge.

Labuhn, I., M. Finné, A. Izdebski, N. Roberts, and J. Woodbridge. 2016. "Climatic Changes and Their Impacts in the Mediterranean during the First Millennium AD." *Late Antique Archaeology* 12 (1): 65–88.

Laes, C. 2011. *Children in the Roman Empire: Outsiders Within*. Cambridge: Cambridge University Press.

Lavan, M. 2019. "Epistemic Uncertainty, Subjective Probability, and Ancient History." *Journal of Interdisciplinary History* 50 (1): 91.

Ledger, M. L., F. Stock, H. Schwaiger, M. Knipping, H. Brückner, S. Ladstätter, and P. D. Mitchell. 2018. "Intestinal Parasites from Public and Private Latrines and the Harbour Canal in Roman Period Ephesus, Turkey (1st c. BCE to 6th c. CE)." *Journal of Archaeological Science: Reports* 21: 289–97.

Leigh, R. 2016. *On Theriac to Piso, Attributed to Galen: A Critical Edition with Translation and Commentary*. Studies in Ancient Medicine. Vol. 47. Leiden: Brill.

Leriche, P. 1986. "Chronologie du rempart de brique crue de Doura-Europos." In *Doura-Europos: Études I*, ed. P. Leriche, A. Mahmoud, E. Will, B. Mouton, G. Lecuyot, S. B. Downey, A. Allara, et al., 61–82. Beirut: Institut Français d'Archéologie du Proche Orient.

Levick, B. 2014. "The Faustinas as Empresses, 138–175." In *Faustina I and II*. Oxford: Oxford University Press.

———. 2001. *Claudius*. Oxon: Routledge.

Lewis, N. 1993. "A Reversal of a Tax Policy in Roman Egypt." *Greek, Roman, and Byzantine Studies* 34 (1): 101–18.

———. 1982. *The Compulsory Public Services of Roman Egypt*. Firenze: Edizioni Gonnelli.

Lewis, N., and M. Reinhold. 1990. *Roman Civilization: Selected Readings*. Vol. 1. New York: Columbia University Press.

Littman, R. J., and M. L. Littman. 1973. "Galen and the Antonine Plague." *American Journal of Philology* 94: 243–55.

Lo Cascio, E. 2018. "Market Regulation and Transaction Costs in the Roman Empire." In *Trade, Commerce, and the State in the Roman World*, ed. A. Bowman and A. Wilson, 117–32. Oxford: Oxford University Press.

———, ed. 2012. *L'Impatto della peste antonina*. Bari: Edipuglia.

———. 2007. "The Early Roman Empire: The State and the Economy." In *The Cambridge Economic History of the Greco-Roman World*, ed. W. Scheidel, I. Morris, and R. P. Saller, 619–47. Cambridge: Cambridge University Press.

———. 1994. "The Size of the Roman Population: Beloch and the Meaning of the Augustan Census Figures." *Journal of Roman Studies* 84: 23–40.

Łuć, I. 2020. "Emperor Commodus' 'Bellum Desertorum.'" *Res Historica* 49: 61–95.

Lukianoff, G., and J. Haidt. 2018. *The Coddling of the American Mind: How Good Intentions and Bad Ideas Are Setting Up a Generation for Failure*. Illustrated edition. New York: Penguin Press.

MacKinnon, M. 2013. "Pack Animals, Pets, Pests, and Other Non-Human Beings." In *The Cambridge Companion to Ancient Rome*, ed. P. Erdkamp, 110–28. Cambridge Companions to the Ancient World. Cambridge: Cambridge University Press.

MacMullen, R. 1983. *Paganism in the Roman Empire*. New Haven: Yale University Press.

Mahoney, A. 2001. *Roman Sports and Spectacles: A Sourcebook*. Indianapolis: Hackett Publishing.

Mangini, A., C. Spötl, and P. Verdes. 2005. "Reconstruction of Temperature in the Central Alps during the Past 2000 Yr from a Δ18O Stalagmite Record." *Earth and Planetary Science Letters* 235 (3): 741–51.

Marciniak, S., T. L. Prowse, D. A. Herring, J. Klunk, M. Kuch, A. T. Duggan, L. Bondioli, E. C. Holmes, and H. N. Poinar. 2016. "Plasmodium Falciparum Malaria in 1st–2nd Century CE Southern Italy." *Current Biology* 26 (23): R1220–22.

Marek, C. 1993. "Die Expedition des Aelius Gallus nach Arabien im Jahre 25 v. Chr." *Chiron* 23: 121–56.

Margaritelli, G., I. Cacho, A. Català, M. Barra, L. G. Bellucci, C. Lubritto, R. Rettori, and F. Lirer. 2020. "Persistent Warm Mediterranean Surface Waters during the Roman Period." *Scientific Reports* 10 (1): 10431.

Martin, L. H. 2013. "The Ecology of Threat Detection and Precautionary Response from the Perspectives of Evolutionary Psychology, Cognitive Science and Historiography: The Case of the Roman Cults of Mithras." *Method & Theory in the Study of Religion* 25: 431–50.

Martín-Chivelet, J., M. B. Muñoz-García, R. L. Edwards, M. J. Turrero, and A. I. Ortega. 2011. "Land Surface Temperature Changes in Northern Iberia since 4000yrBP, Based on Δ13C of Speleothems." *Global and Planetary Change* 77 (1): 1–12.

Martyn, R.E.V., P. Garnsey, L. Fattore, P. Petrone, A. Sperduti, L. Bondioli, and O. E. Craig. 2018. "Capturing Roman Dietary Variability in the Catastrophic Death Assemblage at Herculaneum." *Journal of Archaeological Science: Reports* 19: 1023–29.

Marzano, A. 2021. "Figures in an Imperial Landscape: Ecological and Societal Factors on Settlement Patterns and Agriculture in Roman Italy." In *Climate Change and Ancient Societies in Europe and the Near East: Diversity in Collapse and Resilience*, ed. P. Erdkamp, J. G. Manning, and K. Verboven, 505–31. Palgrave Studies in Ancient Economies. Cham: Palgrave Macmillan.

———. 2013. *Harvesting the Sea: The Exploitation of Marine Resources in the Roman Mediterranean*. Oxford: Oxford University Press.

Mathew, K. S. 2017. *Imperial Rome, Indian Ocean Regions and Muziris: New Perspectives on Maritime Trade*. New York: Taylor & Francis.

Mattern, S. P. 2013. *The Prince of Medicine: Galen in the Roman Empire*. Oxford: Oxford University Press.

Mayor, A. 2020. *Gods and Robots: Myths, Machines, and Ancient Dreams of Technology*. Princeton: Princeton University Press.

McConnell, J. R., M. Sigl, G. Plunkett, A. Burke, W. M. Kim, C. C. Raible, A. I. Wilson, et al. 2020. "Extreme Climate after Massive Eruption of Alaska's Okmok Volcano in 43 BCE and Effects on the Late Roman Republic and Ptolemaic Kingdom." *Proceedings of the National Academy of Sciences* 117 (27): 15443–49.

McConnell, J. R., A. I. Wilson, A. Stohl, M. M. Arienzo, N. J. Chellman, S. Eckhardt, E. M. Thompson, A. M. Pollard, and J. P. Steffensen. 2018. "Lead Pollution Recorded in Greenland Ice Indicates European Emissions Tracked Plagues, Wars, and Imperial Expansion during Antiquity." *Proceedings of the National Academy of Sciences* 115 (22): 5726–31.

McCormick, M. 2013. "What Climate Science, Ausonius, Nile Floods, Rye, and Thatch Tell Us about the Environmental History of the Roman Empire." In *The Ancient Mediterranean Environment between Science and History*, ed. W. V. Harris, 61–88. Leiden: Brill.

McDonald, B. Forthcoming. "The Downturn of Egypt's Eastern Desert in the Middle Roman Imperial Period." *Journal of Egyptian Archaeology*.

———. 2021. "The Antonine Crisis: Climate Change as a Trigger for Epidemiological and Economic Turmoil." In *Climate Change and Ancient Societies in Europe and the Near East: Diversity in Collapse and Resistance*, ed. P. Erdkamp, J. G. Manning, and K. Verboven, 373–410. Palgrave Studies in Ancient Economies. Cham: Palgrave Macmillan.

———. 2020. "Climate Change and Major Plagues in the Roman Period." PhD thesis, University of Oxford.

McGinn, T.A.J. 2004. *The Economy of Prostitution in the Roman World: A Study of Social History and the Brothel*. Illustrated edition. Ann Arbor: University of Michigan Press.

———. 2003. *Prostitution, Sexuality, and the Law in Ancient Rome*. Oxford: Oxford University Press.

McKay, N. P., and D. S. Kaufman. 2014. "An Extended Arctic Proxy Temperature Database for the Past 2,000 Years." *Scientific Data* 1: 140026.

McKenzie, J. 2007. *The Architecture of Alexandria and Egypt, c. 300 B.C. to A.D. 700*. New Haven: Yale University Press.

McMillen, C. W. 2015. *Discovering Tuberculosis: A Global History, 1900 to the Present*. New Haven: Yale University Press.

McNeill, W. 1998. *Plagues and Peoples*. New York: Doubleday.

Merrifield, R. 1996. "The London Hunter-God and His Significance in the History of London." In *Interpreting Roman London: Papers in Memory of Hugh Chapman*, ed. J. Bird, M.W.C. (Mark W. C.) Hassall, and H. Sheldon, 105–13. Oxford: Oxbow.

Millar, F. 2006. *Rome, the Greek World, and the East*. Vol. 3: *The Greek World, the Jews, and the East*. Studies in the History of Greece and Rome. Chapel Hill: University of North Carolina Press.

———. 1993. *The Roman Near East, 31 B.C.–A.D. 337*. Cambridge, MA: Harvard University Press.

———. 1964. *Study of Cassius Dio*. Oxford: Oxford University Press.

Miller, K. M. 1985. "Apollo Lairbenos." *Numen* 32 (1): 46–70.

Miller, P. C. 2020. *Dreams in Late Antiquity: Studies in the Imagination of a Culture*. Princeton: Princeton University Press.

Miller, T. S. 1997. *The Birth of the Hospital in the Byzantine Empire*. Baltimore: Johns Hopkins University Press.

Mitchell, P. D. 2017. "Human Parasites in the Roman World: Health Consequences of Conquering an Empire." *Parasitology* 144 (1): 48–58.

Mitrofan, D. 2014. "The Antonine Plague in Dacia and Moesia Inferior." *Journal of Ancient History and Archaeology* 1 (2): 9–13.

Moorhead, J. 2013. *The Roman Empire Divided: 400–700 AD*. New York: Routledge.

Mordechai, L., and M. Eisenberg. 2019. "Rejecting Catastrophe: The Case of the Justinianic Plague." *Past & Present* 244 (1): 3–50.

Mordechai, L., M. Eisenberg, T. P. Newfield, A. Izdebski, J. E. Kay, and H. Poinar. 2019. "The Justinianic Plague: An Inconsequential Pandemic?" *Proceedings of the National Academy of Sciences* 116 (51): 25546–54.

More, A. F., N. E. Spaulding, P. Bohleber, M. J. Handley, H. Hoffmann, E. V. Korotkikh, A. V. Kurbatov, et al. 2017. "Next-Generation Ice Core Technology Reveals True Minimum Natural Levels of Lead (Pb) in the Atmosphere: Insights from the Black Death." *GeoHealth* 1 (4): 211–19.

Morley, N. 2010. *The Roman Empire: Roots of Imperialism*. London: Pluto Press.

———. 2000. "Trajan's Engines." *Greece & Rome* 47 (2): 197–210.

———. 1996. *Metropolis and Hinterland: The City of Rome and the Italian Economy, 200 BC–AD 200*. Cambridge: Cambridge University Press.

Morony, M. G. 2006. "'For Whom Does the Writer Write?': The First Bubonic Plague Pandemic According to Syriac Sources." In *Plague and the End of Antiquity: The Pandemic of 541–750*, ed. L. K. Little, 59–86. Cambridge: Cambridge University Press.

Morris, I. 1992. *Death-Ritual and Social Structure in Classical Antiquity*. Cambridge: Cambridge University Press.

Moss, C. R. 2012. *Ancient Christian Martyrdom: Diverse Practices, Theologies, and Traditions*. New Haven: Yale University Press.

Mrozek, S. 1994. "Le problème de l'annone dans les villes italiennes du Haut Empire romain." *Publications de l'École Française de Rome* 196 (1): 95–101.

Mühlemann, B., L. Vinner, A. Margaryan, H. Wilhelmson, C. de la Fuente Castro, M. E. Allentoft, P. de Barros Damgaard, et al. 2020. "Diverse Variola Virus (Smallpox) Strains Were Widespread in Northern Europe in the Viking Age." *Science* 369 (6502): eaaw8977.

Mulhall, J. 2021. "Confronting Pandemic in Late Antiquity: The Medical Response to the Justinianic Plague." *Journal of Late Antiquity* 14 (2): 498–528.

———. 2019. "Plague before the Pandemics: The Greek Medical Evidence for Bubonic Plague before the Sixth Century." *Bulletin of the History of Medicine* 93 (2): 151–79.

Munro, D. C. 1904. *A Source Book of Roman History*. Boston: D. C. Heath.

Nappo, D. 2015. "Roman Policy on the Red Sea in the Second Century CE." In *Across the Ocean: Nine Essays on Indo-Mediterranean Trade*, 55–72. Leiden: Brill.

Nash, D. J., G. De Cort, B. M. Chase, D. Verschuren, S. E. Nicholson, T. M. Shanahan, A. Asrat, A. Lézine, and S. W. Grab. 2016. "African Hydroclimatic Variability during the Last 2000 Years." *Quaternary Science Reviews* 154 (December 2016): 1–22.

Needham, J. 2000. *Science and Civilisation in China*. Vol. 6. Cambridge: Cambridge University Press.

Newfield, T. P. 2022. "One Plague for Another? Interdisciplinary Shortcomings in Plague Studies and the Place of the Black Death in Histories of the Justinianic Plague." *Studies in Late Antiquity* 6 (4): 575–626.

Newfield, T. P., A. T. Duggan, and H. Poinar. 2022. "Smallpox's Antiquity in Doubt." *Journal of Roman Archaeology* 35: 1–17.

Newfield, T. P., and I. Labuhn. 2017. "Realizing Consilience in Studies of Pre-Instrumental Climate and Pre-Laboratory Disease." *Journal of Interdisciplinary History* 48 (2): 211–40.

Nicholls, M. 2019. "Galen and the Last Days of Commodus: A Tale of Resilience." In *Galen's Treatise Περὶ Ἀλυπίας (De Indolentia) in Context*, ed. C. Petit, 245–62. Leiden: Brill.

Niebuhr, B. G. 1875. *Niebuhr's Lectures on Roman History*. Vol. 3. London: Chatto & Windus.

Noreña, C. F. 2021. "Imperial Integration on Rome's Atlantic Rim." In *Empire and Religion in the Roman World*, ed. H. I. Flower, 35–70. Cambridge: Cambridge University Press.

———. 2011. *Imperial Ideals in the Roman West: Representation, Circulation, Power*. Cambridge: Cambridge University Press.

Noy, D. 2018. "Social Structure and the Plebs Romana." In *A Companion to the City of Rome*, ed. C. Holleran and A. Claridge, 155–71. New York: John Wiley & Sons.

Nunn, J. F. 2002. *Ancient Egyptian Medicine*. Norman: University of Oklahoma Press.

Nutton, V. 2020. *Galen: A Thinking Doctor in Imperial Rome*. London: Routledge.

———. 2016. "Folk Medicine in the Galenic Corpus." In *Popular Medicine in Graeco-Roman Antiquity: Explorations*, ed. W. V. Harris, 272–79. Leiden: Brill.

———. 2004. *Ancient Medicine*. London: Routledge.

———. 2002. "Medical Thoughts on Urban Pollution." In *Death and Disease in the Ancient City*, ed. V. M. Hope and E. Marshall, 65–73. London: Routledge.

———. 1990. "The Patient's Choice: A New Treatise by Galen." *Classical Quarterly* 40 (1): 236–57.

———. 1983. "The Seeds of Disease: An Explanation of Contagion and Infection from the Greeks to the Renaissance." *Medical History* 27 (1): 1–34.

———. 1979. *On Prognosis*. Corpus Medicorum Graecorum vol. 8, 1. Berlin: Akademie Verlag.

———. 1973. "The Chronology of Galen's Early Career." *Classical Quarterly* 23 (1): 158–71.

Ogden, D. 2013. *Drakōn Gods of Healing*. Oxford: Oxford University Press.

Okamura, L. 1988. "Social Disturbances in Late Roman Gaul: Deserters, Rebels, and Bagaudae." In *Forms of Control and Subordination in Antiquity*, ed. T. Yuge and M. Doi, 288–302. Leiden: Brill.

Oliver, J. H. 1970. *Marcus Aurelius: Aspects of Civic and Cultural Policy in the East*. Princeton: American School of Classical Studies at Athens.

Oliver, J. H., and K. Clinton. 1989. *Greek Constitutions of Early Roman Emperors from Inscriptions and Papyri*. Philadelphia: American Philosophical Society.

Oliver, J. H., and R.E.A. Palmer. 1955. "Minutes of an Act of the Roman Senate." *Hesperia: The Journal of the American School of Classical Studies at Athens* 24 (4): 320–49.

Paine, R. R., and G. R. Storey. 2012. "The Alps as a Barrier to Epidemic Disease during the Republican Period: Implications for the Dynamic of Disease in Rome." In *L'Impatto della peste antonina*, ed. E. Lo Cascio, 179–91. Bari: Edipuglia.

Panagiotidou, O. 2016. "Asclepius: A Divine Doctor, A Popular Healer." In *Popular Medicine in Graeco-Roman Antiquity: Explorations*, ed. W. V. Harris, 86–104. Leiden: Brill.

Parke, H. W. 1985. *The Oracles of Apollo in Asia Minor*. London: Routledge.

Parker, A. J. 1992. *Ancient Shipwrecks of the Mediterranean and the Roman Provinces*. Oxford: British Archaeological Reports.

Parkin, T. G. 2003. *Old Age in the Roman World: A Cultural and Social History*. Baltimore: Johns Hopkins University Press.

———. 1992. *Demography and Roman Society*. Baltimore: Johns Hopkins University Press.

Patterson, H., R. Witcher, and H. Di Giuseppe. 2020. *The Changing Landscapes of Rome's Northern Hinterland: The British School at Rome's Tiber Valley Project*. Oxford: Archaeopress Publishing.

Pavlyshyn, D., I. Johnstone, and R. Saller. 2020. "Lead Pollution and the Roman Economy." *Journal of Roman Archaeology* 33: 354–64.

Perring, D. 2022. *London in the Roman World*. Oxford: Oxford University Press.

———. 2011. "Two Studies on Roman London. A: London's Military Origins. B: Population Decline and Ritual Landscapes in Antonine London." *Journal of Roman Archaeology* 24: 249–82.

Petit, P. 1976. *Pax Romana*. Berkeley: University of California Press.

Pezzullo, A. M., C. Axfors, D. G. Contopoulos-Ioannidis, A. Apostolatos, and J.P.A. Ioannidis. 2023. "Age-Stratified Infection Fatality Rate of COVID-19 in the Non-Elderly Population." *Environmental Research* 216: 114655.

Phang, S. E. 2001. *The Marriage of Roman Soldiers (13 B.C.–A.D. 235): Law and Family in the Imperial Army*. Leiden: Brill.

Phillips, C., F. Villeneuve, and W. Facey. 2004. "A Latin Inscription from South Arabia." *Proceedings of the Seminar for Arabian Studies* 34: 239–50.

Phillips, E. D. 1952. "A Hypochondriac and His God." *Greece & Rome* 21 (61): 23–36.

Platts, H. 2019. *Multisensory Living in Ancient Rome: Power and Space in Roman Houses*. London: Bloomsbury Publishing.

Pollard, N. 2000. *Soldiers, Cities, and Civilians in Roman Syria*. Ann Arbor: University of Michigan Press.

Prowse, T. L., H. P. Schwarcz, P. Garnsey, M. Knyf, R. Macchiarelli, and L. Bondioli. 2007. "Isotopic Evidence for Age-Related Immigration to Imperial Rome." *American Journal of Physical Anthropology* 132 (4): 510–19.

Quenemoen, C. K. 2013. "Columns and Concrete." In *A Companion to Roman Architecture*, 63–81. New York: John Wiley & Sons.

Raoult, D., O. Dutour, L. Houhamdi, R. Jankauskas, P.-E. Fournier, Y. Ardagna, M. Drancourt, et al. 2006. "Evidence for Louse-Transmitted Diseases in Soldiers of Napoleon's Grand Army in Vilnius." *Journal of Infectious Diseases* 193 (1): 112–20.

Rathbone, D. 2007. "Roman Egypt." In *The Cambridge Economic History of the Greco-Roman World*, ed. W. Scheidel, I. Morris, and R. P. Saller, 698–719. Cambridge: Cambridge University Press.

———. 2006. "Poverty and Population in Roman Egypt." In *Poverty in the Roman World*, ed. M. Atkins and R. Osborne, 100–114. Cambridge: Cambridge University Press.

———. 1997. "Prices and Price Formation in Roman Egypt." In *Économie antique: Prix et formation des prix dans les économies antiques*, ed. J. Andreau, P. Briant, and R. Descat, 183–244. Saint-Bertrand-de-Comminges: Musée Archéologique.

Rathbone, D. 1983. "The Weight and Measurement of Egyptian Grains." *Zeitschrift für Papyrologie und Epigraphik* 53: 265–75.

Rathbone, D., and S. von Reden. 2015. "Mediterranean Grain Prices in Classical Antiquity." In *A History of Market Performance: From Ancient Babylonia to the Modern World*, ed. R. J. Van der Spek, J. L. van Zanden, and B. van Leeuwen, 149–235. London: Routledge.

Raymond, I. W. 1936. *The Seven Books of History against the Pagans; The Apology of Paulus Orosius.* New York: Columbia University Press.

Rebillard, É. 2009. *The Care of the Dead in Late Antiquity*. Trans. E. T. Rawlings and J. Routier-Pucci. Ithaca: Cornell University Press.

Reff, D. T. 2004. *Plagues, Priests, and Demons: Sacred Narratives and the Rise of Christianity in the Old World and the New*. Cambridge: Cambridge University Press.

Renberg, G. H. 2006. "Public and Private Places of Worship in the Cult of Asclepius at Rome." *Memoirs of the American Academy in Rome* 51/52: 87–172.

Retsö, J. 2003. "When Did Yemen Become 'Arabia Felix'?" *Proceedings of the Seminar for Arabian Studies* 33: 229–35.

Reynolds, P. 2017. "The Supply Networks of the Roman East and West: Interaction, Fragmentation, and the Origins of the Byzantine Economy." In *Trade, Commerce, and the State in the Roman World*, ed. A. Wilson and A. Bowman, 353–95. Oxford: Oxford University Press.

Rickman, G. E. 2002. "Rome, Ostia and Portus: The Problem of Storage." *Mélanges de l'école Française de Rome* 114 (1): 353–62.

———. 1980. "The Grain Trade under the Roman Empire." *Memoirs of the American Academy in Rome* 36: 261–75.

Ritner, R. 1998. "Egypt under Roman Rule: The Legacy of Ancient Egypt." In *The Cambridge History of Egypt*. Vol. 1: *640–1517*, ed. C. F. Petry, 1–33. Cambridge: Cambridge University Press.

Rives, J. B. 2020. "Animal Sacrifice and the Roman Persecution of Christians (Second to Third Century)." In *Religious Violence in the Ancient World: From Classical Athens to Late Antiquity*, ed. C. R. Raschle and J.H.F. Dijkstra, 177–202. Cambridge: Cambridge University Press.

———. 2011. "The Persecution of Christians and Ideas of Community in the Roman Empire." In *Politiche religiose nel mondo antico e tardoantico: Poteri e indirizze, forme del controllo, idee e prassi di tolleranza*, ed. G. A. Cecconi and C. Gabrielli, 199–217. Bari: Edipuglia.

———. 2007. *Religion in the Roman Empire*. New York: Wiley.

———. 1999. "The Decree of Decius and the Religion of Empire." *Journal of Roman Studies* 89: 135–54.

Rizzo, G. 2018. "Ostia, le anfore e i commerci mediterranei: Un bilancio preliminare." *Archeologia Classica* 69: 223–66.

Roberts, A., and J. Donaldson, eds. 1868. *The Ante-Nicene Christian Library*. Trans. S. Thelwall. Vol. 7. Edinburgh: T & T Clark.

Robin, C. J. 1992. "Guerre et épidémie dans les royaumes d'Arabie du Sud, d'après une inscription datée (IIᵉ s. de l'ère chrétienne)." *Comptes rendus des séances de l'Académie des Inscriptions et Belles-Lettres* 136 (1): 215–34.

Roselaar, S. T. 2016. "State-Organised Mobility in the Roman Empire: Legionaries and Auxiliaries." In *Migration and Mobility in the Early Roman Empire*, ed. L. de Ligt and L. E. Tacoma, 138–57. Leiden: Brill.

Ross, J. C., and S. R. Steadman. 2017. *Ancient Complex Societies*. London: Taylor & Francis.

Rossignol, B. 2012. "Le climat, les famines et la guerre: Éléments du contexte de la peste antonine." In *L'Impatto della peste antonina*, ed. E. Lo Cascio, 87–122. Bari: Edipuglia.

Rossignol, B., and S. Durost. 2007. "Volcanisme global et variations climatiques de courte durée dans l'histoire romaine (Ier s. av. J.-C.–IVème s. ap. J.-C.): Leçons d'une archive glaciaire (GISP2)." *Jahrbuch des Römisch-Germanischen Zentralmuseums Mainz* 54 (2): 395–438.

Roth, J. P. 1999. *The Logistics of the Roman Army at War: 264 B.C.–A.D. 235*. Leiden: Brill.

Routson, C. C., C. A. Woodhouse, and J. T. Overpeck. 2011. "Second Century Megadrought in the Rio Grande Headwaters, Colorado: How Unusual Was Medieval Drought?" *Geophysical Research Letters* 38 (22): L22703.

Rowan, C. 2012. *Under Divine Auspices: Divine Ideology and the Visualisation of Imperial Power in the Severan Period*. Cambridge: Cambridge University Press.

Rowan, E. 2017. "Bioarchaeological Preservation and Non-Elite Diet in the Bay of Naples: An Analysis of the Food Remains from the Cardo V Sewer at the Roman Site of Herculaneum." *Environmental Archaeology* 22 (3): 318–36.

———. 2016. "Sewers, Archaeobotany, and Diet at Pompeii and Herculaneum." In *The Economy of Pompeii*, ed. M. Flohr and A. Wilson, 111–34. Oxford: Oxford University Press.

Roxan, M. M. 1986. "Observations on the Reasons for Changes in Formula in Diplomas circa AD 140." In *Heer und Integrationspolitik: Die Romischen Militardiplome als Historische Quelle*, ed. W. Eck and H. Wolff, 265–92. Cologne: Bohlau.

Roymans, N. 2019. "Conquest, Mass Violence and Ethnic Stereotyping: Investigating Caesar's Actions in the Germanic Frontier Zone." *Journal of Roman Archaeology* 32: 439–58.

Russell, B. 2013. *The Economics of the Roman Stone Trade*. Oxford: Oxford University Press.

Russell, S. J., D. Babovic-Vuksanovic, A. Bexon, R. Cattaneo, D. Dingli, A. Dispenzieri, D. R. Deyle, et al. 2019. "Oncolytic Measles Virotherapy Does Not Legitimize Opposition to Measles Vaccination." *Mayo Clinic Proceedings* 94 (9): 1834–39.

Sabatier, P., L. Dezileau, C. Colin, L. Briqueu, F. Bouchette, P. Martinez, G. Siani, O. Raynal, and U. Von Grafenstein. 2012. "7000 Years of Paleostorm Activity in the NW Mediterranean Sea in Response to Holocene Climate Events." *Quaternary Research* 77 (1): 1–11.

Sabraa, T., and S. Borsch. 2016. "Plague Mortality in Late Medieval Cairo: Quantifying the Plague Outbreaks of 833/1430 and 864/1460." *Mamluk Studies Review* 19: 115–48.

Salesse, K., E. Dufour, M. Lebon, C. Wurster, D. Castex, J. Bruzek, and A. Zazzo. 2014. "Variability of Bone Preservation in a Confined Environment: The Case of the Catacomb of Sts Peter and Marcellinus (Rome, Italy)." *Palaeogeography, Palaeoclimatology, Palaeoecology* 416: 43–54.

Sallares, R. 2007. "Ecology." In *The Cambridge Economic History of the Greco-Roman World*, ed. W. Scheidel, I. Morris, and R. P. Saller, 13–37. Cambridge: Cambridge University Press.

———. 2002. *Malaria and Rome: A History of Malaria in Ancient Italy*. Oxford: Oxford University Press.

———. 1991. *The Ecology of the Ancient Greek World*. Ithaca: Cornell University Press.

Saller, R. 2022. *Pliny's Roman Economy: Natural History, Innovation, and Growth*. Princeton: Princeton University Press.

———. 2012. "Human Capital and Economic Growth." In *The Cambridge Companion to the Roman Economy*, ed. W. Scheidel, 71–86. Cambridge: Cambridge University Press.

Salmon, P. 1974. *Population et dépopulation dans l'Empire Romain.* Collection Latomus vol. 137. Brussels: Latomus.

Sánchez-Moreno Ellart, C. 2009. "Las Declaraciones de Defunción en el Imperio Romano: El caso de Egipto." In *Formae mortis: El tránsito de la vida a la muerte en las sociedades antiguas,* ed. F. Marco Simón, F. Pina Polo, and J. Remesal Rodríguez, 217–52. Barcelona: Universitat de Barcelona.

Scheffer, M. 2009. *Critical Transitions in Nature and Society.* Princeton: Princeton University Press.

Scheidel, W. 2019. *Escape from Rome: The Failure of Empire and the Road to Prosperity.* Princeton: Princeton University Press.

———. 2017. *The Great Leveler: Violence and the History of Inequality from the Stone Age to the Twenty-First Century.* Princeton: Princeton University Press.

———. 2013. "Disease and Death." In *The Cambridge Companion to Ancient Rome,* ed. P. Erdkamp, 45–59. Cambridge Companions to the Ancient World. Cambridge: Cambridge University Press.

———. 2012a. "Physical Well-Being." In *The Cambridge Companion to the Roman Economy,* ed. W. Scheidel, 321–33. Cambridge: Cambridge University Press.

———. 2012b. "Roman Wellbeing and the Economic Consequences of the Antonine Plague." In *L'Impatto della peste antonina,* ed. E. Lo Cascio, 265–95. Bari: Edipuglia.

———. 2010. "Coin Quality, Coin Quantity, and Coin Value in Early China and the Roman World." *American Journal of Numismatics* 22: 93–118.

———. 2008. "Roman Population Size: The Logic of the Debate." In *People, Land, and Politics: Demographic Developments and the Transformation of Roman Italy, 300 BC–AD 14,* ed. L. de Ligt and S. J. Northwood, 17–70. Leiden: Brill.

———. 2007a. "A Model of Real Income Growth in Roman Italy." *Historia: Zeitschrift für Alte Geschichte* 56 (3): 322–46.

———. 2007b. "Demography." In *The Cambridge Economic History of the Greco-Roman World,* ed. W. Scheidel, I. Morris, and R. P. Saller, 38–86. Cambridge: Cambridge University Press.

———. 2003. "Germs for Rome." In *Rome the Cosmopolis,* ed. C. Edwards and G. Woolf, 158–76. Cambridge: Cambridge University Press.

———. 2002. "A Model of Demographic and Economic Change in Roman Egypt after the Antonine Plague." *Journal of Roman Archaeology* 15: 97–114.

———. 2001a. *Death on the Nile: Disease and the Demography of Roman Egypt.* Leiden: Brill.

———. 2001b. "Progress and Problems in Roman Demography." In *Debating Roman Demography,* ed. W. Scheidel, 1–81. Leiden: Brill.

———. 1996. "Finances, Figures and Fiction." *Classical Quarterly* 46 (1): 222–38.

Schneider, H. 2007. "Technology." In *The Cambridge Economic History of the Greco-Roman World,* ed. W. Scheidel, I. Morris, and R. P. Saller, 144–71. Cambridge: Cambridge University Press.

Schott, J. M., trans. 2019. *The History of the Church: A New Translation.* Oakland: University of California Press.

Scobie, A. 1986. "Slums, Sanitation, and Mortality in the Roman World." *Klio* 68 (2): 399–433.

Scott, S., and C. J. Duncan. 1998. *Human Demography and Disease.* Cambridge: Cambridge University Press.

Scrimshaw, N. S., C. E. Taylor, and J. E. Gordon. 1968. "Interactions of Nutrition and Infection." *Monograph Series, World Health Organization* 57: 3–329.

Sedov, A. V., and Salles, J.-F. 2010. *Qāni': Le port antique du Ḥaḍramawt entre la Méditerranée, l'Afrique et l'Inde: Fouilles russes 1972, 1985–89, 1991, 1993–94* (Indicopleustoi). Turnhout: Brepols.

Seeck, O. 1897. *Geschichte des untergangs der antiken welt.* Berlin: Siemenroth & Troschel.

Segre, A. 1947. "The Byzantine Colonate." *Traditio* 5: 103–33.

Seland, E. H. 2014. "Archaeology of Trade in the Western Indian Ocean, 300 BC–AD 700." *Journal of Archaeological Research* 22 (4): 367–402.

Sessa, K. 2019. "The New Environmental Fall of Rome: A Methodological Consideration." *Journal of Late Antiquity* 12 (1): 211–55.

Shchelkunov, S. N. 2011. "Emergence and Reemergence of Smallpox: The Need for Development of a New Generation Smallpox Vaccine." *Vaccine* 29 (Suppl. 4): D49–53.

Sheldrick, N. 2021. *Building the Countryside: Rural Architecture and Settlement in Tripolitania during the Roman and Late Antique Periods.* London: Society for Libyan Studies.

Sidebotham, S. E. 2019. *Berenike and the Ancient Maritime Spice Route.* Berkeley: University of California Press.

Sigl, M., M. Winstrup, J. R. McConnell, K. C. Welten, G. Plunkett, F. Ludlow, U. Büntgen, et al. 2015. "Timing and Climate Forcing of Volcanic Eruptions for the Past 2,500 Years." *Nature* 523 (7562): 543–49.

Siler, N., Y. Kosaka, S.-P. Xie, and X. Li. 2017. "Tropical Ocean Contributions to California's Surprisingly Dry El Niño of 2015/16." *Journal of Climate* 30 (24): 10067–79.

Silk, M. J., and N. H. Fefferman. 2021. "The Role of Social Structure and Dynamics in the Maintenance of Endemic Disease." *Behavioral Ecology and Sociobiology* 75 (8): 122.

Silver, M. 2011. "Antonine Plague and Deactivation of Spanish Mines." *Arctos* 45: 133–42.

Simmonds, A., N. Marquez-Grant, and L. Loe. 2008. *Life and Death in a Roman City: Excavation of a Roman Cemetery with a Mass Grave at 120–122 London Road, Gloucester.* Oxford: Oxford Archaeology.

Singer, P. N., ed. 2014. *Galen: Psychological Writings: Avoiding Distress, Character Traits, The Diagnosis and Treatment of the Affections and Errors Peculiar to Each Person's . . . of the Body.* Cambridge: Cambridge University Press.

Smith, P., and G. Kahila. 1992. "Identification of Infanticide in Archaeological Sites: A Case Study from the Late Roman-Early Byzantine Periods at Ashkelon, Israel." *Journal of Archaeological Science* 19 (6): 667–75.

Song, S., Z. Peng, W. Zhou, W. Liu, Y. Liu, and T. Chen. 2012. "Variation of the Winter Monsoon in South China Sea over the Past 183 Years: Evidence from Oxygen Isotopes in Coral." *Global and Planetary Change* 98–99: 131–38.

Speidel, M. 2014. "Roman Army Pay Scales Revisited: Responses and Answers." In *De l'or pour les braves! Soldes, armées et circulation monétaire dans le monde romain,* ed. M. Reddé, 53–62. Bordeaux: Ausonius.

———. 1992. "Roman Army Pay Scales." *Journal of Roman Studies* 82: 87–106.

Spurr, M. S. 1986. *Arable Cultivation in Roman Italy, c. 200 B.C.–c. A.D. 100.* Journal of Roman Studies Monographs no. 3. London: Society for the Promotion of Roman Studies.

Stark, R. 1996. *The Rise of Christianity.* Princeton: Princeton University Press.

Stathakopoulos, D. 2012. "Death in the Countryside: Some Thoughts on the Effects of Famine and Epidemics." *Antiquité Tardive* 20: 105–14.

———. 2004. *Famine and Pestilence in the Late Roman and Early Byzantine Empire: A Systematic Survey of Subsistence Crises and Epidemics*. Burlington, VT: Ashgate.

Symonds, R. P. 2008. "Terminus Post Quem: Datation systèmatique et la représentation numérique et graphique de la chronologie des céramiques." *Société Française de l'étude de La Céramique Antique en Gaule (SFECAG)*: 607–19.

———. 2006. "The Pottery." In *Development on Roman London's Western Hill: Excavations at Paternoster Square, City of London*, 81–86. MoLAS Monograph 32. London: Museum of London Archaeology.

Szabó, C. 2020. "Religious Appropriations and the Antonine Plague." *Brukenthalia* 10: 807–20.

Tacoma, L. E. 2016. "Migration and Labour." In *Moving Romans*. Oxford: Oxford University Press.

Tainter, J. 1988. *The Collapse of Complex Societies*. Cambridge: Cambridge University Press.

Talbert, R.J.A. 1987. *The Senate of Imperial Rome*. Princeton: Princeton University Press.

Talty, S. 2009. *The Illustrious Dead: The Terrifying Story of How Typhus Killed Napoleon's Greatest Army*. New York: Crown.

Tan, J. 2017. *Power and Public Finance at Rome, 264–49 BCE*. Oxford: Oxford University Press.

Tchernia, A. 2016. *The Romans and Trade*. Oxford: Oxford University Press.

Temin, P. 2013. *The Roman Market Economy*. Princeton: Princeton University Press.

———. 2006. "The Economy of the Early Roman Empire." *Journal of Economic Perspectives* 20 (1): 133–51.

Țentea, O. 2003. "Legion XIII Gemina and Alburnus Maior." *Apulum* 40: 253–65.

Terpstra, T. 2015. "Roman Trade with the Far East: Evidence for Nabataean Middlemen in Puteoli." In *Across the Ocean: Nine Essays on Indo-Mediterranean Trade*, 73–94. Leiden: Brill.

Terpstra, T. T. 2013. *Trading Communities in the Roman World: A Micro-Economic and Institutional Perspective*. Leiden: Brill.

Thatcher, D. L., A. D. Wanamaker, R. F. Denniston, Y. Asmerom, V. J. Polyak, D. Fullick, C. C. Ummenhofer, D. P. Gillikin, and J. A. Haws. 2020. "Hydroclimate Variability from Western Iberia (Portugal) during the Holocene: Insights from a Composite Stalagmite Isotope Record." *The Holocene* 30 (7): 966–81.

Thèves, C., E. Crubézy, and P. Biagini. 2016. "History of Smallpox and Its Spread in Human Populations." *Microbiology Spectrum* 4 (4).

Thonemann, P. 2021. *Lucian: Alexander, or The False Prophet*. Clarendon Ancient History Series. Oxford: Oxford University Press.

Tomber, R. 2018. "Egypt and Eastern Commerce during the Second Century AD and Later." In *Trade, Commerce, and the State in the Roman World*, ed. A. K. Bowman and A. Wilson, 531–55. Oxford: Oxford University Press.

Toner, J. 2015. *The Day Commodus Killed a Rhino: Understanding the Roman Games*. Baltimore: Johns Hopkins University Press.

———. 2013. *Roman Disasters*. Oxford: Polity Press.

Tran, N. 2020. "Boatmen and Their Corpora in the Great Ports of the Roman West (Second to Third Centuries AD)." In *Roman Port Societies: The Evidence of Inscriptions*, ed. P. Arnaud and S. Keay, 85–106. British School at Rome Studies. Cambridge: Cambridge University Press.

Tucci, P. L. 2008. "Galen's Storeroom, Rome's Libraries, and the Fire of A.D. 192." *Journal of Roman Archaeology* 21: 133–49.

Twitchett, D., and M. Loewe, eds. 1986. "Postscript to Chapter 16." In *The Cambridge History of China.* Vol. 1: *The Ch'in and Han Empires, 221 BC–AD 220,* 873–78. Cambridge: Cambridge University Press.

van Minnen, P. 2001. "P. Oxy. LXVI 4527 and the Antonine Plague in the Fayyum." *Zeitschrift für Papyrologie und Epigraphik* 135: 175–77.

Varlik, N. 2015. *Plague and Empire in the Early Modern Mediterranean World.* Cambridge: Cambridge University Press.

Varone, A. 2015. "Newly Discovered and Corrected Readings of Iscrizioni 'Privatissime' from the Vesuvian Region." In *Inscriptions in the Private Sphere in the Greco-Roman World,* ed. R. Benefiel and P. Keegan, 113–30. Leiden: Brill.

Virlouvet, C. 1997. "Existait-il des registres de décès à Rome au Ier siècle ap. J.-C?" *Publications de l'École Française de Rome* 230 (1): 77–88.

Viste, E., and A. Sorteberg. 2013. "Moisture Transport into the Ethiopian Highlands." *International Journal of Climatology* 33 (1): 249–63.

Vlach, M. 2022. "The Antonine Plague: Evaluation of Its Impact through Epidemiological Modelling." In *Simulating Roman Economies: Theories, Methods, and Computational Models,* ed. T. Brughmans and A. Wilson, 69–108. Oxford: Oxford University Press.

———. 2020. "The Antonine Plague and Impact Possibilities during the Marcomannic Wars." In *Marcomannic Wars and the Antonine Plague: Selected Essays on Two Disasters That Shook the Roman World,* ed. M. Erdrich, B. Komoróczy, P. Madejski, and M. Vlach, 23–36. Brno: Czech Academy of Sciences.

Waebens, S. 2012. "Reflecting the 'Change in AD 140': The Veteran Categories of the Epikrisis Documents Revisited." *Zeitschrift für Papyrologie und Epigraphik* 180: 267–77.

Walker, B., C. S. Holling, S. Carpenter, and A. Kinzig. 2004. "Resilience, Adaptability and Transformability in Social-Ecological Systems." *Ecology and Society* 9 (2).

Walker, D. R. 1978. *The Metrology of the Roman Silver Coinage: From Pertinax to Uranius Antoninus.* Vol. 3. Oxford: British Archaeological Reports.

Wallace-Hadrill, A. 1994. *Houses and Society in Pompeii and Herculaneum.* Princeton: Princeton University Press.

Walzer, R. 1949. *Galen on Jews and Christians.* Oxford: Oxford University Press.

Webster, G. 1998. *The Roman Imperial Army of the First and Second Centuries A.D.* Norman: University of Oklahoma Press.

Weisweiler, J. 2021. "Capital Accumulation, Supply Networks and the Composition of the Roman Senate, 14–235 CE." *Past & Present* 253 (1): 3–44.

Wesson, R. G. 1967. *The Imperial Order.* Berkeley: University of California Press.

Whitehorne, J.E.G. 1977. "Was Marcus Aurelius a Hypochondriac?" *Latomus* 36 (2): 413–21.

Whittaker, C. R. 1964. "The Revolt of Papirius Dionysius A.D. 190." *Historia: Zeitschrift für Alte Geschichte* 13 (3): 348–69.

Wickham, C. 2005. *Framing the Early Middle Ages: Europe and the Mediterranean, 400–800.* Oxford: Oxford University Press.

Wilkes, J. J. 1999. "The Roman Army as a Community in the Danube Lands: The Case of the Seventh Legion." In *The Roman Army as a Community*, ed. A. Goldsworthy and I. Haynes, 95–104. Supplementary Series 34. Portsmouth, RI: Journal of Roman Archaeology.

Wilkins, J. 2015. "Medical Literature, Diet, and Health." In *A Companion to Food in the Ancient World*, ed. J. Wilkins and R. Nadeau, 59–66. London: John Wiley & Sons.

Williams, D. H. 2020. *Apology as Dialogue and Appeal: Defending and Defining the Faith*. Oxford: Oxford University Press.

Wils, T.H.G., I. Robertson, Z. Eshetu, M. Koprowski, U.G.W. Sass-Klaassen, R. Touchan, and N. J. Loader. N.d. "Towards a Reconstruction of Blue Nile Baseflow from Ethiopian Tree Rings." *The Holocene* 20 (6): 837–48.

Wilson, A. 2011. "City Sizes and Urbanization in the Roman Empire." In *Settlement, Urbanization, and Population*, ed. A. K. Bowman and A. Wilson, 161–95. Oxford: Oxford University Press.

———. 2009. "Indicators for Roman Economic Growth: A Response to Walter Scheidel." *Journal of Roman Archaeology* 22: 71–82.

———. 2007. "The Metal Supply of the Roman Empire." In *Supplying Rome and the Empire: The Proceedings of an International Seminar Held at Siena-Certosa Di Pontignano on May 2–4, 2004, on Rome, the Provinces, Production and Distribution*, ed. E. Papi and M. Bonifay, 109–25. Portsmouth, RI: Journal of Roman Archaeology.

———. 2002. "Machines, Power and the Ancient Economy." *Journal of Roman Studies* 92: 1–32.

Woodson, A. L. 2014. "A Record of Holocene Climate Change from the Sunda Shelf, South China Sea." Master's thesis, East Carolina University.

Woodson, A. L., E. Leorri, S. J. Culver, D. J. Mallinson, P. R. Parham, R. C. Thunell, V. R. Vijayan, and S. Curtis. 2017. "Sea-Surface Temperatures for the Last 7200 Years from the Eastern Sunda Shelf, South China Sea: Climatic Inferences from Planktonic Foraminiferal Mg/Ca Ratios." *Quaternary Science Reviews* 165: 13–24.

Woolf, G. 2000. *Becoming Roman: The Origins of Provincial Civilization in Gaul*. Cambridge: Cambridge University Press.

Woytek, B. E., K. Uhlir, M. Alram, M. Schreiner, and M. Griesser. 2007. "The Denarius under Trajan: New Metallurgical Analyses." *Numismatic Chronicle* 167: 147–63.

Wright, W. 1882. *The Chronicle of Joshua the Stylite: Composed in Syriac A.D. 507*. Cambridge: Cambridge University Press.

Yarrow, L. M. 2012. "Antonine Coinage." In *The Oxford Handbook of Greek and Roman Coinage*, ed. W. E. Metcalf, 423–52. Oxford: Oxford University Press.

Yeh, H.-Y., R. Mao, H. Wang, W. Qi, and P. D. Mitchell. 2016. "Early Evidence for Travel with Infectious Diseases along the Silk Road: Intestinal Parasites from 2000-Year-Old Personal Hygiene Sticks in a Latrine at Xuanquanzhi Relay Station in China." *Journal of Archaeological Science: Reports* 9: 758–64.

Young, G. K. 2001. *Rome's Eastern Trade: International Commerce and Imperial Policy, 31 BC–AD 305*. London: Routledge.

Zanker, P. 1990. *The Power of Images in the Age of Augustus*. Ann Arbor: University of Michigan Press.

Zaroug, M.a.H., E.a.B. Eltahir, and F. Giorgi. 2014. "Droughts and Floods over the Upper Catchment of the Blue Nile and Their Connections to the Timing of El Niño and La Niña Events." *Hydrology and Earth System Sciences* 18 (3): 1239–49.

Zelener, Y. 2012. "Genetic Evidence, Density Dependence and Epidemiological Models of the 'Antonine Plague.'" In *L'Impatto della peste antonina*, ed. E. Lo Cascio, 167–77. Bari: Edipuglia.

———. 2003. "Smallpox and the Disintegration of the Roman Economy after 165 AD." PhD diss., Columbia University.

Zuiderhoek, A. 2009. "Government Centralization in Late Second and Third Century Asia Minor: A Working Hypothesis." *Classical World* 103 (1): 39–51.

INDEX

Aelius Aristides: on disease, 81, 121–123, 142, 199; on Rome 1, 3–5; *Sacred Tales* of, 74, 142

Alexander of Abonuteichos, 100, 125–131

Alexandria, 29, 63–64, 117–119; coins of, 163–164; and disease, 64; grain fleet of, 27, 51–52, 162; soldier recruitment in, 149

Annona, 37, 43, 45, 47–49, 52–53, 156, 216, 219–221

Antioch, 56, 72; disease in, 42, 82, 84, 126; food shortage in, 21–22

Antonine plague: in the countryside, 97–106; cures for, 123–129, 198, 200–201; duration, 217; emergence, 57–58, 65–66, 69–74; epigraphic evidence for, 99–101, 161–162, 130–131, 189–192; genetic evidence for, 90–93; immunity, 94–96, 140, 218; livestock deaths during, 122, 198–200; mortality, 93–94, 105–106, 214–216, 227–228; and population density, 97–99, 106, 117–118, 189; at Rome, 86–90, 94–95, 104, 107, 109; seasonality of, 81, 122; symptoms of, 91–92, 121–123, 142, 169–170

Antoninus Pius, 19, 31, 56–57, 68, 134

Apollo: association with Commodus, 206, 209; association with epidemics, xiv, 70–74, 121–122, 125–127, 137; oracles of, 75; 100–101, 113, 133, 142; worship of, 126–127, 234

Aquileia: armies in, 84, 107; epidemic in, 107–111, 115, 123–124, 142, 171

Arabia: epidemic in, 57–60, 62, 69; Roman expeditions into, 67–68; and trade, 1, 59–61, 65;

Armenia, 56, 123

Artemis, 73, 131

Asclepius: appearance in dreams, 114, 129; as healer of disease, 116, 125–126, 129, 235; temples of, 11, 121

Athens, 10; associations with the Antonine plague, 115–116, 186; fifth-century BC plague in, xvii, 72–74, 79, 113–114, 116, 140, 200, 206

Augustus, 100; conquest of Egypt, 27–30; invasion of Arabia, 67, 218; Tiber flood under, 24

aVARV. *See* smallpox

Avidius Cassius: invasion of Parthia, 70–72, 82–83, 218; liberation of Alexandria, 119; rebellion of, xv, 119, 144–145, 166–171, 179

banditry. *See* brigandage

bathhouses, 6, 10, 13–15, 134

Berenike, 57, 60–61, 63, 68

Black Death. *See* bubonic plague

brigandage, 169, 173–182, 189, 196–197, 213, 217, 219; in Egypt, 117–121, 164, 166

Britain, 66, 70, 100–103, 126–127, 146, 155–158

bubonic plague, 15–16, 80–82, 92, 226–227, 239; under Justinian, 25, 94

burials: correlated with epidemics, 86–87, 101–103; genetic analysis of, 16, 44–45, 101–103; of infants, 10; laws concerning, 86–87

Cassius Dio: on the AD 190 Roman epidemic, 81, 94, 177, 198–202; on Commodus's character, 187, 194–196, 204–207, 211–212; on the death of Marcus Aurelius, 185–187; on epidemics, 108; on events under Augustus, 30

cereals. *See* grain

China: epidemics in, 103–105, 170; Roman contact with, 61–63

Christians, 120, 131–141; persecution of, 113, 131–132, 161, 233–239

Claudius: grain shortage under, 30–31; infrastructure improvements of, 53, 162

Cleander, 196–967, 201–206

climate: xx, 25–29, 34–41, 54

coins: of Commodus, 207, 219–220; debasement of, 49, 162–164, 173, 175, 179–180, 225–228; and epidemics, 87–89, 101, 115, 125–128, 156; and the Nile, 31; non-Roman, 59; and violence, 167–168, 178–180

Commodus: accession of, 114, 185–189, 193–194; "African Fleet" of, 37, 219–221; childhood of, 167, 170–171, 187; death of, 180, 212–213; elite hostility toward, xix, 177; epidemic at Rome under, 94, 115, 122, 124, 193, 198–204, 217; megalomania, 195–196, 204–212; unrest under, 177–179, 194–195, 201–204, 217

Coptos, 57, 63

corpses: accumulation of, 10–12, 24–25, 86, 116, 140; counting of, 94; disposal of, 17, 102, 106

covid-19. *See* SARS-CoV-2

Ctesiphon, xiii, 56, 71–72, 82, 218

Cyprian of Carthage, 137, 140–141, 236–239

Cyprianic plague, 138, 139–140, 219, 233–239

Deserters' War, 178–181, 206

diarrhea, 13, 25, 85, 91

drought: in Antioch, 21; and cereal harvest, 41, 45; and the Cyprianic plague, 236; in Edessa, 42; in Egypt, xvii, 33–36, 119, 162–163; ENSO-related, 29, 33–36; in Europe, 38, 54

Dura-Europos, xiii, 66, 71–72

dysentery, 25

Edessa, 42, 46, 72, 82

Egypt: coinage of, 162–164; depopulation in, xvii, 117; disease in 62–64, 74; eastern desert, 63; economy of, 94, 117–118, 158–159, 164–166, 222–228; grain production in, 3, 6, 27–37, 40–41, 47, 49, 51–52, 192, 219–222; soldiers stationed in, 67–70; trade via, 65, 216; violence in, 118–121

El Niño–Southern Oscillation, 34–36

Ephesus, 83–84, 130–131

Equatorial East Africa, 28–29, 34–36, 68

Ethiopia. *See* Equatorial East Africa

Eusebius, 46, 50, 88, 134, 161

famine: deadliness of, xx, 192; economics of, 20, 49–50, 219–222; in Egypt, 27, 29–30, 32, 156–157, 162, 166, 173, 192; during epidemics, 42, 50, 81, 108–109, 176, 198–202, 205, 228–230; following food shortages, 45–46; frequency of, xvi, 46; and migration, 20–22, 181–122, 197; mitigation of, 18–19, 30, 41, 104, 206; due to storms, 38; and violence, 21; and volcanic eruptions, 25.

Farasan Islands, 68–69

floods: 10, 24–37, 108, 133, 156–159, 162–164, 219

food shortage. *See* famine

Galen: early career of, 77–79, 85; on Commodus's childhood sickness, 170–171; cures and medicines of, 123–125, 167; descriptions of disease and epidemics, 79–81, 90–92, 103–105, 107–110, 114–115, 122, 142, 169–170, 192; on food, 43–47; on health and sanitation, 12–14; immunity to disease, 95–96; relationship with Marcus Aurelius, 114, 144; on religion, 121, 129, 131; suffering of, 90, 142, 206, 210–211

Gaul, 37, 59, 70, 73, 98, 134–135, 159, 161, 178, 218, 221, 231

gladiators, 134, 142, 149, 159–160, 174–176

Glycon, 125–128. *See also* Alexander of
    Abonuteichos
grain: contamination, 44; cultivars, 41–44;
    distribution, 17, 20, 22, 27, 30, 39–40, 45, 48,
    50, 83, 87, 156; imports to Rome, 3, 30–31, 37,
    50–53, 169, 209, 219–222; prices, 220–222,
    229; production, 27–30, 156, 162–164;
    shortages, 21, 32–33, 38, 45–47, 108–109,
    162, 181, 192, 200–206; storage, 20, 49, 162;
    subsidies, 40, 48; taxes and tribute of, 19,
    188, 221–222, 230; transportation of, 31, 37,
    50–53, 156–157, 162, 216, 219, 229
graves. *See* burials; corpses

Hadrian, 14, 19, 31–32, 51, 56, 68
Han Empire. *See* China
Herculaneum, 44
Herodian: on the AD 190 Roman epidemic,
    124, 197–204; on Commodus, 171, 189,
    194; on violence, 178–179, 223
Hispania, 100, 151, 158–160
hospitals, 116

India, 1, 6, 59–60, 68, 81
Indian Ocean: climate, 28, 36; trade 59–66, 69
inflation, 49, 225–228
Italy: agriculture in, 37–38; epidemics in, 25,
    106–111, 123, 144, 147, 182, 197–199; late
    second-century AD distress in, 178–182;
    soldiers in, 84, 149, 178–181, 218

Julius Caesar, 25, 29, 48, 159
Justinianic plague. *See* bubonic plague

Kushan Empire, 62–63

La Niña. *See* El Niño–Southern Oscillation
labor: seasonal, 8, 22; shortage of, 158–159,
    164, 229–230
Lake Tana, 28, 36
Londinium. *See* London
London: second-century decline of, 126–127,
    155, 235; and smallpox epidemics, 81, 102,
    105

Lucian of Samosata, 72, 82, 125–129, 131
Lucius Verus: and the first Antonine plague
    epidemic in Rome, 85–89; character
    of, xviii, 56, 88–89; death of, 109–111,
    119, 127, 143, 186; laws of, 53, 86; in
    Parthia, 24, 56–57, 70, 73–74, 82, 95, 107,
    171, 218

malaria, xvi, 8, 14–15, 22, 25, 64
malnutrition, 15, 41–48, 54, 81, 219. *See also*
    famine
Marcia, 201–205, 212
Marcomannic Wars: and disease transmis-
    sion, 107, 114, 143–147, 189, 218; and
    economic disruptions, 149, 156–159;
    recruitment for, 147–150, 174; treaties to
    end, 172, 188–189, 193
Marcus Aurelius: and Christians, 132–135;
    death of, 114, 185–188, 205; fiscal crisis
    under, 150–151; on health, 13; laws of, 53,
    86–88, 156, 160–161, 176–177; *Meditations*
    of, 114, 137, 142, 167, 176, 186; propaganda
    of, 150–151, 159, 167–168; response to
    epidemics, 86–90, 99–101, 109–110, 115–116,
    127, 147; sicknesses of, 145, 166–167,
    170–171, 185–187, 205; Tiber flood under,
    24–25, 77–78; travels of, 169, 172–173;
    unrest under, xv, 143–144, 175–176; war
    policies of, 147–151, 157, 172–175
Maternus. *See* Deserters' War
measles, 80, 90, 95
miasma theory, 114
migration, 16, 21–23, 38, 54, 57, 85, 111, 114–121,
    156, 169, 181–182, 193, 197, 200
military, Roman. *See* soldiers
mines: of Alburnus Maior, 151–152, 158; and
    disease transmission, 151–154; flooding
    of, 157; of Rio Tinto, 151; work stoppages
    at, 142, 225, 236
Mithraism, 73, 189–191
Mons Claudianus, 157, 200

Nero: Great Fire under, 17, 154, 205–206;
    reputation of, 31, 188

Nile: delta, xvii–xviii, 64, 117–118, 121; flooding of the, 27–37, 133, 158, 162, 219; and trade, 57, 63–64, 229

nilometers, 29, 31

Nisibis, 42, 71–72, 82

Noricum, 107, 145, 189–190

North Africa, 27, 30–31, 37, 59, 98–99, 158, 219

parasites, 5, 9, 13–16, 25, 44, 62

Parthia: Roman wars against, 24, 56–57, 65–74, 81–85, 89, 95, 107, 149–152, 168, 217–218; and trade, 61–63

Periplus of the Erythraean Sea, 60

Pliny the Elder, 14, 29, 64, 78

Pliny the Younger, 18–20, 31, 52, 131, 135

praetorian guard, 108, 147, 150, 178, 180, 196–197, 201, 203, 211

predation, 17, 19, 47, 173–174, 228

Puteoli, 52, 161–162, 229

quarries, 154–159, 200, 236

Red Sea, 26, 36, 56–68

refugees. See migration

resilience, 5–6, 23, 27, 93, 214–216, 230–231

Roman Climate Optimum, 26

SARS-CoV-2, xv–xvi, 80, 93

scapegoating rituals, 113, 116, 130, 141, 212

sea surface temperature, 34–37

Seleucia, xiii–xv, 56, 70–72, 82

senators, 4, 8, 29, 48, 83, 122–123, 142, 160, 172, 177, 194–197, 201–202, 206, 209–212

Seneca, 8, 29, 31, 115

Septimius Severus, 175, 218, 222–224, 231

Sicily, 27, 37

Silk Roads, 62, 65

skeletons. See burials

slaves: abandonment of, 11, 139; daily life of, 12, 22; health of, 9, 48, 90; in the military, 149, 159; runaway, 145, 173–181, 189

smallpox: associations with the Antonine plague, xv, 90–92, 122–123; in the early modern period, 80–81, 96–97, 102, 105–106, 239; in pre-modernity (including aVARV), 42–43, 91–92, 199–200, 217, 227

Smyrna, 74, 81, 121–122

sodales Antoniniani, 95

soldiers: diplomas of, 147–149, 175; desertion of, 145, 167–169, 173–182, 189; disease transmission via, 57, 65–74, 83–86, 107–108, 116, 145–146, 172–173, 189, 217–218; epidemics among, 80–82, 109, 114, 142–147; payments to, 150–151, 160, 174–175, 179–180, 223–225; shortage of, 146–149, 174

Spain. See Hispania

speleothems, 26

storms, 28, 30–31, 38–39, 45, 50–51

Syria, 42, 65–66, 68, 70, 73–74, 82, 124, 218, 231

Tacitus, 4, 31

taxes: and corruption, 18–19; flight from, 32–33, 111, 119–120, 164, 174; on gladiators, 160; in grain, 44, 162–163, 192, 221–222, 230–231; on trade, 65, 67–68; 223

theriac, 123–124, 167

Tiber River, 11, 24–25, 28, 31, 49, 51, 78, 115, 133

Titus, epidemic under, 17, 87, 94

Trajan, 30–31, 53, 65, 67, 70, 78, 125, 218

Trajan Decius, 234

transportation: maritime, 31, 39–40, 50–52, 59–62, 65, 156–157, 219–220, 229; overland, 46, 52, 62, 65, 103

tree rings, 26, 35–38

volcanic eruptions, 25–26, 28, 44

Vologases IV, 56

wheat. See grain

Yemen. See Arabia

Yersinia pestis. See bubonic plague